European Union Public Health Policy

Ranging from influence over world trade laws affecting health to population health issues such as obesity to the use of comparative data to affect policy, the EU's public health policies are increasingly important, visible, expensive and effective. They also provide an invaluable case study for those who want to understand the growth and impact of the EU as well as how states can affect their populations' lives and health.

European Union Public Health Policy capitalizes on extensive new research, providing an introduction to the topic and indicating new intellectual directions surrounding the topic. An introductory section and extended conclusion explore the meaning of public health, the relationship of EU public health policy to health care policy, and the place of public health in the study of European integration and Europeanization. Focusing on health system transformation, global health governance and population health, the chapters address:

- relevant policy issues and EU policies;
- effects of the EU policies on practice or outcomes;
- an explanation of the policy trajectory;
- current issues and likely future directions or conflicts.

Drawing together an international and multidisciplinary selection of experts, this volume is an important contribution for all those interested in public health policy, EU health policy and EU governance.

Scott L. Greer is Associate Professor of Health Management and Policy at the University of Michigan's School of Public Health, USA, and Honorary Senior Research Fellow at LSE Health, London School of Economics and Political Science, UK.

Paulette Kurzer is Professor of Political Science in the School of Government and Public Policy at the University of Arizona, USA.

Routledge Advances in European Politics

European Union Public Health Policy

Regional and global trends

Edited by Scott L. Greer and Paulette Kurzer

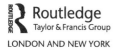

Routledge
Taylor & Francis Group

LONDON AND NEW YORK

First published 2013
by Routledge
2 Park Square, Milton Park, Abingdon, Oxfordshire OX14 4RN

Simultaneously published in the USA and Canada
by Routledge
711 Third Avenue, New York, NY 10017

First issued in paperback 2016

Routledge is an imprint of the Taylor & Francis Group, an informa business

British Library Cataloguing in Publication Data
A catalogue record for this book is available from the British Library

Library of Congress Cataloging in Publication Data
European Union public health policy : regional and global trends / edited
by Scott L. Greer and Paulette Kurzer.
    p. ; cm. — (Routledge advances in European politics ; 90)
    Includes bibliographical references.
    I. Greer, Scott L.   II. Kurzer, Paulette, 1957-   III. Series: Routledge
advances in European politics ; 90.
    [DNLM: 1. European Union.   2. Health Policy—trends   Europe.
3. International Cooperation—Europe.   4. Public Health
Administration—Europe.   5. Public Health Practice—Europe.
WA 530 GA1]
    362.1094—dc23
                                                        2012024222

ISBN 13: 978-1-138-68611-3 (pbk)
ISBN 13: 978-0-415-51664-8 (hbk)

Typeset in Times New Roman
by Swales & Willis Ltd, Exeter, Devon

Contents

Figures

Tables

Contributors

François Briatte, University of Grenoble, France.

Elize Massard da Fonseca, Center for Metropolitan Studies, Brazilian Center for Analysis and Planning (CEM/CEBRAP), São Paulo, Brazil.

Heather Elliott, Department of Health Management and Policy, School of Public Health, University of Michigan, USA.

Scott L. Greer, Department of Health Management and Policy, School of Public Health, University of Michigan, USA.

Sébastien Guigner, Institute of Political Science, Centre Emile Durkheim, University of Bordeaux, France.

Boris Hauray, CNRS-INSERM-EHESS, Université Paris 13, France.

Holly Jarman, Department of Health Management and Policy, School of Public Health, University of Michigan, USA.

Loes Knaapen, Social Studies of Medicine Department, McGill University, Canada.

Paulette Kurzer, School of Government and Public Policy, University of Arizona, USA.

Wolfram Lamping, Institute for Political Science, Technical University of Darmstadt, Germany.

Jenny Cisneros Örnberg, Centre for Social Research on Alcohol and Drugs (SoRAD), Stockholm University, Sweden.

Donley T. Studlar, Department of Political Science, West Virginia University, USA.

1 Introduction

What is European Union public health policy?

Scott L. Greer

Defining European Union public health policy is hard: because the place of public health in the EU is new and still under debate; and because the borders and meaning of public health are less agreed than its scholars and practitioners might think. This introductory chapter first addresses the problem of defining public health. The second section addresses the issue of public health policy in the European Union, identifying it and separating it from the very substantial economic policies associated with the EU that also have economic effects. It argues that the public health policies of the EU are concentrated in three areas: the EU as a global actor (with repercussions inward on the EU itself); the EU as a supporter of health systems; and the EU as a public health regulator in its own right. The third section presents the chapters in the book.

What is public health policy? A plea for empirical definitions

At its most abstract, public health is the health of the population: their freedom from disease, incapacity, and avoidable death. Public health policy is that range of policies that contribute to such an end—from injury prevention to anti-smoking campaigns, to health systems strengthening, to microbiological research. Public health stands in relation to society like the doctor in relation to the patient: charged with diagnosing, prescribing, and treating its ills. In other words, public health is affected by almost every policy in government, and almost every policy in government could potentially be seen as more or less successful public health policy. And just like medical diagnoses, prescription, and influence over patients are highly imperfect, the influence of public health diagnoses, advice, and influence over states and peoples are highly imperfect.

We see the confusion in the endless definitional conversations that afflict public health. They are sparked by practical organizational requirements (such as degree accreditation or reorganization of a ministry), by professional self-definition (such as the border wars between medicine, nursing, and public health), by disagreement about whether a public health policymaker should be attending a given government meeting, or by simple disagreement about what topics are fit for public health scholars. The particularly neuralgic definitional divide is between public health and medicine; stances range from outright opposition (the argument that prevention and public health, rather than clinical medicine, save lives) to a variety of tangled syntheses that mirror the tangled relationships between public health and medically trained people in governments, practice, and scholarships.

The first problem for scholarship in particular is conceptual overreach. It arises when the impact of every policy on public health becomes a warrant for public health advocates to intervene in any and all areas of public health. On one hand, the odds are good that their expertise is either irrelevant (as with many discussions of social and health care services policy within public health) or very partial (epidemiology can say something about almost any topic in society, but not necessarily something other scholars and policymakers will find useful or want to hear). On the other hand, basic politics suggests that the expertise, connections, and coalitions of public health policymakers, like any other policymakers, have limits. The problem of integrating public health into the thinking of other policymakers, aka "Health in all policies," has scarcely been solved (Ståhl et al. 2006; Geyer and Lightfoot 2010; Greer 2012b).

The second problem arises when the difficulty of discussing public health's nature and borders leads to unreflective definitions that mix the quintessence of public health with the organization and preoccupations of any one country. It is a basic methodological mistake to confuse the field of action (public health) with the people acting on the field (whatever corps of people have "public health" in their job description) (Bourdieu 2012, p. 334). Public health's definitional debates are particularly prone to go wrong when participants cross borders; every one of the small number of studies comparing public health in Europe reveals major differences in the form and content of public health organization and activity (Mereckiene et al. 2010; MacLehose et al. 2001; Reintjes et al. 2007; Reintjes 2012; Elliott et al. 2012; Mounier-Jack and Coker 2006; Coker and McKee 2008; Brand 2012).

It stands to reason that the starting point of a conversation in the UK, where public health is dominated by highly trained medical specialists, will take a different course from conversations in the United States, where the two-year Masters of Public Health is the dominant degree, or from the numerous countries of continental Europe where there is no particularly prestigious degree or profession associated with the field. Furthermore, the big differences between polities matter and might not be easy to explain. Historical research, by far the dominant kind of scholarly research into public health politics and organization, has so far found path-dependent and otherwise patternless variation, a challenge to social scientists of all kinds (Baldwin 2005a,b). It has also made it clear just how different "public health" looks from different standpoints (Solomon et al. 2008)—and how often a writer's assumptions about "how it is done" turn out to actually mean "how it is done in my country."

The way out of these two problems—overreach and parochialism—is to abandon such "legislative" definitions, in which the academic observer determines the nature and scope of the topic. Instead, we should examine the scope of the policies—and the definitional debates—in different jurisdictions. Searching for the true nature of public health, or public health policy, is an activity best left to philosophers and advocates. Those from the social sciences who wish to understand the dynamics of public health policymaking would probably be better off starting with the policies, and understandings, of the participants in the system they are studying. In the case of the European Union, this means understanding two separable issues: the effects of the EU on public health, which are mostly from its role as an economic actor, and the set of policies that, as a practical question of EU politics, *do* involve the justifications and people associated with public health. The former might constitute a challenge to public health systems and advocates, and something they can use their participation in government to attack; the latter is what they are accustomed to doing.

What is the European Union? A public health policy approach

The European Union is a distinctive organization in world politics. Its institutions and politics are like those of many other polities, but as a whole it resembles little else. It began as a club of six countries that agreed to pool sovereignty over coal and steel, and later share atomic energy—and, fatefully, then, to form a common market with supranational institutions. Over decades it grew in both territorial expanse and the power of its law and institutions. Sometimes extension was due to great interstate bargains such as the ones that relaunched the internal market for 1992, admitted the post communist states of central Europe, or founded the currency union. Often, though, the deepening of integration was the work of the institutions: the entrepreneurial executive Commission and the European Court of Justice, which between them created many a *fait accompli* of integration that states found they could only accept. Later, the European Parliament would start to become a credible voice, heard in many of this book's chapters.

The EU might have distinctively powerful and entrepreneurial institutions, but its powers are theoretically enumerated in treaties, the most recent of which is the Lisbon Treaty. Like the constitutions of most federations, the treaties enumerate the powers of the EU. Where there is no "treaty base," there is no basis for EU action. But like the constitutions of many federations, this restriction has proven more able to channel than to prevent the expansion of EU power. The mechanism is simple: the EU might not have treaty bases authorizing significant action in the area of health care, for example, but it is firmly within its rights (as defined and expanded over the years by the Court of Justice) when it regulates the internal market that includes the patients, doctors, providers, devices, and money of a health system.

The activity of these institutions then drives further European integration in a process known as spillover, in which integration essentially begets integration. Sometimes integration creates a demand for integration—if European integration allows farmers to buy and sell cattle across borders, it creates demands, come a crisis, for somebody to certify the quality of meat. Such spillover creates pressure for integration in the form of a nexus for cross-border coordination, and in the geopolitical and institutional environment of Europe it works (Knab 2011). Sometimes integration operates in a largely political sense: once the Court has created a right to health care across borders, everybody with an interest in health care has a reason to flock to Brussels and populate a new and once-unthinkable European Union health policy community (Greer 2006b). Both kinds of integration process are at work in this book.

The logic of integration instills its own biases, however. The powerful treaty bases have actually given rise to the "constitutional principles" of the European Union, known as the "four freedoms" in an appropriation of a phrase first coined for more inspiring ends by Franklin Delano Roosevelt. The four freedoms are the freedom of movement of goods, services, capital and people within the EU. A policy that interferes with such freedoms needs a powerful justification in theory, and a strong coalition in politics, to survive.

A European Union with a derisory budget, powerful legal system, and "constitutional" commitment to freedom of goods, services, capital and people is a perfect example of a regulatory state. Its principal policy tool is regulatory: setting the conditions under which others, including states, may make their decisions and ensuring that they do not interfere with the four freedoms in the internal market. Regulatory states can be infuriating because they make others pay for their policy goals; the Court can enunciate a right to health care, but member states must pay for it. Policy advocates in the EU often spend much of their time developing forums, programs, and initiatives that will help them counteract the information deficits, democratic deficits, and distrust such an organization creates among those it regulates.

Once European integration has taken place in a policy area—once the EU has an acknowledged role—the problem becomes one of action and impact. After integration comes EU policymaking and Europeanization. Those topics involve asking what combination of lobbying, institutions, entrepreneurship and luck explains EU agendas and policy decisions, and then, what impact it has and why.

What this all means is that the EU has two kinds of impact on public health. One comes through its role as an economic actor. The other is through policy justified by and intended to improve Europeans' health. The latter is the focus of this book, but the former is the crucial context.

The EU: Economic actor

The EU is first and foremost an economic actor; it is no accident that it was called an "Economic Community" until 1992. The economic influence of the EU on public health comes through two routes. One is the regulatory agenda of the internal market. This is the core business of the main EU institutions: Court, Commission, Council and Parliament. They are engaged in developing law and policy that broadens and deepens economic integration. Policy in this area suffers from the "constitutional asymmetry" that Fritz Scharpf identified (Scharpf 2002). The Treaties enable more liberalization ("negative integration," the removal of barriers to trade within Europe) than promoting new EU-wide standards and proposals ("positive integration," the creation of programs that raise standards, regulate, or compensate losers). In health care, this has meant the Court making a series of deregulating decisions that Lamping discusses in Chapter 2. For public health, it means that the meaning of "public health" in EU law is primarily a basis for a limited exception to liberalization on the grounds that it would endanger somebody's health. The EU's constitutional asymmetry is visible here: public health does not mean positive, forward-looking policies; it means a limited set of exceptions to the market integration that is the core business of the EU. The public health policies in this book come from and through those institutions, but must operate with weaker treaty bases and less legal support.

The other way the EU influences public health as an economic power is through its role as a macroeconomic actor. It began with Eurozone accession, which involved retrenching and stabilizing government finances in most countries to meet the criteria. A few countries also, of course, misrepresented their finances. Once inside the Eurozone, the very different economies of the EU lost their monetary sovereignty to the European Central Bank (ECB). Losing their monetary sovereignty deprived them of the ability to adapt to economic mismatches by letting their currencies appreciate or depreciate, and caused them to lose autonomy over interest rates and a measure of financial regulation. Interest rates became the responsibility of the ECB. The ECB is easily as powerful as any other EU institution, and less accountable than any of them. The price of bringing Germany into the Eurozone was a one-sided Treaty obligation to promote price stability, unmodified by other objectives such as promoting employment.

The financial crisis that started in 2008 brought together the macroeconomic and regulatory faces of the EU. While the salvation—or not—of the Eurozone lay in the hands of the ECB, possibly with assistance from the bickering heads of state, the Commission and the right governments that dominate the European Union in those years set out to use their market-regulating policies to reform markets through more forceful application of EU regulation. The global center-right, which very much includes the Commission nominated by Europe's mostly right-wing governments, has a profound tendency to address macroeconomic crisis with microeconomic initiatives that deregulate and shift the costs of economic change onto labor (usually known as flexibility). These are ideas that have been recurrently proposed by liberalizers for decades, with mixed application and results. It is far from obvious why a Commission proposal to invent a new patent system or rewrite the Posted Workers Directive (as discussed by Jarman in her chapter) is the solution to a macroeconomic crisis. The truly consequential actions involving the Commission have been the austerity agreements that are reshaping peripheral Eurozone economies and thereby social determinants of population health such as education, inequality, and employment (Fahy 2012; Bradley *et al.* 2011; Stuckler *et al.* 2010b). The other implication of this microeconomic shift among Europe's top policymakers was an unpropitious environment for further regulatory activity justified by health concerns. Health may be wealth, as the Tallinn Charter[1] would have it, but in the short term it has become harder to justify new health policy initiatives that might interfere with industry interests.

European Union: Public health policymaker

The flip side of constitutional asymmetry is that Europe is much worse at promoting public health—positive integration—than it is at market-making—negative integration—or fiscal policy. That theme shows throughout this book: the EU powers over public health are weak, derived from some other power (e.g., trade policy, consumer protection), or both. It is not striking that such policies are weak. It is, rather, striking how they sometimes work and gain coherence (Brand 2010, Greer 2011). These policies are diverse, and public health policy might be the most diverse area of EU policy intervention precisely because the treaty bases for public health action are so weak.

In general, there are three kinds of power: law (ultimately, coercion); resources, such as expert staff; and money. The structure and focus of EU health policy comes from the different availability and uses of those resources.

The most obvious and most powerful tool is law (Greer *et al*. forthcoming 2012). Law has compelling and obvious virtues as a tool of public health. It must be followed: there are penalties for a firm that violates tobacco labeling law or a state that neglects to implement that law, and the courts will enforce those penalties. The fact that cases can be brought under EU law, including the Treaties themselves, by the Commission or by a wide range of other actors, and then decided and enforced by member state courts, means that EU law is both powerful and likely to keep growing in influence (Kelemen 2011). EU patient mobility law, discussed by Lamping in Chapter 2, is largely a story of single people bringing cases about their own personal problems—and thereby leading member state and EU courts to develop a far-reaching integrationist and deregulatory jurisprudence (also Greer 2009a).

The EU has a variety of legal bases with which to pass legislation on public health. Title XIV of the TFEU, dedicated to public health, is not the place to look. While it is a striking confirmation of public health policy's rise to prominence in an EU whose treaty did not even mention public health until 1992,[2] Title XIV does not contain many authorizations or competencies for EU actions. Instead, the place to look is in Title I and the treaty articles concerned with the creation and maintenance of the internal market. There we find broad competencies, for example Title 26:

1   The Union shall adopt measures with the aim of establishing or ensuring the functioning of the internal market, in accordance with the relevant provisions of the Treaties.
2   The internal market shall comprise an area without internal frontiers in which the free movement of goods, persons, services and capital is ensured in accordance with the provisions of the Treaties.

This is a tremendous competency. In short, if the market needs it, and nothing else in the Treaties forbids it, then it is a plausible policy. There is no such equivalent in health or social policy, where the Treaties carefully circumscribe actions taken in the name of those policy fields. The constitutional asymmetry that Scharpf noted, with the EU far better at negative than positive integration, is obvious. That said, there is scope for the EU to adopt legislation under these and similar articles that promotes health. The logic is that there must be some level of harmonization within a single market, so that safety, information, and product standards are similar and countries cannot create negative externalities for each other. Thus, for example, the EU has the ability to pass legislation on food, cigarette, and alcohol labels (see Kurzer, Chapter 11; Cisneros Örnberg, Chapter 12; and Studlar, Chapter 13). Some articles, of course, do forbid meaningful harmonization or public health policy, as in the tightly written treaty articles blocking harmonization of taxation policy and therefore most uses of taxes to discourage use of legal but harmful substances.

Law also includes the impressive set of competencies that the EU has in certain areas. Notably, the EU is a powerful actor in trade law, and trade (as Guigner, Jarman and Massard da Fonseca argue in Chapters 7, 8 and 9). This area of policy is intricate and easy to ignore or caricature. But it is very important because the EU is a key player in the global negotiations and bilateral treaties that shape the regulation of the world economy—which goes far beyond the simplistic discussions of "free trade" that dominate public discussions. The WTO and its associated agreements are setting the framework for commerce in a very broad sense, from the mobility of doctors to patent protections on medicines and the rules governing health insurance, and the EU is a powerful policy actor and potential veto player.

What the EU does not have is money or resources for major health policies. The EU might be a powerful legislative and judicial machine, but it is also very thinly resourced. The EU budget is capped at around 1 percent of the EU's GDP, and much of that money is spent on agricultural subsidies and regional aid. While the sums of money are impressive, and there is a case that both could be spent with better or worse health consequences,[3] the kind of money needed to make big public health interventions such as shared vaccine pools, healthy infrastructure, or almost anything to do with the operation of health care services is missing. Instead, the EU has developed a habit of very carefully targeting the small amount of money it can spend on any one policy field, such as health. It cannot use its money to make much policy—but it can affect politics.

A classic use of the small EU budget is networking. The promotion of European networks on a given topic, with support for academic and NGO activity to formulate demands, simultaneously creates a constituency for European integration and gives a voice to under-resourced interests who might not appreciate the combination of single market policies and business lobbies that otherwise dominates EU politics (Greenwood 2007). The cycle that networks engage is hardly original to health policy (Brodscheid and Coen 2003; Pollack 2003)—the EU initiative, taken in the name of something obviously good (e.g., less cancer mortality, see Briatte in Chapter 4), funds the creation of networks and data collection enterprises, which then start to demand further EU actions to address problems they found and support work they started.

Another classic use of EU budgets is research. EU-funded research brings money to countries with very small budgets, but can be spectacularly ineffective at actually selecting worthwhile projects or producing or disseminating knowledge (Galsworthy *et al.* 2012; Ernst *et al.* 2010; Charlesworth *et al.* 2011). But is it fair to see EU investment in research as a device to produce knowledge? Research spending might better be viewed as a device for producing EU networks and Europeanization by subsidizing networks.

When it is more than a hit-or-miss subsidy to EU-centric networks, research often works best by promoting comparable data sets (See Elliott, this volume). These work by first setting standards for data—for example, categories for identifying people with HIV—(Steffen 2012) then collecting the data, and then seeing how different countries stand. When a country does badly, as with the Dutch on perinatal mortality (EURO-PERISTAT 2008) or the English with cancer (Briatte, this volume), then there is an opportunity for advocates in that country to make the case for action. EU money works by broadening expert networks to include more countries, and deepening them by giving them more resources and expertise, as in communicable disease control (Greer, this volume; Greer 2011).

But, as Knaapen argues in her chapter, network development as a European Union policy tool has a way of producing unexpected effects. She details how efforts to improve, rationalize, and standardize medical care by funding guideline projects did not produce guidelines on medical care. Instead, the networks involved produced guidelines for good guideline writing.[4] Her chapter stands as a reminder of how all policies, and in particular ones dependent on professional networks, can produce unexpected effects.

A final strategy to maximize Europeanization per Euro is to support and integrate partners in Brussels. At its most basic, this means more or less overt subsidies to NGOs. Research on EU lobbying (e.g., Coen 2007; Coen and Richardson 2009) makes it clear that many non-business interests are subsidized by the Commission through direct grants or contracts to do work such as publicity, hotlines, and capacity building (i.e., to research good strategy to shape politics). Supporting NGOs helps make the EU seem like less of a business-dominated political system and more like one that listens to less organized interests in society. The result is that EU-wide platforms for diffuse interests such as consumers, the elderly, caretakers or youth get assistance and inclusion that their raw political strength would never get for them. Europe, in theory, benefits from non-business viewpoints and from the organization of yet more interests at the EU level. Once they exist, then they can become included in the penumbra of the political process. In health, this is particularly likely to mean the platform or forum strategy, in which the EU (the Commission) brings together different parties to debate an issue such as obesity (Sanchez-Salgado 2007). Investment in friendly interest groups is both an agenda-setting mechanism and a way to gain information (Jarman 2011a; See Kurzer and Cisneros Ornberg, this volume). Platforms give some, mostly in industry, an opportunity to show their social responsibility. It gives others, mostly NGOs, an opportunity to learn, and others in all three an opportunity to keep an issue on the agenda when the politics are otherwise hostile.

Resources are the last source of power. Resources are things like physical premises or communications systems (like the European surveillance system TESsY) but above all trained staff. They are lagged indicators of money, but unlike money they are not fungible and can neither be created at a moment's notice nor abandoned easily. The EU is notably weak in this kind of resource, not just because of its tiny budget, but also because the member states have resolutely kept the size of the Commission capped (and half of its staff works in support areas, mostly translation). The result is that while the Commission has thousands of employees capable of initiating and supporting policy and legislative agendas, it has almost nobody who could directly provide much support in running a state. That is not the Commission's job, and the member states' approach to funding keeps it from becoming the Commission's job.

The obvious route around government budgetary constraint is, of course, to create an agency. One of the reasons to create an agency is that it becomes easier to argue for a larger budget—perhaps not what the original theorists of new public management intended, but a widely noted phenomenon. Even the tiny European Centre for Disease Control and Prevention (ECDC, Greer, Chapter 10), with over 300 employees, is a significant increase in the EU's public health resources—the whole Directorate-General for Health and Consumer Protection ("DG Sanco") has slightly less than a thousand staff to cover its huge policy fields. Likewise, the European Medicines Agency has about 750 staff and the European Food Safety Agency (Grant 2012) about 450[5]—so those three agencies have more staff than the whole of DG Sanco. The resource multiplier is greater still because the agencies create demand for domestic agencies and often provide capacity building—a large part of the ECDC's work amounts to creating opportunities and pressures for member state governments to invest more in communicable disease control, and a similar dynamic is visible in EFSA and EMA (Krapohl 2008; Hauray 2006; Hauray and Greer, Chapters 6 and 10). Furthermore, member states are very aware that giving the Commission power or money means encouraging its integrationist entrepreneurialism. Their solution is often agencies, for which member states can write more detailed job descriptions and be reasonably sure that they will not engage in the kind of political entrepreneurship associated with the Commission (Pollack 2003). Agencies, at least in theory, are more likely to have greater autonomy, adhering to the implicit contract in their establishing legislation, and also to develop reservoirs of technical expertise that the Commission cannot establish under its existing budget or civil service rules.

A neofunctionalist regulatory state

We have, then, a very distinctive kind of polity in the EU. It has an enormously powerful legal system unmatched by taxing or spending abilities. It has an executive that is very experienced in the use of grants, research money, and contracts to shape politics—politics, after all, is cheaper than policy. And it has nugatory resources, though its associated agencies have specialist staff less equipped for political entrepreneurialism than for addressing concrete problems. The EU is a regulatory state in that it regulates rather than spends (Majone 1994). Its underlying regulatory asymmetry is not simply towards liberalization, but also towards the use of law rather than money or resources. Even when it does have resources, as with the three agencies associated with DG Sanco, they are about regulation (EFSA, EMA) or information (ECDC) rather than direct action. Such a state externalizes the costs of its actions:

> The efficiency of the EU politico-administrative system derives to a significant degree from the fact that it externalizes the massive costs of governing the Union to member states. The EU is cheap and effective in part, because, of those involved in devising, drafting, and applying EU legislation, EU officials are probably only a minority.
>
> (Page 2001, pp. 148–9)

It is not hard to see why this might bother member state policymakers who are unimpressed by the EU's tendency to spend the member states' money on EU priorities—especially when, as in much health care law, they were never even invited to vote, but rather saw the Court develop a whole jurisprudence without member states' support. Needless to say, international trade law is even more completely regulatory, with no money at all to counteract the costs and redistribution it imposes, and the EU rather than a democratically elected member state government often speaks for Europe in its development.

So the EU is a regulatory state, and its most effective public health policies are the ones that invoke law. But what happens when it does spend money on health? It spends on shaping politics. This means grants, contracts, research, forums and other mechanisms that all share a tendency to build capacity among networks of academics and NGOs who will then support more EU action, as well as the kind of cognitive Europeanization we see when the EU becomes the frame for comparative studies.

Such investment in building European public health politics is part of a broader dynamic in studies of European integration known as neofunctionalism (Niemann 2006; Stone Sweet 2004; Haas 1958).[6] While there have been quite a few debates about neofunctionalism, many of which caricature or misapply it (Greer 2012a), its core insight is sound and often maps onto the arguments in this book. In short, integration promotes integration. One mechanism, which we might call social neofunctionalism, highlights the way policy problems spill over. It is visible, for example, in the argument that free movement of goods and products in the internal market creates a demand for common regulation. If people move, then their infections move too, and we have a prima facie case for the ECDC. Another, though, focuses on the ability of the EU institutions themselves to create policy problems that then can only be resolved through more EU activity—the case, it seems, with EU health care law (Lamping, this volume; Greer 2006b).

The book: Health systems, global health, and public health policies

Much literature on EU health policy has focused on health care services. This book focuses on the broad range of public health, a topic it shares with and picks up from Steffen (2005) as well as, to a lesser extent, Randall (2001) and Mossialos *et al.* (2010).

There are three major areas where the EU influences public health policies and even outcomes, and where public health is recognized as a major issue in policy-making. They are the role of the EU in strengthening, weakening, and shaping the context of health systems; the role of the EU in global health, where its role as a major actor in trade policy means it shapes and is shaped by global rules that affect health care; and the role of the EU in directly addressing public health issues such as obesity, alcohol, or smoking.

These topics still exclude much, from illegal drugs policy to technical assistance with sanitary and phytosanitary standards in states neighboring the EU. We excluded topics that fit into their own self-contained policy worlds such as environmental policy, foreign aid, labor law, or, in most cases, the macroeconomic policy decisions that are so consequential for health. They affect the health of the public, but few would recognize them as "public health" issues. We might wish it otherwise, but all that means is we might wish that future scholars conduct a study of the intellectual and political mobilization that make macroeconomics or environment a "public health" issue. We still had to exclude topics as diverse as blood and blood products, a self-contained policy area; the commercial manipulation of "wellness" (Kickbusch, and Payne 2003), which is interesting but lacks much of a political warrant on the EU level; and occupational health and safety, which is not really regarded as a public health issue in EU law.[7]

Each chapter identifies the characteristics of the policy area and the EU competencies it addresses, then discusses what the EU has done over time, and tries to identify the extent of Europeanization in the policy area. Each chapter then concludes with a discussion of tensions and future directions in the policy area.

The EU and health services

Health care is part of public health, and the EU has increasingly shaped health care systems through direct and indirect policy measures. Part I starts with Wolfram Lamping's chapter (Chapter 2) on the best-known area of EU health policy, the law and politics of patient mobility and associated issues such as the influence of competition and public procurement law on health care systems. Health care is a major part of population health, and the most visible EU policies in health have focused on health care. Furthermore, the dynamics of constitutional asymmetry are very clear: Lamping leads with autonomous courts using their latitude to expand internal market law, while most other chapters detail policies that bog down in the EU legislative process.

The next four chapters discuss more subtle ways in which the EU shapes health systems. In Chapter 3, Heather Elliott discusses the seemingly boring comparative health data that suffuses health policy discussions. She points out that EU policy can be a lever of policy change in member states. Funding comparative studies at the detailed clinical level that influences networks produces the kind of detailed data that embarrasses health care elites and lends itself to concrete actions. The result is that the provision of data—and the shock to countries that find their results comparatively poor—can impel policy action. François Briatte, in his chapter on cancer care (Chapter 4), discusses the oldest and perhaps most successful case of such indirect EU policy. He traces the development and institutionalization of EUROCARE, the program on comparative cancer outcomes that has made it possible to compare European states' cancer outcomes while weaving a network of cancer care advocates and elites. Then Loes Knaapen (Chapter 5) discusses a less-known EU policy in an area of great importance to health care workers and reformers: the efforts of the EU to shape guidelines that would standardize, rationalize, and thereby improve health care across Europe. She shows that while the EU can successfully empower expert networks, it is not always able to predict what they will Europeanize.

Boris Hauray addresses another area of EU power, and an increasingly controversial one—the regulation of medicines and medical devices. In Chapter 6 he explains the gradual unification of both regulation and networks into a "Europe of medicines," albeit one whose failings and biases are all too publicly on display in a recent series of scandals that are pushing further integration. He stresses the extent to which networks constitute and created European medicines regulation, which is part of the reason for its opacity and industry-friendliness.

The EU and global health governance

Part II focuses on the public health policies that come from the EU's established powers in the international system, especially the world trade system. The EU might not be a powerful geopolitical actor in a way that attracts attention in the world's defense or foreign ministries, but it certainly attracts attention among international lawyers, trade negotiators, and all the advocates and lobbyists interested in global public health. This is because of its considerable formal and informal powers—no other international organization is, for example, a member of the G-20.

The three chapters in this section present the EU as an actor in international health. Sébastien Guigner, in Chapter 7, asks the basic question: when is the EU an actor? His chapter presents what the EU does and the variability in its actions and effects on the international stage over time. In Chapter 8, Holly Jarman focuses on how the European Union's law and policy is reshaping health as an object of trade, and how the EU is grappling with the consequences. Her chapter shows how health care has been redefined as a tradable service in politics and law, and the ability of pro-liberalizing forces to use the EU has increased. Solidarity and the public good are exceptions to a liberalizing bias in both EU law and the international law the EU shapes. Elize Massard da Fonseca (Chapter 9) then discusses intellectual property and access to medicines, one of the hottest topics in public health but one that is all too often drawn as a simple moral tale. After showing the influence of pharmaceutical firms on EU intellectual property law—down to the ability to block shipment of medicines from India to Latin America—she discusses the tensions when the EU tries to export this preference to the global environment. The EU might have a strong lobby for access to medicines, but she concludes that the pharmaceutical industry has a stronger role in policymaking than other actors, and it shows in the European approach to intellectual property rights.

The EU and population health

Finally, there are a variety of positive policies in the areas where existing EU policies have contributed to public health problems. The oldest area of public health policy is communicable disease control, and it is an area of longstanding (if often very disappointing) international cooperation. In part III, Scott L. Greer (Chapter 10) shows how the European Union came to be an actor, in a nearly perfect case of spillover. Between crises, funding wove networks of European communicable disease elites and advocates; during crises, network members could suggest European communicable disease policies to match the cross-border threats within the EU itself. Paulette Kurzer, in Chapter 11, addresses the newer but more common and dangerous threats of non-communicable diseases through policy on food, nutrition, and physical activity. In this area, action seems unlikely in an EU with weak competencies and a right-wing majority, but there is nonetheless a thriving policy debate and a variety of platforms that have taken root. In Chapter 12, Jenny Cisneros Örnberg focuses on another major threat to public health—alcohol. She explains the origins of EU policy in the convergence of European drinking patterns on an alarmingly bibulous model. As with nutrition, the result is an EU policy where it would be reasonable to expect none, but one that does not use the most powerful tools the EU wields. Donley Studlar (Chapter 13) discusses EU policy on tobacco, showing how the EU came to oppose tobacco (with strong Treaty amendments and signature of the Framework Convention on Tobacco Control, among other things) while finding its actions limited by a strong pro-tobacco contingent led by a major tobacco industry player, Germany.

Conclusion: Permissive dissensus and public health policy

Liesbet Hooghe and Gary Marks, in an influential early 2009 article, argued that the European integration has moved from a permissive consensus to a constraining "dissensus"—that as the EU has become politicized and democratized, it has lost the protective cocoon of an elite consensus on the desirability of integration and has to justify itself with policies that gain popular support. Public health policy in the European Union has grown up in what they call the era of "constraining dissensus" in which "elites . . . must look over their shoulders" (p. 5).

But in the area of public health, old politics have worked quite well.[8] The language of traditional integration theory, particularly neofunctionalist accounts of spillover and supranational entrepreneurship, work surprisingly well. Stories in which the Commission and the Court are major actors, or in which the EU states empower the Commission to gain a bigger voice in international politics, fit comfortably in the classic stories scholars tell about the EU. Newer stories also show the flexibility and effectiveness at integration of newer methods of European integration such as funding for networks or provision of data. They collectively tell a story of successful European integration, with EU institutions and policy advocates finding ways to create an EU policy agenda and mechanisms even in a policy area like tobacco, obesity, or health care law where the competencies of the EU are strong and most member states reluctant to cede sovereignty.[9]

Public health politics in the EU, in other words, is the politics of a permissive dissensus. If member state leaders were to be of one mind, perhaps they could be the ones who shape EU public health policy. Instead, they are diverse, they disagree, and they are all too easy to trap with all the old and new mechanisms of European integration. There was little support anywhere, including the Commission, for an obesity policy, and yet there is one. There was almost no support for a health care services policy, and yet there is one. And while it might seem hard to object to research on cancer, it should not be hard to ask what business it is of the EU to finance cancer and other research or advocacy networks whose demands member states are supposed to meet.

The EU is undoubtedly under pressure from voters, but much of its work is carried out by people with only vague democratic accountability, far out of sight of heads of state or voters. In the bureaucratic world, the machinery of integration is running quite well. Policy advocates (many of them financed by the EU institutions), the Court and its associated European legal elite, the Commission, and all manner of expert networks are formulating policy and developing agendas that slowly expand the reach and effectiveness of EU policy. Their work is hidden in plain sight, in endless web pages of plans, platforms, proposals, strategies, reports and evaluations. It is not because of secrecy or superb political tactics that they have done so much to integrate Europe at a time when integration was supposed to be slowing; it is because the agenda is so often set in narrow circles of advocates and experts. The result is the wide range of EU policies in this book that would have been unimaginable, or laughable, a few decades ago, from coordinated medicines licenses to a trade policy on medical tourism to a policy on alcopops.[10] European integration, and Europeanization, have enjoyed a permissive dissensus in which the fragmentation of opponents permits all sorts of policies.

This account might look strange to the many frustrated advocates of European public health policies. They can point to a cavernous gap between what the EU does, and what it could do, in all of the areas that we discuss in this book. It protects health care services from world trade law, as Jarman notes—but it also creates markets within the EU and makes solidarity an exception rather than a rule. It no longer subsidizes tobacco farmers, but any anti-tobacco advocate could point out what it does not do. It has an ECDC that is legally and practically sidelined when it comes time for states to buy vaccines for their people. Its pharmaceutical industry enjoys fast approval times, opacity about conflicts of interest, and a leading role in shaping intellectual property policy, as Hauray and Massard da Fonseca show. More insidiously, many of its actions are areas where government and industry can see mutually acceptable outcomes—and so the EU focuses on food labels and safety while the CAP goes unreformed, while alcohol and tobacco policies focus on areas industry can tolerate such as advertising to children or preventing drunken driving. The EU does not take up some of its most powerful weapons in these struggles.

All too often, the effective policy instrument would involve countering industry interests, and the EU instead compromises with industry through a mix of commitments that do not address the basic problems (e.g., portion size or marketing to children) and shifts the focus of policy to undesirable side effects. A policy about obesity turns into McDonalds financing exercise facilities next to its restaurants, and a policy to deal with alcohol abuse turns out to be a policy against drunk driving. Drunk driving is bad, and exercise is good, but those initiatives put the onus on the individual (to sober up after drinking, to exercise after eating fast food) and leave the company's business model intact.[11] These measures have public health value, but they clearly represent a compromise.

That disappoints many. But the fact is that there is a wide range of European public health policy to discuss, as the authors do in this book. The diverse policies and issues have different histories, but each has been touched by European integration in a way that would have been hard to imagine in 1980. More and more often, we have not a politics of European integration in health, but a politics of EU public health policies. The chapters in this book detail the transformation, effects, and future of these policies.

Notes

1 The Tallinn Charter: Health Systems for Health and Wealth, www.euro.who.int/document/e91438.pdf, accessed March 3, 2012.
2 Before that, and in both EU and international trade law to this day, "public health" usually constitutes a permitted exception to trade liberalization rather than a justification for a policy in itself. See Jarman, Chapter 8.
3 As the EU did when it started subsidizing tobacco farmers in 1970, and then again when it stopped doing so. See Studlar, Chapter 13.
4 The transformation she details—from EU policies that try to produce a harmonized European Way, to EU rules for making divergent national policies—is interestingly common as a way of dealing with diversity in EU politics. See Greer and Sokol, forthcoming.
5 From the three agencies' websites, accessed March 3, 2012, with all three showing numbers that correspond to their 2010 annual reports. For our purposes it does not pay to examine these numbers too closely because they vary with consultants, secondments, and temporary staff.
6 And also, arguably, Scheingold (1971).
7 For a more comprehensive review of EU actions in health, see Greer, Elliott, Wismar and Palm, forthcoming.

8   Judging by Google Scholar's list of works citing the article, responses focused on the structure of EU party politics and votes far outnumber work testing their propositions about what happens to policy and policymaking.

9   For a particularly good study of the resilience of European law, and how the mechanisms that helped created it then help to sustain it, see Vauchez (2012).

10   In 1953, a French politician proposed many of them, and they were indeed considered laughable (Parsons 2003, p. 32, pp. 86–88).

11   See Lewin *et al.* (2006) for an analysis of how leading food companies structure and comply with their commitments.

Part I

The EU and health systems

2 European Union health care policy

Wolfram Lamping

> It is clear that Europe does have an effect on health systems. We need to consider
> how we can manage this impact to ensure that it is a positive one for health.
>
> (Former Commissioner for Health and Consumer Protection,
> David Byrne, SPEECH/03/315; June 2003)

Introduction

In the spirit of Kittel (2002, p. 17) one could ask, "Who would have thought only a decade ago the EU would have created a (formally) borderless European health care market?" In the past ten years, the EU has opened the once-sealed world of territoriality and insurmountable administrative thresholds in favor of patients. EU members have gone beyond the exclusive institutional arrangements of their home health care systems, and let patients/consumers or providers experience the EU (almost) as if it were a single country. The result is that the borders of the national health care states, protected by social law, surrounded by barriers to enter and separated from each other, (at least legally) are becoming less significant. Indeed, step by step and by small degrees, health policy has been "nudged" into Europeanization, even though most member states' health authorities have rejected the idea conceptually and still regard health care as a core national issue.

European Union and European integration impact health policy in multiple ways, although there is not yet a singular, formalized EU health policy. Examining the EU treaty, Hervey (2007, p. 1) concludes that, at first glance, there is "nothing (which) would touch national health policies or their fundamental values and principles"; therefore there is reason to assume that health policy is the "less likely policy field" (Martinsen 2005, p. 1036) for discussing Europeanization effects. Is health policy, then, an appropriate example for exploring the impact of "Europe"? Yes, in so far as it is one of the best examples of demonstrating how EU institutions have successfully made a non-topic one of its most popular and challenging future policy fields (Lamping and Steffen 2009). As differential, patchy, accidental and discontinuous as health policy integration has been, member states nonetheless constitute part of a multi-level, multi-tiered and multi-governance system of European health policy that is unique. It is a policy field created by judges and by markets rather than politics—though it is not necessarily unsystematic in its architecture. Health policy in the EU is mirroring what is politically possible, not what might be normatively desirable.

This chapter briefly introduces the issues, arenas, and EU powers in this policy area in the second section. The third section systematizes the "health care puzzle" by reviewing the history of EU health care policies, including the judicial and legislative history, and identifying driving forces. Subsequently, conflicts, opportunities, and the future direction of travel will be outlined in the forth section. Here the main argument will be that European health care, still a gatecrasher in the member states, is a textbook example of a tug-of-war of powers between EU bureaucracy and member governments. Notably, most of the latter are unwilling to accept this kind of "uninvited Europeanization" (Greer 2006b). Although the ability of EU institutions to create EU powers in health care against political opposition is remarkable and should not be underestimated, the effects of EU health care policies on the ground are still limited due to a lack of supporters in the national bureaucracies, in national health care organizations, and not least in member state politics (cf. Greer 2009b, 2011).

Health care and European integration: Formally national and well-protected

There is a momentous difference between public health and health care at EU-level: Unlike public health, where the DG Health and Consumers (DG Sanco) has provided considerable political leadership over the years drawing on a direct, robust treaty base, EU authority and influence in health care are much more fragile, subtle and indirect, that is, they are mainly strategically deduced from other treaty mandates and dependent upon the "serendipity" (Randall 2000) of ECJ jurisdiction (cf. Steffen and Lamping 2009). It comes as no surprise that until recently there has been no genuine EU health care law or EU health care policy concerned with the regulation, organization, financing, and provision of health care. The explanation for this is part of the secret of EU health care integration and part of the "magic formula" which—to a large extent—helps to explain the success of this new EU policy field. In other words: In order to understand the peculiarity of the relationship between integration and health care, we have to understand both the limited competence of the EU in the field of health care and the EU institutional strategies, inertia, momentum, and creativity that addresses health care integration at the supranational level. Those interested in the history of health care integration will be particularly attuned to the constraints on EU policymaking and the ability of EU institutions to occasionally (try to) use their powers for unexpected purposes.

The puzzling picture of European health care integration results from, on the one hand, the particular characteristics of the health care sector as a highly regulated market for services, goods and professionals/patients. On the other hand, given the cross-cutting nature of health care, ambiguous treaty provisions allow EU institutions to play the famous "treaty base game" (Rhodes 1995), that is, to transfer topics and co-opt legitimization from treaties not related to health per se.

EU health policy is, for the most part, a question of establishing common ground with other areas of politics, in particular the EU's internal market regime. More directly stated, the logic and rationality of the health policy integration processes can only be sufficiently understood if one does *not* take the social policy jurisdiction norms of the EU treaty into account.

Given this context, member governments' marginal interest in health care integration issues and the low relevance of EU health policymaking in national debates is in some ways understandable. The EU founding Treaties provide the EU with only restricted responsibilities and competencies in marginal areas of health policy, granting member states exclusive health policy rights. Article 168 TFEU (ex Art. 152) famously concedes that "Union action shall respect the responsibilities of the Member States for the definition of their health policy and for the organisation and delivery of health services and medical care." Direct influence of the EU on financing and delivery of medical care, that is on the core of the national health care states, is still formally excluded from the policy mandate of the Union. In this respect, the Lisbon Treaty does not differ significantly from the previous one. Moreover, Art. 153 TFEU (ex-Art. 137, 1) still rules that qualified majority voting is the standard method in most policy fields—with the exception of, inter alia, "social security and social protection of workers," which are formally still well protected by unanimity (and governments' self-interests) in the Council. In these exceptional areas, national policies are coordinated or standardized by agreements at the European level, but national governments remain in full control of the decision process, and none of them can be bound without consent.

Explicit exceptions include cross-border social security rules, which are under the competence of the Union (Art. 48 TFEU; ex Art. 42). Art. 5 No. 3 TFEU entitles the EU to take initiatives to ensure coordination of member states' social policies, and Art. 4 and 9 TFEU, like Art. 3 TEU (Treaty on European Union), raises the protection of health ("well-being") to the rank of a Community objective to be considered in all EU policies. The EU Charter of Fundamental Rights, which is legally binding since its incorporation in the Lisbon Treaty, states that "everyone has the right of access to preventive health care and the right to benefit from medical treatment" (Art. 35). The overall impression of the Lisbon Treaty is that it respects national sensibilities to legislate in the health care area and emphasizes the competence of member states—but it does not give up the secondary target of increasing the compatibility of member states' health care systems. The Treaty's explicit objective is to strengthen cooperation and coordination between member states and to establish the EU as a benchmarking and monitoring agency on member states' political "radar screen," by applying procedures such as the Open Method of Coordination (OMC) to health care (Art. 168, 2 TFEU).

Member governments' originally nonchalant attitudes toward the role of the EU in health care can be explained by both a fallacious sense of being (formally) protected from any substantial impact of the EU on this policy field, as well as "poverty of imagination," or unwillingness to believe the EU could be influential in national health care regimes. This attitude might account for governments that very often seem to be surprised by supranational policy initiatives or jurisdiction, but are at the same time unwilling (or unable) to politically react on the EU initiatives. The ECJ jurisdiction on patients' rights in cross-border health care is a good example of this dynamic.

Governments' attitudes, however, seem to be in line with citizens' expectations. According to the results of the Eurobarometers (See Standard Eurobarometer 73, Spring 2010, pp. 205 and 214),[1] "health" is among the six areas in which a majority of European respondents, on average, would prefer decisions to be taken at national level. Twenty of the 27 countries would prefer decisions on health to be taken at national level, with a European average of 62 percent. Note that there is a divergence between old and new member states on this topic. Compared to the old member states, the scores of those in favor of decisions taken at EU level are slightly higher in almost all 12 new member states (except Hungary).

The politics of health care integration: On detours, the search for backdoors and neo-functionalisms in the making

Leibfried and Pierson (Leibfried 2005; Leibfried and Pierson 2000) distinguish between three different "pressures" through which European integration affects the national social welfare states. These include (a) the "direct pressures of integration" in the form of "positive" EU initiatives/Community legislation, (b) the "direct pressures of integration" in the form of "negative" integration policies, and (c) the "indirect pressures of integration" as flexible alignment measures undertaken on the part of the national welfare states in order to accommodate the (feared or actual) wide-ranging effects of economic integration (single market; intra-European competition) and the Economic and Monetary Union (fiscal self-bindings, etc.). A fourth category should also be included at this point: (d) the Open Method(s) of Coordination (OMC), the Europeanizing effects of which, if there are any, are clearly different from the other three "pressures." In what follows, I examine in more detail modes (a), (b) and (d).

Direct positive pressures of integration

The *direct positive pressures* of integration result from political decision making at the supranational level, via regulatory policies. These include direct health policy initiatives of the Union that member states have to adopt and implement, as well as health policy programs, which aim at harmonizing and coordinating member states' actions in areas in which the EU has a robust policy mandate. At first glance these supranational initiatives have social purposes explicitly envisaged to limit or correct market effects. The rationale for intervening is an economic one since most of the programs can be understood as removing potentially unfair competitive advantages, which are also barriers to an ideally functioning integrated market. The EU prescribes concrete institutional requirements and an institutional model with which member states' policies have to comply. Although the EU's scope for "positive" initiatives is restricted to specific policy areas, in health care the completion of the internal market as well as the consumer protection/public health-mandate of the Commission allowed for some important Community regulations. Examples include the common regulatory framework for medicinal products in the area of market entry (Directive 2001/83/EC), the free movement of pharmaceuticals within the single market, and the certification and registration of medical devices. The recognition of professional qualifications (Directive 2005/36/EC) aims to facilitate the free movement of EU citizens by making it easier for (health) professionals qualified in one member state to practice in another (currently under revision; see COM 2011/367). Additionally, the EU developed a system of coordination of national social security systems and health insurance coverage within the Community, which is governed by Council Regulations 1612/68, 1408/71, 574/72, 3095/95 and 118/97 (among others). These binding regulations are motivated by the need to adopt social security measures necessary initially to technically facilitate the mobility of (migrant) workers and members of their families and subsequently to guarantee the free movement of EU citizens. The 1408/71-regime made sure "that the new exit options opened up by the common market were actually matched by corre-sponding entry options" (Ferrara 2003, p. 630). This regulation, setting out the conditions under which individuals have access to health care when they move within the EU (see also well C-9/74 and C-20/85), has currently been refined with regard to cross-border health care.

Directive 2011/24/EU of 9 March 2011 titled the "Application of Patients' Rights in Cross-border Healthcare" applies to individual patients who decide to seek health care in a member state that is not their home country. At least formally, the Directive has ushered in a new phase of common EU regulation in the field of patients' mobility and cross-border care within the EU. It was (and still is) govern-ments' attitude of rejection and political contumacity vis-à-vis the ECJ's jurisdic-tion over cross-border health care which finally forced action on the issue. Such a situation might have provided the Commission with a strong legitimacy to act— and it actually took the opportunity and the ECJ decisions as source of legitimacy and inspiration. In this case, ECJ and the Commission acted in tandem driving on neo-functionalist roads—true to the maxim that "the solution to European policy is European policy" (Greer 2006b, p. 134).

The patients' directive is the first attempt to collectivize and codify patients' rights (and member states' responsibilities). The aim has been to promote the idea of a borderless European health care market, to provide clarity and certainty as to the application of free-movement principles to health services, and to specify the rights of consumers and patients' in terms of quality and safety standards. Despite huge opposition from member governments as well as from the vast majority of members of the European Parliament, who repeatedly claim that the Commission's initial conception (COM 2008/414) was going too far and that unrestricted freedom of mobility for patients and health services will lead to a loss of control over health budgets, the directive was finally approved by the European Parliament in January 2011 and subsequently by the Employment, Social Policy, Health and Consumer Affairs Council in February 2011 after a complex political procedure of almost six years. This directive is a striking example of both the political limits of the Commission's overambitious health care blueprints, and of conflicts of interest among member states coming to the fore. These became particularly contentious as the EU initiative approached national "red lines" or had identifiable financial implications for single member states.

The new directive, which according to the Council's opinion is based on the internal market *and* the health policy mandate of the treaty alike, still allows governments to pull the emergency brake, as they keep important cost control instruments in their hands. They define which health care is to be reimbursed and the level of financial coverage provided, since patients are *entitled* to reimbursement for planned health care in other member states *if* the same or similar health care would have been paid for by the social security system in the home country. Moreover, reimbursement is made up to the amount that would have been paid if the same or similar treatment had been provided in the home country—although there is the possibility for member states to go beyond this threshold. In the case of hospital care, the member state of affiliation can also introduce a system of prior authorization for reimbursement—but only under specific conditions defined in the directive (such as the financial stability of the health care system; questionable quality and safety of treatment; or whether the treatment can be provided in the member state of affiliation within a medically justifiable time limit). Finally, member states have to establish national contact points for cross-border health care in order to provide citizens with information on their entitlement to seek health care abroad—not least with regard to the new European reference centers/ networks to be institutionalized in order to provide highly specialized health care.

The phalanx of member government was divided during the many Council negotiations. Smaller and economically poorer member states (such as Portugal, Poland, Lithuania or Romania) expressed their fear that the directive could have a negative impact on their health systems given the possibility of a large outflow of patients or medical specialists to other member states. The same group of countries raised concerns about the impact of a massive inflow of patients from wealthier member states—this could lead to a double disadvantage: to an under-supply for the domestic population (waiting lists, waiting times, etc.) since patients from wealthier countries are much more profitable for domestic providers, while at the same time patients from poorer countries will hardly be able to "enjoy" treatment in expensive health care systems (such as in Austria, France, or Germany) given the fact that providers in these countries are to be remunerated according to the fee schedule in the poorer countries.

Others, among them many new member states, were in favor of a stricter limitation of health treatments that would be reimbursed under the new regime, fearing negative financial repercussions on their health systems. The richer member states, for obvious reasons (cost control, etc.), insisted on a strict application of the prior authorization procedure whenever possible and appropriate. Meanwhile the Commission, in line with the ECJ "philosophy," argued for prior authorization to be the exception and for a reversal of the burden of proof because, "the introduction of a prior authorisation scheme . . . will limit the exercise of rights conferred upon the citizens directly by the EC Treaty, [and] must be proportionate and justified by imperative reasons as those mentioned in the same case-law" (COM 2008/414, 14).

No matter how one interprets the final directive, from a political perspective it can be characterized as a typical EU compromise in health care trying to find the balance between the respect for the ECJ jurisdiction (and as such trying to avoid further "shattering" case-law based on internal market law), the respect for the right (and obligation) of member states to organize, run and manage their health care systems, and the right of patients' hoping for more harmonization, clarity and legal certainty. This section of the new patients' directive is characteristic for member governments' perspective on this new EU law:

> Notwithstanding the possibility for patients to receive cross-border healthcare under this Directive, Member States retain responsibility for providing safe, high quality, efficient and quantitatively adequate healthcare to citizens on their territory. Furthermore, the transposition of this Directive into national legislation and its application should not result in patients being encouraged to receive treatment outside their Member State of affiliation.
>
> (Directive 2011/24/EU; no. 4)

The future role and relevance of the ECJ in health care is very much dependent upon how and to what extent member states are willing to transpose this directive into national social law.

Direct negative pressures of integration

Negative integration policies eradicate national norms at times. Negative integration policies can be denoted as *explicit* spillover effects, that is, externalities associated with economic integration and market building. They define conditions for market access and market functioning and aim at containing legal prohibitions against national regulations that might otherwise function as obstacles and barriers to free movement or as distortions of competition between member states within the community.

While the four "market freedoms" (Art. 26-37 and 45-62 TFEU) aim at restrictions on the free movement of goods, services and persons within the EU's internal market, the competition law focuses on the liberalization of the internal market creating a regime of undistorted competition on the EU market through the ban on cartels (Art. 101 TFEU), the prohibition of any abuse of a dominant market position (Art. 102 TFEU), and the prohibition of subsidies or other aid granted by the state that might distort competition (Art. 106–108 TFEU). These tools allow coordination between EU internal market regulations and national social security policies since their rationality and *raison d'être* are different in many ways. EU law's supremacy over domestic law in case of conflict over norms means that national institutions have to adjust their systems, which is challenging given that the EU does not precisely define what exactly an EU-compatible national model should be. There are exceptions to the strict application of the EU competition regime, at least with regard to the so-called "services of general economic interest" (Art. 14 TFEU, Art. 106 No.2 TFEU and in the Protocol No. 26 on Services of General Interest). Although the concrete meaning and scope is still contentious and dependent on each individual case, these Treaty provisions should not be understood as merely symbolic.

The logic of EU free movement and competition law as well as its application to law on health systems had been a new and unfamiliar (let *al*one an unwanted) experience for EU member governments. Confronted with unexpected "attacks" from the ECJ and the Commission, member states sometimes have to justify policies that had been unchallenged and therefore assumed to be legitimate at national level and under their social law regimes. The Court decisions, in particular those on patient mobility, which were a step forward in the rights of European citizens (they gave citizens a wider choice for seeking medical care), set in motion an exigent and inescapable dynamic among governments and health policy actors. The delivery of health services and medical care to patients had been thought to be largely unaffected by European integration politics. The ECJ rulings were internal market rulings and by no means health or social policy rulings, but their implications have been inherently political and have had an impact on health policy. The ECJ did not interpret the fundamental freedoms extensively; rather, it interpreted them systematically, despite the hopes of member states. It is no longer possible to ignore that health care is an essential part of SEM and that the influence of the so-called "four fundamental freedoms" is especially significant. These freedoms include: the *freedom of movement for persons* (labor market for professionals; mutual/automatic recognition of national qualifications and diplomas, especially in the health professions; Union-wide access of EU citizens to medical care), *goods* (e.g., the market for pharmaceutical products and medical technology), *services* (e.g., cross-border delivery of services and the choices available to patients; freedom of establishment) and *capital* (e.g., in hospital investment) within the emerging European health care market.

Against firm opposition from the majority of national governments and health insurance schemes, in its jurisdiction the ECJ has harmonized rights and established patients' rights to seek out-patient care in another member state, with reimbursement from the home institution. It also specified the conditions under which reimbursement from the home institution could be claimed for in cases of in-patient care. Meanwhile much has been written on the ECJ case law on the delivery of health care cases. The most important cases include the famous Kohll (C-160/96) and Decker (C-120/95) cases via Vanbraekel (C-368/98) and Geraets-Smits and Peerbooms (C-157/1999) to (inter alia) Watts (C-372/04) and others. Perhaps even more influential has been the EU harmonization legislation articulating the aforementioned directive on patients' rights in cross-border health care.

The "Watts-"decision (C-372/04 of May 2006) is both typical and remarkable in at least five respects: First, it should have come as no surprise for member states, although it did for Britain, that the obligation to reimburse costs of treatment in another EU member state applies also to systems where treatment is provided free of charge (benefits-in-kind). Second, in order to calm governments' nerves, the Court confirmed that national authorities are entitled to institute a system of waiting lists in order to manage supply and to set priorities on the basis of resources availability. It conceded that maintaining financial balance can be a justification for requiring prior authorization for medical treatment abroad, particularly in systems with waiting lists. But, third, since governments quite obviously refused to learn from previous ECJ jurisdiction on health care, the Court made perfectly clear that prior authorization cannot be refused if treatment in the country of affiliation is not available *within an acceptable time as determined by the medical circumstances*. This was a slap in governments' faces after a series of "warning shots." Fourth, and against this background, the Watts ruling can be interpreted as a social-political one because in its core it is about defining acceptable degrees of pain, limiting strain imposed by physical suffering, and it is about improving quality of life in times of disease. Fifth, the decision emphatically points to a shift in which the ECJ no longer treats EU citizens from an economic perspective as simple "consumers" on the European health care market—but as patients from a genuine social-policy perspective.

It is therefore not surprising that most member state governments perceived the ECJ-rulings in Watts and similar cases as a source of disturbance, and adopted a negative and defensive stance towards the ECJ jurisdiction (cf. Obermaier 2009; Greer 2009b). And, as the Commission discovered, member states ultimately rejected the rulings as an "attack on their right to organize their health and social security systems in their own way under *subsidiarity*" (COM 2001/723:11). This holds true also for the EU competition regime.

The financial, structural, and practical consequences of the internal market's four freedoms seem to be in inverse proportion to the "crisis scenarios" in national health policy debates. The effect of the single market competition regime remains an underestimated dimension. In case of incompatibility, the EU competition law might effectively pressurize member states' institutional, regulatory and normative frameworks. Meanwhile, the "rules of the game" are slowly becoming clearer. As soon as social security institutions act "economically" according to the quite liberal interpretation of the ECJ, they lose their national privileges. Following the Court's stepwise attempts to legally specify the relationship between national social policy institutions and European competition regime, much depends on how these institutions are internally constructed, how they are normatively justified, and finally what specific function they have in the institutional arrangement of each welfare state.

Without going into detail (cf. Lamping 2005; Mossialos *et al*. 2010), one peculiarity should be kept in mind when debating the applicability and (possible) impact of the internal market law on health care and health care organizations. European competition law distinguishes between (i) the *function* of an organization and (ii) its real *activity* on a specific market. In other words, whenever an entity acts economically it is legally treated as an undertaking *regardless of its legal status or the way in which it is financed or the profit/non-profit question* (see, e.g., C-118/85; C-41/90, paragraph 21; or C-160/91, paragraph 17).[2] At the same time, in a 1977 ruling (C-13/77; re-confirmed in the 2006 FENIN ruling C-205/03), the ECJ declared that "any abuse of a dominant position within the market is prohibited [. . .] even if such abuse is encouraged by a national legislative provision," as in the case of social health insurance schemes or national health services.[3]

Political pressures of integration: Much ado about nothing?

The Open Method(s) of Coordination (OMC) is an attempt to politically coordinate the shift in specific policy areas among member states and to channel them as similarly as possible. Via the OMC and at a communal level, policy areas in which the EU has no legal access are to be developed. The result is a post-regulatory approach and a sort of experimental governance, referred to and embedded in EU debates on new forms of governance. Within the scope of the OMC, (non-binding) aims in the form of guidelines are formulated, while both qualitative and quantitative indicators are designated in benchmarking and self-commitment processes. Governing competences and capacities remain entirely at the national level since the general guidelines and the more detailed recommendations for each member state lack compulsory character. Voluntariness is the price the Commission has to pay in order to motivate member states to take part in these new procedures. But the Commission is well aware of the fact that once the OMC has proved to be an effective instrument, voluntariness could turn into moral, and thus de facto, obligation. In health policy, however, current politics are still far away from this scenario.

At the 2002 European Council of Barcelona, the Commission was assigned with the task of discussing and examining aspects of cross-border health care and service arrangements. These included questions of "access" (guarantee of general access to health provision), "quality" (guarantee of a high quality of provision), and the "financial stability" (guarantee of long-term financial stability) of member states' health care systems on the basis of performance indicators and benchmarking. Meanwhile, with regard to the identification of "best" or "better practices," the EU gathers and compares a wide range of health-related data (see the chapters by Briatte, Knaapen, and Elliott, this volume). Given the institutional and policy differences between employment and pension policy on the one hand and health care on the other, it is not surprising that the application of the OMC to health care is still contentious, especially when it comes to measuring health systems' performance. Given the sensitivity of health care, most member states' health authorities resist attempts to evaluate and rate their systems, to improve transparency, and to make them comparable, and are afraid of coming off badly, "Member States do not want to be given grades. They do not agree on qualitative and quantitative indicators because their results might be used against them" (Stein 2003, p. 24). In other words, governments' self-confidence and openness to learning from each other and to trying to resolve problems commonly is quite low in this policy field.

Exclusive, inner circles of pro-EU health experts are busy collecting evidence and constructing indicators in order to better compare practices and measure progress toward common objectives, there is reason to assume that the OMC has little, if any, significant effect on national health care politics and national health care settings—although causality or correlation with national policy change is hard to detect. For most member governments, the OMC is a sort of obligatory exercise, and in no way an "affair of the heart." The OMC can theoretically promote learning from differences and through the definition of common values. But what if governments do not want to learn? What if it is only the national health policy experts, sent from their national ministries to the OMC working groups, who, already socialized to the Brussels "game" and familiar with "Euro-speak," learn and support the OMC? In their home countries, these administrative experts often live the life of outsiders within their ministries of health. Whether or not the OMC will have any effect on the ground largely depends on the role these bureaucrats are able to play in their respective ministries of health. As yet, however, there is still a lack of reliable empirical evidence of the practical effects of OMC in health care in the "old" member states. This is also true for Central and Eastern EU member states that are still in the process of "catching-up" in health care as well as in other areas. According to the Eurobarometer, these countries also find themselves in a situation where their populations seem to be more in favor (though not at all enthusiastic) of decisions on "health" being taken at EU level than do the "older" member states (here: Standard Eurobarometer 73, Spring 2010, pp. 205–14).

Conflicts, tensions, and the future direction of travel

As yet unparalleled in the world, the EU is a laboratory for an experiment with a number of debatable, if not unwanted, policy outcomes and unintended consequences of trends such as services liberalization, the expansion of cross-border trade and competition in health services, and patients seeking treatment in other EU member states. One of the main findings of research is that health care integration is still tightly constrained by governments' (legitimate) self-interests and the dominant market character of European integration. It is still far from being a stable policy concern of and within the EU. Governments still disapprove of further integration of health care, especially with regard to unrestricted patient mobility, a borderless competitive European market for health care providers, and further application of internal market law on their health systems. One should bear in mind that European health care policy is not produced in a vacuum, but rather in a space filled with social, political, and economic forces in which member states mobilize considerable self-interest, and responsibility and expectations of security are traditionally directed toward the nation (member) states. Given these dynamics, it comes as no surprise that European health care integration is predominately the result of the ECJ applying internal market law to national health systems and the Commission. The shaping of European health policy illustrates the juridification of governance, for the Court's decisions function as a policy surrogate.

European health care integration is a striking example for what Weiler (1982) and Haltern (2004) called "integration through law." In sum, European health care integration consists predominately of ECJ decisions often followed by Commission initiatives, both partners in a circle of self-reference and referral.[4] "Integration through law" might not be a problem as long as EU projects can rely on permissive consensus among the addressees (output legitimacy).

Much of the EU market-making policies seem to be in favor of patients—as long as the patients are able and willing to exploit the new opportunities. Yet, we also see that among the majority of member governments this sort of permissive consensus is less pronounced, if it exists at all. There was little, if no, demand among member states for European initiatives in the health care sector. The unwillingness, and the inability, of national health ministers to engage in health policy integration was partly compensated by the active role of the ECJ, which did not hesitate to interfere with member states' social law regimes. In this respect, EU health care integration is probably one of the EU's boldest ventures in pushing through "Europeanization" (i.e., liberalization)—ironically without disposing of the competencies at EU level.

As part of its own push for the establishment of a common market for health care, the ECJ has driven a wedge through the middle of the welfare states ("regulatory dichotomy"; Lamping 2005). The states are still able to shape the demand side of their health care systems, that is, the groups affected, the payout criteria, or the service catalogues; however, the ECJ is continually liberalizing the production side of services. The ECJ has precisely defined the conditions under which institutions fall under the jurisdiction of EU competition law, and under which they have portfolio protection, that is, when institutions may keep their privileges and special rights. In case of doubt, it is the ECJ that acts as border (and market) patrol.

Divided regulation in the European health care arena

One important aspect of European market integration is that governments have slowly become aware of potential incompatibilities between national and supranational legislation. However, regulatory capacities of national governments have not been abolished—they have simply changed. Furthermore, European integration does not merely restrict national policy choices, it simultaneously enhances strategic policy options of governments and private actors (domestically and via "Brussels"). There is undoubtedly no *general* pressure to liberalize or privatize institutional health care arrangements, even though one can observe a strong tendency to adjust to greater market conformity in certain sectors as well as the salience of competition as a rationale for the emerging European health care market. Also, processes of "privatization"—and sometimes processes of de-regulation—are simultaneously processes of denationalization, shifting regulatory social-policy competences to the supranational level. There are, thus, many roads on which the EU can drive within the member states, but sometimes it is still the member states which are able to stop the EU by changing the traffic lights to red.

Regarding the problem of health care integration there is certainly no lack of juridical dominance and technocratic rationality, but there is a notable lack of politics. Bringing politics back in, however, is a complex issue when governments are unwilling to act (not to mention the unwillingness to react) politically. This reticence is due to a bundle of factors, and in particular the differential impact of the EU on national health care systems as well as different degrees of national concerns. Differences across countries depend largely on the institutional arrangements of national health systems (which at least partly explains why member states often are "lone fighters" in EU health care politics and more concerted action is complicated and unlikely), and on the cleavages among EU health care states (such as old/large vs. small/new; winners/losers, etc.). On the one hand, given the problem of collective action, it is fairly complicated for governments to form large political coalitions. On the other hand, the difficulty of organizing coordinated action by member states makes it easier for the Commission to prevent concerted member states' action against its initiatives.

Since the late 1990s, DG Sanco has shown determination in agenda setting and problem framing, and in confronting governments with elaborate policy proposals against national authorities. The Commission, especially in health care, is very dependent upon supporting coalitions at all levels of the policy process (analyzed by Greer 2011). This is at once a strength in its engagement of key stakeholders, as well as the Achilles' heel of the Commission's policy initiatives. Health care is a striking example of the Commission's capacity to become a network organization, working with and through public and private bodies within the member states and at EU level. This is particularly valuable when conflicts with governments occur, like in the wake of the OMC or during the negotiations of the patients' directive. An EU-level pro-integration health-policy community and (directly or indirectly Commission-financed) pro- and pan-European platforms have rapidly grown. This expanding supranational health-policy collectivity has led to a gradual trans-nationalization of policy discourse and goal setting at both administrative and scientific levels. Less action has been seen at political, *let al*one public, levels.

Apart from politics, there is ample criticism on the effect of European integration on health care—both that integration has gone too far, and that it has not gone far enough, in health care. For the former, the many obstacles patients face when they try to travel as European consumers of health care to get treatment abroad point to the still striking health inequalities within EU member states and across the EU. It comes as no surprise for those in favor of greater integration and more EU harmonization that member governments are the bêtes noires, sticking to their authority in an irrational manner. The proponents of further health policy integration complain that governments tend to ignore the many opportunities and benefits European integration could provide for health care actors and the health care sector (both by cross-border synergies and by "de-frosting" domestic institutions that are well-protected by entrenched lobby interests and marked by strong path-dependencies). Those who are pro-integration contend that governments underestimate the added value of harmonization and Europeanization to health care systems (borderless European market, economies of scale, access to high-quality treatment for all EU citizens, and the like).

Those who argue that integration has gone too far emphasize the de-stabilizing and de-structuring effects of integration in general and of the ECJ jurisdiction in particular. They also point to the Commission's overambitious attempts to integrate this sensitive policy area and especially on the lack of evaluation, that is, a lack of knowledge on the real effects of EU integration initiatives in national health care systems. Since this research line is more related to the here and now, I will concentrate on briefly highlighting some of these concerns.

We may assume that health care systems could develop problems with health service planning as a result of the mobility of professionals. There is some work on the effects of increasing health professional mobility on the performance of health systems, especially since the enlargements in 2004 and 2007 (cf. e.g., the seminal work on health professional mobility in Europe by Wismar *et al.* 2011a). The conclusion that can be drawn from these studies is that there is still a lack of knowledge about the scope and consequences of this phenomenon, that is, the impact of mobility of health professionals on both their own health systems and the labor market in the country of destination. There is, however, reason to worry about health systems in low- and middle-income countries in danger of being further weakened by losing health workforce (Glinos 2012).[5]

Scientific studies into the size and the characteristics of health care tourism, the financial effects for countries whose citizens receive care abroad (insurers, local pharmacies, etc.), and the effects for health care systems in countries that are typical destinations for health tourists still remain widely lacking (as an exception the recent study by Wismar *et al.* 2011b). In the long run, however, a rising number of EU citizens crossing borders for effective and high-quality health care could raise further questions about differences in quality (treatments, services, etc.), about patient safety, but especially about creating an insurance-based common "standard benefits package." However, member states have spent on average no more than 1 percent of public spending on health care for cross-border health care. This estimate includes unplanned cross-border health care (such as emergency care). This indicates that while patient mobility has become a relevant issue on the EU's agenda, it is not in the "real life" of health systems. In other words, the EU is trying to meet a need that has not yet been demanded by a relevant number of EU citizens, let *al*one purchasers and providers of health care.[6] This is a typical example for a solution seeking a problem.

Adapting to the rights and demands of the "European patient" could be a future challenge for health care organizations and could lead them to adapt to the European market and to think differently about how they plan, finance and provide health care.[7] This will only occur once there is a significant increase in the number of patients/insured seeking treatment abroad and a qualitative change in the demand for specific treatment (such as treatment in highly specialized hospitals or in European reference centers).

As seen in this chapter, the ECJ case law and the Commission's initiatives of positive legislative polices have created rights-based "commodification" (EU citizens/patients as consumers) and have de-bordered the national health care markets. This has led to the growing body of ECJ jurisdiction in the field of patients' mobility and patients' rights (see above), which Scharpf (2008) describes as "individual rights against national solidarity" (my translation). The EU has been willing and able—in the words of Greer (2009b)—to transform "secret gardens" into "public parks." But while patients/consumers are allowed to stroll in these parks (provided that they are able to pay the "entrance fee") and providers to pass by the open gates (following the internal market regulations), member states still are the major attendants in their respective park (provided that states behave in conformity with EU law).

Moreover, governments are still able to basically "tame" the effects of patient mobility, at least in the sense that it is they who define the national benefits catalogue while medical treatment in other member states is reimbursed. With regard to the member state level, Greer (2011, p. 198) argues that "policymaking with little or no supporting coalitions is a good . . . demonstration of power but it is not a route to effective implementation." In health care, consequential changes in patient, market, or administrative, *let al*one political, behavior, are far from being clearly visible. There are limits to what the ECJ can do to change policy, according to Greer's 2009 study of "old" and large EU health care states. It comes as no surprise that the result of, on the one hand, a fairly unspecific EU impact on health care systems (regulatory framework; internal market; OMC) and, on the other, member states' *surface compliance*,[8] is that the impact of European integration on health care structures, the mobility of patients, and financial stability has been manageable in most countries. Moreover, as Greer (2009b) and Greer and Rauscher (2011a) have shown, the question of whether EU market-making in health care automatically means the creation of common markets, is a tricky one. They provide sobering, but not surprising, evidence (drawn from the UK and Germany) that it is questionable that EU attempts to remove barriers to cross-border activity are creating any kind of market in health care: They found almost no behavior by states or stakeholders that was both competitive and attributable to EU policy.

Whether all this—be it the minimalist implementation of EU health care law on the ground or the stepwise liberalization of the European health care market despite its debatable side-effects—is good or bad, is in the normative eye of the beholder. At the same time, much research remains to be done in order to analyze and better understand the different implementation/compliance patterns of member states in health care and the causal mechanisms underlying these different trajectories. Comparative studies of the impact of EU law are still rare (cf. the work done by Obermaier 2009 and Greer and Jarman 2012).

Conclusions: Destination Europe for national health care systems?

> In truth, the impact of European law is neither as positive nor as negative as it is often described. The free movement of health services does raise issues, certainly.

> But the provisions of the Treaties are not going to change the world of healthcare on their own.
>
> (Former Commissioner for Health and Consumer Protection,
> David Byrne, SPEECH/03/315; June 2003)

There is still no clear dividing line between the member-state arena and the European arena in health care. How could there be one given the dynamics of European integration and the unwillingness to discuss questions of *finalité*? The contours of a cross-level EU health care compound are slowly becoming visible, marked by a new and complex overlapping of responsibility and jurisdiction between the national and supranational levels and plural locations of decision making. Within this compound, a rights-based "European health care citizenship" community without trans-national solidarity and without effective cooperation and coordination at supranational level is emerging. The effects of this kind of integrated health care that provides unequal access to health care abroad despite formally equal rights or regionally imbalanced labor markets for professionals will certainly call for further supranational activity in the years to come.

As demonstrated in this chapter, there are definitive loopholes for further integrating health care—but they seem to be politically highly contested, particularly when national competencies and national financial resources are at issue. Whether European integration is "killing national health and insurance systems but healing patients" (Hatzopoulos 2002) remains to be seen in the years to come. In the meantime we should not expect European institutions to take up basic health care functions, such as the financing and delivery of care, nor should we expect member states to give up these competencies.

Notes

1 The question was: "For each of the following areas, do you think that decisions should be made by the (national) government, or made jointly within the European Union?"
2 Cf. C-180/98 to C-184/98C-218/00; see also C-41/90 and C-244/94).
3 Cf. C 123/83; C-41/90; C-35/96; C-180/94 to C-184/98; also C 67/96, C 219/97, C 115/97-C117/97 and C 180/98-184/98).
4 EU influence on health care stands as an example of the traditional neofunctionalist paradigm: The process of health care integration is mainly fueled by functional and institutional spillovers. In this respect, Greer (2006b) demonstrates that neofunctionalism still provides a convincing explanation of the ongoing, unintended (at least from the member states' standpoint) expansion of EU competencies.
5 Much lesser than even the competition law dimension is the impact of the fast-growing field of EU public procurement rules on health and national steering instruments discussed by Hatzopoulos (2008) and Hatzopoulos and Stergiou (2010). Public procurement rules are a concrete expression of the fundamental freedoms, in particular the free provision of services. More recently, freedom of establishment cases are challenging health care systems and will be of utmost importance in the near future—most notably with regard to hospitals and pharmacies.
6 According to a study conducted by one German health insurance company (Techniker Krankenkasse) in 2010 (Wagner *et al.* 2010), nearly 90 percent of a sample of 40,000

insurees did not know anything about the Directive on Patients' Rights. Since the implementation of the entitlement for cross-border care in 2004, the demand has remained at a steady level—around 1 per cent of all insurees of the Techniker Krankenkasse per year were seeking treatment in another EU member state.

7 See, for example, Zanon (2011) with respect to the implications for the NHS.

8 That is, an implementation which can at best be described as minimalist—the effects of which are tamed (or absorbed) and transformed in policies that do not really "harm" national health systems (financially, power equilibriums, institutional figurations, etc.) (cf. also Greer and Rauscher 2011b)—but which still runs the risk of bringing the ECJ into play.

3 European Union health information infrastructure and policy

Heather Elliott[1]

Rudolph Virchow once noted that "Medicine is a social science, and politics nothing but medicine at a larger scale" (Virchow 1848). While this may have been true in the late nineteenth century, this observation holds little validity in the politically infused environment of European Union (EU) public health. As David Stuckler and colleagues noted, Virchow's statement could now be read as "Social Science is medicine, and medicine is nothing but politics at a larger scale" (Stuckler *et al.* 2010a). The politics of health and public health policy are not only impacted by politics, but are intertwined within the EU institutions that produce them. Public health policy is inherently a political exercise and every new health program that is budgeted for is subjected to the same political environment and constraints as other policies in the EU. The development of a health information infrastructure at the EU level is no exception. This is particularly true for official sources of information, such as from national statistical offices; and even more so for comparisons between states, such as between the member states of the EU. Still very much a work in progress, however, this infrastructure reflects the technical complexities of international comparisons in health, as well as broader political choices and priorities.

It is clear that health information and the development of a standardized health data structure within the EU has become an area of active infrastructure development within the Community. This is, however, technically difficult; health indicators are challenging to standardize and measure within single countries, *let al*one between countries with different political, cultural, and economic institutions. An awareness of the politics behind the development of the EU health information infrastructure, how the infrastructure came to be, as well as its capacity, is a critical step to understanding the greater public health environment in the EU—especially as the data and information drawn from that system can play a pivotal role in shaping wider EU public health debates. This chapter presents the development of health information infrastructure and policy in the EU and discusses some of the challenges associated with such an endeavor.

History of European health information and policy development

Health policy was not part of the European Union's formal mandate until 1992. Up until that point, EU treaties provided no specific Treaty article for health, although progress was made on specific areas (e.g., cancer), and health was integrated elsewhere in the Treaties as part of other policy objectives. EU health regulations and policy may seem commonplace in 2012; however, these frameworks had to be built as situations and crises arose. A telling example of the pressure for data comes from the related field of food safety and animal health. The bovine vCJD catastrophe in the UK created a crisis because no record of trade in animals or animal products was in place in the EU. As a result, several countries closed their borders to UK beef products, interrupting not only agricultural trade, but also the market infrastructure of the EU. While this example refers to food safety issues, which are distinct from public health data and information systems, it illustrates that regulations were created in response to crises. The vCJD crisis indirectly exposed the feeble public health infrastructure and prompted the development of several EU-level regulations, including public health measures such as the regulation of blood, organs, and tissues. These are some of the earliest examples of the creation of a EU public health and health policy competency.

Following the Treaty of Rome in 1956 and the Single Europe Act in 1986, both of which included aspects of health in the EU treaties, the 1992 Maastricht Treaty provided the first specific legal basis in the area of health by creating a limited European Community competence for public health (Article 129). This was the first time that health data and indicators (along with other areas, such as epidemiological surveillance and control of communicable diseases) were formally designated as an area of action by the European Union (or more accurately, the European Community, at the time). European action on health data and indicators was developed, in part, due to the need for common standards, as well as cooperation that would enable the comparison of health information, data, and indicators between European countries. In order to initiate the process of establishing standardized indicators and health measures between member states, the High Level Committee on Health established the Working Party on Community Health Data and Indicators (Working Party). This group was made up of high-level officials in the Ministries of Health in the EU who were charged with assessing the comparability of EU health data, the feasibility of creating standardized data measures and information systems in the EU, and assessing what other actions could be taken at the EU level to develop a community health information system (Brender *et al.* 1996).

The first concrete focus for work on health information was the health monitoring program.[2] This program aimed to establish a Community health monitoring system that would:

(a) measure health status, trends and determinants throughout the Community;
(b) facilitate the planning, monitoring and evaluation of Community programs and actions; and

(c) provide member states with appropriate health information to make comparison and to support their national health policies.[3]

Apart from the detailed aims and work areas of the health monitoring program (which are described in the Annex to the program itself), there are three aspects in particular worth noting.

First, the budget; the entire budget for this five-year program was set at 13.8 million European Currency Unit (ECU), so only around 2.76m ECU each year. From the start, therefore, this severely constrained the ability of the health monitoring program to develop health data collection at European level. Although the detailed objectives and actions set out in Annex 1 of the program included objectives such as support for the routine collection of a set of Community health indicators and the use of Community-wide surveys, in practice the very limited budget made such ambitions unrealistic. The practical way forward was rather to focus on technical means of ensuring comparability between the data already collected by the member states, and encouraging the adaptation and completion of such data collection where necessary (McKee and Ryan 2003). While this was a successful response to the challenge presented by the health monitoring program and made much progress, it made Community health information very much dependent on what information national authorities chose to collect and the timescales on which they collected it and passed it on to the European level. The result was limited data and delays of several years in its availability, which still affect the European health information system today.

Second, the scope, and in particular the absence of collecting any data on the "elephant in the room"—the health systems of the member states. Although the overwhelming bulk of national resources and political attention in health was focused on the health systems of the different countries, the Community health monitoring program conspicuously omits comparisons between health systems from its scope. This reflects the clear orientation of the Treaty mandate for Community action on health, which makes it clear that European action should focus on public health, not health systems or health care. Nevertheless, given the resources allocated to health systems and their impact on health, it is noteworthy that they are not included in this health information system—again, a structural choice that has affected all subsequent work. As an aside, it is worth noting that in the end, this omission has not prevented comparative international information on health systems from being collected and analyzed, as has been shown by the work of the Organization of Economic Co-Operation and Development (OECD) in particular[4]—it has just ensured that this has been done independently from the formal framework of health information of the European Union.

The third key element was the structure of this program as a stand-alone program on health monitoring. This was one of eight different programs that were established as part of the initial strategy for putting in place action on public health at European level. However, several of the other programs included strong information dimensions, such as those on communicable diseases, cancer, rare diseases, injury prevention and drug prevention.[5] This structure created both coordination and integration of health information challenges, with different information systems being developed for different issues under these eight separate programs. This illustrates the reason for the shift to an "integrated" approach with the first (2003–2008) health program, which brought all these different areas of action together into a single integrated program.

Improving "information and knowledge for the development of public health" was in fact given as the first of the three core objectives of the first health program. The budget was also somewhat increased, with the overall budget for the program of €312m equating to about €21m per health for the health information strand. However, the ambition of the health information activities had also increased, with the central aim of

> developing and operating a sustainable health monitoring system to establish comparable quantitative and qualitative indicators at Community level on the basis of existing work and of accomplished results, and to collect, analyse and disseminate comparable and compatible age- and gender-specific information on human health at Community level concerning health status, health policies and health determinants, including demography, geography and socioeconomic situations, personal and biological factors, health behaviours such as substance abuse, nutrition, physical activity, sexual behaviour, and living, working and environmental conditions, paying special attention to inequalities in health.
>
> (Annex, paragraph 1.1)

Alongside the raft of other health information objectives, the budget still seems remarkably limited and clearly still constrained the ability to achieve these objectives in practice. The picture did not substantially change with the second health program; although health information was again one of the central three objectives of the program, the fundamental difficulties of making progress in the area remained.

The extent to which these constraints limit the development of the health information system overall is illustrated by the resources allocated where the EU has made Europe-wide information a priority. Two examples are particularly relevant, as they concern areas that relate to the overall health information aims: drug dependence and communicable diseases. The European Monitoring Centre for Drugs and Drug Addiction (EMCDDA) was established in 1993 in order to provide evidence and data concerning drugs and drug addiction.[6] This is carried out through a combination of methods for data collection including specific surveys to ensure comparable Europe-wide data, with an annual budget of over €16m in 2012. The European Centre for Disease Prevention and Control (the ECDC) was established in 2004 to monitor the specific area of infectious diseases, and has a budget of over €58m in 2010. The comparative paucity of resources for the overall area of health information illustrates the structural difficulties in developing this area at European level.

Like many important policy areas, the development of health information and data structures is politically sensitive. With any survey or quantitative measure of health, one runs the risk of reducing complex health phenomena to simple rankings. This can been seen in the variability and inconsistency in health indicators that provide data on quality of health care, health promotion, and aspects of the provision and use of health care services (Kilpeläinen *et al.* 2012).[7] While politically charged, it is clear that the Commission is working to develop an infrastructure for data collection and dissemination within the EU.

Growth of health information infrastructure

The question remains, therefore, as to how the Commission will be able to build a sustainable health information infrastructure within these constraints. The European Union has a developing health strategy, part of which includes producing comparable health information and indicators for use by public health authorities, policymakers, health professionals, and wider stakeholders. However, a major question is just how politically stable is this strategy and is it a high priority for the Commission? In 1993, there was no concept of a complete and all-encompassing EU public health strategy (Birt 2008). There were a few uncoordinated disease-prevention programs, and member states operated their own health information systems. That being said, one of the current goals of EU health information systems is to develop coherence and compatibility of national systems, not replace them; however, a significant amount of work has been done at the EU level to define health indicators, improve the consistency of reporting of health status, as well as the collection of health data in member countries. As discussed above, health information is far from apolitical. Political jockeying and budget priorities played a large part in the creation of this strategy and the implementation of it. While professionals and practitioners in the public health field often sanctify these programs, it does not mean these programs are prioritized in the greater policy environment. This strategy is smaller than originally intended; however, it has produced several working programs and developed a working infrastructure.

Harmonization of health data and information systems can be seen in other areas as well, particularly in the areas of rare diseases and cancer. The "Europe Against Cancer" programs (1987–2000) were EU-level programs that aimed to reduce the expected number of deaths due to cancer by 15 per cent by the year 2000. Between 1987 and 2000, expected cancer deaths dropped by 9 per cent (European Public Health Alliance 2003). While information systems and data collection may not be directly responsible for this reduction, understanding cancer inequalities and incidence can only be done through a solid data and information infrastructure. Given the results of "Europe Against Cancer" thus far, the Commission has continued to support member states in reducing cancer deaths and has set a goal to reduce cancer incidence by 15 per cent by 2020.

Efforts to help those with rare diseases in Europe have also been against a backdrop of health information infrastructure. In the EU, any disease that affects fewer than five people in 10,000 is considered rare (European Commission, Directorate General Health and Consumers 2012b). In order to combat these diseases, the EU is attempting to pool fragmented and scarce resources from member states to share information and expertise across borders. Due to the low prevalence, and thereby limited dispersion of professional expertise on these diseases throughout the EU, many patients must travel to seek health care services when expertise is unavailable in their own country. Ensuring that medical information and knowledge is accessible to patients and other medical professions, and that these diseases are coded and traceable within morbidity and mortality information systems will encourage adequate recognition of these diseases, both politically and economically. Information systems will continue to provide vital data and will highlight the harmonization efforts in place as well as ones that are needed in the future.

Current state of affairs

The current EU health information and data infrastructure system does not consistently provide timely and/or useful data. There has been a large push in the EU over the last several years to improve the development of these systems and these efforts are largely reflected in the current EU health surveys, European Community Health Indicators, the communicable disease infrastructure in the EU, as well as in the regulations at the Community level. These areas are all active policy areas that are being developed. A particular emphasis has been placed on developing a framework based on an agreed set of international classifications (such as the International Classification of Diseases, the International Classification of Health Accounts, etc.), as well as the development of operational systems to collect data on the health of populations, and the creation of summary measures and population health indicators (European Commission, Directorate General Health and Consumers 2012a). The Commission currently presents health data in several different databases[8] and relies heavily on the EU health surveys, ECHIs, and member state data collection infrastructures.

The European Community Health Indicators were developed under the Health Monitoring Programme and the Community Public Health Programme (European Commission, Directorate General Health and Consumers 2012c). While the main list of indicators were developed between 2003 and 2008, work on the development of a EU health information system started as early as 1994 (Kilpeläinen *et al.* 2008). Multiple stakeholders were involved in the creation of the ECHI, including the Commission, the ECHI project groups, and member states. The development of indicators that were valid and comparable across member states was a large component of the second phase of the ECHI Project. These indicators were ultimately approved by the Network of Competent Authorities (NCA) of the member states after extensive discussions with the Working Parties and the NCA. As of 2012, there are 88 health indicators with over 40 core ECHI indicators. The European Commission provides the extensive list of indicators; however, they are grouped under five main headings (European Commission, Directorate General Health and Consumers 2012c). The following are the main group of indicators with examples of the type of events they are capturing:

- demographic and socio-economic situation: population, birth rate, total unemployment
- health status: infant mortality, HIV/AIDS, road traffic injuries
- health determinants: regular smokers, consumption/availability of fruit
- health interventions—health services: vaccination of children, hospital beds, health expenditure
- health interventions—health promotion: policies on healthy nutrition.

There have been multiple phases and working groups, as well as the development of shortlist ECHIs. The most recent project that was designed to continue the work of the ECHI and ECHIM projects is the European Community Health Indicators and Monitoring joint action. This three-year project is funded by the European Union Second Programme of Community Action in the Field of Health 2008–2013. The main objective of the most recent ECHIM project is to "consolidate and expand the ECHI Indicator system towards a sustainable health monitoring system in Europe" (Kilpeläinen *et al.* 2008). By working with multiple stakeholders, including member sates, the Commission, Eurostat, the WHO, the OECD, and other organizations, the project members aim to improve and maintain the current list of ECHI indicators while facilitating the development and implementation of future indicators at the member state, regional, and EU-levels.

While one of the goals of the ECHIM project is to implement health data collections that are valid, comprehensive, and comparable across member states, this has yet to take place. One of the only studies to date on the ECHI in Europe found that while the ECHI indicators are available in all EU countries, no country has a full list of indicators available (Kilpeläinen *et al.* 2012). In most countries, many of the ECHI indicators can be drawn from data systems that are already in place. Mortality and morbidity data, as well as other routinely collected data including demographic information and hospital discharge information, is available in almost every member state. Several countries lack ECHI indicators on more intricate and complex concepts such as health determinants and the quality of health care. This discrepancy lies within a country's data system infrastructure, as well as the broader institutional landscape of the member state. As Kilpeläinen *et al.* noted, many European countries are not able to link information on individuals' socio-economic status to any specific health status indicators. Not only is this a problem for data comprehensiveness, effectiveness, and comparability across states, but public health systems will not be able to provide data to policymakers, citizens, and other stakeholders at the state, regional or EU level.

The lack of comparability and implementation of all the ECHI indicators is of no surprise given the EU institution landscape in health. As was found with specific areas such as communicable disease institutions (largely those in the ECDC), there is fragmentation of these data systems, with some countries performing better than others. Several Community projects have been developed to help member states gather the information needed for all the ECHI indicators: the European Health Interview Survey (EHIS), which is being conducted by

Eurostat, and the possible future European Health Examination Survey (EHES), for which a pilot study has been funded by the Commission (Kilpeläinen *et al.* 2012).

While standardizing European Community Health Indicators across fragmented health information systems and member states is a feat to be sure, it is necessary for evidenced-based policy implementation at all governmental levels in the EU. The next step, which will ensure standardized, comprehensive, and comparable indicators, is to further standardize measurement instruments and collection methods in the EU. A coordinated health data infrastructure would also provide information on a variety of EU policy areas, such as mobility of professionals, free movement of goods, agriculture, environment, transportation, and education, among others. Most areas of local, regional, and EU spending affect health, and many EU-level policies will influence population health. Strong data systems will help fill the data and information need for Health in All Policies.

It is interesting to note as well that the data infrastructure around communicable diseases has been considered a success among some in the EU. This is the only area where original monitoring of diseases developed into both a legal require-ment as well as a central European agency (the European Centre for Disease Prevention and Control). The development of the ECDC in 2005 was spurred by the aim to strengthen Europe's ability and capacity to deal with infectious diseases. This decision was no doubt a part of the desire to form more cohesive European health networks, but was also linked quite heavily to the political visibility of communicable diseases and specific crises such as the Severe Acute Respiratory Syndrome (SARS) in 2003, as well as the H1N1 flu in 2009. While the ECDC is similar in theory to the United States' Centers for Disease Control and Prevention, it relies much more on national authorities (termed Competent Bodies by the ECDC), than on an EU authority exclusively. Given the fragmentation and different disease profiles within countries, this seems rather reasonable. However, the communicable disease networks and institutions within the EU are quite fragmented and lack the capacity to act in a coordinated fashion against a European-wide health threat (Elliott *et al.* 2012). Although this is due, in part, to institutional factors, it is also because of a lack of data harmoni-zation and infrastructure. Organizations that are responsible for communicable disease surveillance within member states may not be able to share data and health information on an intra-state level, leastwise with other member state competent bodies.[9] While the communicable disease information systems are much more advanced in individual member states, EU-level systems are still being harmonized and coordinated in order to produce complete, comprehensive, and standardized data sets.

The development of EU law and action in health more generally has brought with it specific information requirements and regulations for cells and tissues, blood, tobacco advertising, as well as cross-border health care. Comparative European data on the prevalence of these issues will be critical on developing law at the supranational level, as well as at the member state level. Further work is being developed in these areas, especially through the recently adopted (in 2008) framework regulation on public health statistics. This framework will have to be put into practice through the implementation of existing legislation, as well as those currently being developed. Understanding what this legislation covers will be critical to understanding the future of health information in the EU, as well the development of a health information infrastructure.

Improving health information has been a Community goal for well over a decade. The desire to develop new systems of data collection that provide information related to communicable diseases, injuries, tobacco use, morbidity, and mortality is a Community priority and will continue to be of the utmost importance in the evolving EU health agenda. Additionally, new and/or improved information systems can provide policymakers, researchers, health professionals, and Community members information about the cost, structure, efficiency, effectiveness, and reliability of health systems throughout the EU.

Future developments

Comparative European information on health clearly can have a substantial impact. This has been shown in areas such as cancer, where benchmarking of comparative cancer data has had a substantial and continuing effect on national cancer programs (Coleman *et al.* 2008; Briatte, this volume). Likewise, comparable and timely European surveillance data for communicable diseases have proved vital in underpinning a Europe-wide response to major communicable disease threats such as SARS and H1N1 (ECDC 2010), as well as for ongoing work on conditions such as tuberculosis.

Nevertheless, these areas remain unusual in having such a direct impact, and many challenges still remain in order to realize the potential impact of comparative European health information. This section outlines some potential issues and ways forward.

Providing timely and relevant data

The first challenge in building a European health information system was methodological—a collective exercise of identifying what health topics were relevant for comparative European data, analyzing what different data were available from what different sources within countries or at European level, and on that basis developing definitions and methodologies for European data and indicators. The scale and complexity of this challenge should not be underestimated. A great deal of work is required for any given indicator in order to be able to use data from different national systems in a comparable way, for example. European comparability, for example, requires reviewing all the different national definitions of a given indicator in order to arrive at shared definitions—even core measures such as mortality statistics can be coded quite differently in different places. This could be due to different formal coding systems of different countries (i.e., use of different versions of the International Classification of Disease, or different systems again), or just different practices (Johansson 2008). The precise methods of collecting data need to also be compared, or a Europe-wide data collection tool developed which will generate relevant and comparable data. This could prove to be quite difficult, however, given these tools would appear in 23 different official languages, for example. Enormous progress was made on this under the health monitoring program, and then under the health information strands of the health programs (European Commission 2004c). Although there is always more such developmental work to be done, a good basis has successfully been built up for the core set of European Union Health Indicators.[10]

The central challenge now is the fundamental one of providing relevant data for health policy on a timely basis for public authorities and wider stakeholders. Timeliness is a key issue. Much of international health data is woefully out of date, in policy terms. Even for such core data as mortality, European data are only published several years later—typically two to three years later. For example, at the time of writing in 2012, the most recent data on causes of death available from Eurostat is from 2009—and for some countries, even earlier; 2008 for France and Italy, and 2005 for Belgium.[11] This reduces the potential impact these data have on policymaking. Additionally, given the relatively short mandate period of a health minister, any comparative health data that is generated will only become available after the health minister has left. This makes such data much less effective in steering policy. This time gap also contrasts with the timeline of availability of other areas of data, such as data about the economy or the labor market. However, even within the area of health, some data become available quite rapidly. For example, data on some communicable diseases such as influenza or measles are typically made available quite quickly, even within days or weeks. This demonstrates that it is technically feasible to provide health data much more rapidly, and on a timescale that would make it much more relevant for influencing policy. Accomplishing this, however, will remain a central challenge for the European health data infrastructures and systems.

Easily accessible, centralized data

Many of the European indicator projects that were developed were a highly efficient and effective way of bringing together specific experts in a given field across Europe. However, projects are necessarily (under the EU's financial rules) time-limited, which creates problems of continuity. Moreover, even if successive projects in given areas are funded, the results are fragmented across the different teams involved.

The exception, as is often the case, is communicable diseases. The ECDC has established a central operational capacity and a centralized database at the European level which serves as a "one-stop shop" for data. This means that there is formalized capacity at the European level to bring together data from across Europe, such as the ECDC's "The European Surveillance System" (TESSy) database.[12] The Commission has been making efforts to address this more generally. These include the establishment of a mechanism for "on-call" data collection and analysis on particular topics, although it is too soon to assess how effective this tool is in practice.[13] The Commission is also developing a European health Wikipedia in order to bring together the results of different projects into an integrated European resource. This also includes a centralized database and data viewer and extraction tool,[14] which may be able to provide comparative European data from different sources and projects in a single place. This would make these data more accessible and usable in practice. As for the official data collated by Eurostat, access to the data facilities have been improved somewhat.[15] It remains to be seen how effective these efforts by the Commission are in practice, given that users tend to be more familiar with the longer-established and user-friendly data sources of the WHO European Health for All database and/or the OECD health data.[16]

Regional data

In describing these efforts on comparative European health data, the unit of comparison has typically been the member state. From a legal and historical perspective, this is to be expected; the participating entities of the European Union are its member countries, which make them the logical unit of comparison.

However, this has hit up against the trend for regionalization of health decision making across Europe in recent decades. The primary decision-making and organizational level for health and health systems is now at the regional or local level in most EU countries. The ISARE projects[17] have mapped an appropriate level of health decision making within the different member states, and their results show the appropriate sub-national entities for health decision making, and the availability (or lack of it) of health indicators for those regions.

This regionalization, together with the wide degree of internal variation within most member states (EUROSTAT 2009) suggests that aggregate comparisons of health data at the country level may actually be of limited use, and highlight the importance of being able to make such comparisons at the regional level. However, this does not obviate the need for European comparisons. On the contrary, the European dimension is essential to making regional comparisons, precisely because the most comparable regions may well be in other countries.

In principle, regional level data are probably already available for many health indicators within countries. Sometimes it is already provided with a regional breakdown to Eurostat, such as mortality data, which is available down to the local (NUTS2) level. However, this even has limitations, with regionalized data not provided for Scotland, for example. In other areas it is either not provided at the European level, or not collected in a way that allows regional breakdowns in the first place by member states.

This is not only a technical issue. The regionalization of powers within countries has political implications too, with different political parties in power in different regions, for example. Enabling regional comparisons has potentially sensitive implications for internal politics, which may also affect the willingness to provide the data enabling such comparisons at the European level.

Inequalities

The persistent and widespread issue of health inequalities is a central concern of EU health policy (European Commission 2009c), as well as more widely (Marmot *et al.* 2008). In order to support this policy objective, it is important to be able to address inequalities as part of overall health indicators, whether by specific indicators, or simply by being able to break down existing whole-population indicators by socio-economic group. However, at a technical level, doing this may require linking two different data sets, such as that for the indicator in question and one for the socio-economic status of the people involved. This raises both technical challenges (e.g., has the data been collected in a way that allows this to be done?) and legal ones (e.g., although the EU's data protection framework allows this to be done, does the national implementing legislation?). Being able to provide EU health information in a way that supports work towards overcoming health inequalities may therefore require both technical and legal action.

Specific conditions

There are also striking differences in the extent to which data are available at the European level on the principal burdens of disease. For example, although cardiovascular disease and strokes are the single largest cause of death in the European Union, the infrastructure for data is not as well developed as it is for cancer, a leading cause of death in Europe (The status of health in the European Union 2008). In terms of morbidity, mental illness represents a heavy burden of disease throughout Europe (The status of health in the European Union 2008), but is not correspondingly well served with data, either about the disease burden itself or about the process and outcomes of European health systems in responding to it (OECD 2011).

Technology and innovation uptake in health systems

A central issue for sustainability of health system finances is uptake of innovations and good practices. There are wide variations within and between European countries in terms of cost (Fahy *et al.* 2011) and in terms of outcomes (OECD 2010). This suggests that there is scope for substantial gains in efficiency in the health sector, at least in principle. This suggests that it is vital to be able to monitor how well health systems (and their different parts) are adopting innovations and improving productivity. Yet this is not well measured. For example, leading estimates of the contribution of technology to overall changes in health system expenditure have taken the approach of calculating the effect of technology indirectly, as a residual after other effects were accounted for, rather than measuring it directly (OECD 2004). There is comparable data on major items of equipment such as magnetic resonance imaging units, plus some disease-specific analysis (OECD 2011), but given the central contribution of technology to overall health system performance, this area remains a key challenge.

E-health

Linked to this (and one of the key technological changes in and of itself) is the move to information technology systems within hospitals and health systems. While these systems will hopefully directly help improve efficiency and quality of care, such information technology systems open up the possibility of generating new sources of data. There are several potential advantages of extracting data directly from these systems: it minimizes the need to have separate parallel structures for data collection alongside care provision because the data collected as part of care provision can be used directly; additionally, it could vastly improve the timeliness of such data.

Moreover, as such data have the potential to elucidate the details of the care process, it also opens up the possibility of being able to access much more detailed information, potentially illustrating differences in practices.

Of course, such an approach has its own challenges in terms of how accurate and reliable such data are, because they are being collected not only for statistical purposes, but for immediate patient care. Nevertheless, this potentially offers a change in European collection and provision of data on health. Moreover, momentum for linking up different systems may be supported by the implementation of the directive on patients' rights in cross-border healthcare (Directive 2011/24/EU 2011). This includes both provisions to support cooperation on e-health at the European level, and creates a need for data flows between different administrations. While the actual volume of such cross-border healthcare remains marginal in terms of overall national volumes, the momentum generated by this new framework may help to support e-health more widely.

Data protection

This topic in turn links to issues around data protection. Within the EU, personal data are rightly regarded as particularly sensitive, and given particular protection in the existing laws (Directive 95/46/EC 1995). For example, although there is scope to share data between health professionals when they are all under an equivalent guarantee of secrecy, this is only for the purposes of the immediate care of the patient concerned. Being able to link up care episodes to see the overall performance of the system, for example, requires being able to share data more widely for the purpose of producing public health statistics. Although this can be allowed by member states, the lack of a clear basis for this at European level in the relevant legislation creates a patchwork of different rules which hinder the generation of accurate data (Verschuuren *et al.* 2008). This is also not what citizens want—provided that personal data are not made public before being anonymized, citizens have supported the idea of data sharing to enable health improvement more generally (Barrett *et al.* 2006).

The European Commission has recently published proposals for revision of the EU's data protection rules, which work toward ensuring the potential processing of data for such public health objectives (European Commission

2012b). It remains to be seen how these proposals will develop during their revision by the European Parliament and the Council of Ministers, and how far the resulting framework enables the sufficient linkage of different data sets for public health in practice.

Well-being

This chapter has focused principally on the past and future of indicators addressing health. The disadvantage of such indicators, though, is that actors outside health tend not to pay much attention to them. This is a characteristic of most sectoral indicators, of course, but it is a particular problem for health, given that so much of health (and so many of the problems that health systems end up dealing with) is shaped by influences far beyond the health sector. These include influences from the education, employment, housing, transport, and environmental sectors, among others.

The concept of well-being can provide a measurable focus for inter-sectoral collaboration around a shared objective; an objective, moreover, that is a formal core objective of the EU itself. Health has been identified as a central part of overall assessments of individual and population well-being.[18] There are projects underway at the EU level and elsewhere that seek to develop measurements of well-being that integrate different definitions and understandings of well-being (European Commission 2009b). It would seem vital for health to be included as one dimension of well-being in these measurements, both for recognition of the relevance of the health sector itself, and potentially as a platform for engagement with other policy sectors around this common objective.

Conclusions

Providing comparative information on health across the countries of the European Union has been one of its most substantial and unique areas of added value in health, as described above. Nevertheless, the work is far from done, with substantial challenges remaining in order to realize the full potential of this information. The ability of policymakers, health professionals, and others to utilize comparative information to improve health depends on resources for further development, especially in regards to the improvement in both the relevance and timeliness of data. The Commission's proposal for the next program is the first time since the introduction of the health mandate and the health monitoring program when there will not be a specific program or strand on health information (European Commission 2011c). Rather, health information and evidence has been "mainstreamed" throughout the proposed program. It is not clear what the impact of this will be in practice, but it will help demonstrate how relevant and effective the EU is in health more broadly.

European data matters because governments, having been part of the process of providing it, then have to take notice of what it says. Some of the most effective areas of European leverage on health have depended crucially on comparative

European information, as described above. As the European health information area now has a solid core of well-developed indicators, realizing the potential of those indicators for improving health will depend on investing the resources to ensure that the relevant data are available in a timely and sustained manner in the coming years.

Notes

1 I would like to thank Nick Fahy for his extensive comments and invaluable advice; all errors remain mine.
2 Decision No 1400/97/EC of the European Parliament and of the Council of 30 June 1997 adopting a programme of Community action on health monitoring within the framework for action in the field of public health (1997 to 2001); OJ L 193/1 of 22.7.97.
3 Ibid., Article 1.2.
4 In particular through the Health Data series of the OECD; see: http://www.oecd. org/document/30/0,3746,en_2649_37407_12968734_1_1_1_37407,00.html (accessed September 11, 2012).
5 See: http://ec.europa.eu/health/programme/policy/eight_programmes/index_en.htm (accessed September 11, 2012).
6 See its website: http://www.emcdda.europa.eu/index.cfm (accessed September 11, 2012).
7 For a complete list and discussion see Kilpeläinen *et al.* (2012).
8 These databases are the following: the European Community Health Indicators (ECHI) and other European health indicators, the Heidi data tool, the injury database, the sustainable development indicators-data collection, the food demographic, and socio-economic data collection, as well as Eurostat.
9 In November of 2010, the Management Board of the ECDC decided to designate one Competent Body (termed the Coordinating Competent Body (CCB)) in each member state to coordinate the official relationship between the ECDC and the other Competent Bodies within the member states. The goal behind this restriction is to create more transparency, efficiency and simplicity between the ECDC and member states.
10 See: http://ec.europa.eu/health/indicators/echi/list/index_en.htm (accessed September 11, 2012).
11 See: http://epp.eurostat.ec.europa.eu/statistics_explained/index.php/Causes_of_death_statistics (accessed September 11, 2012).
12 See: http://ecdc.europa.eu/en/activities/surveillance/tessy/pages/tessy.aspx (accessed September 11, 2012).
13 See: http://ec.europa.eu/eahc/health/tenders_H01_2010.html (accessed September 11, 2012).
14 See: https://webgate.ec.europa.eu/sanco/heidi/index.php/Main_Page (accessed September 11, 2012).
15 See: http://epp.eurostat.ec.europa.eu/portal/page/portal/health/public_health/data_public_health (accessed September 11, 2012).
16 See: http://www.oecd.org/health/healthdata and http://www.euro.who.int/en/what-we-do/data-and-evidence/databases/european-health-for-all-database-hfa-db2 (accessed September 11, 2012).
17 See: http://www.isare.org/rapports.asp (accessed September 11, 2012).
18 See: www.oecd.org/progress.

4 The politics of European public health data

François Briatte

Introduction

This chapter examines the effect of public health data on European policymaking. Political stakeholders of all kinds and at all levels of government are frequently observed making non-trivial use of public health data, often in the form of indicators such as mortality rates or expenditure levels.[1] Virtually all forms of strategic reasoning and communicative action are infused with such indicators, most of which have become increasingly available to decision makers through national and supranational administrative units, academic research centers and third parties like think tanks or international organizations. Nothing about public health data might therefore be deemed entirely new, but their widespread diffusion within and across borders suggests that their political effects may increase.

Given the essential role of the European Union (EU) as a venue for cross-national policy learning, it is then necessary to ask how public health data translate into public health politics when European-wide indicators are used as benchmarks of policy success—or failure. The political valence of public health data cannot be discounted as merely anecdotal insofar as death rates or percentage points of gross domestic product are easily transmogrified into sources of fame or shame for the governments that account for them. Specifically in the context of public health, where numbers frequently stand for either sick or dying populations, the symbolic weight of aggregate measures such as prevalence or survival rates can carry the same psychological impact that pain and death induce at the level of individuals (Jennings 1999). In that respect, there is nothing trivial about a mortality table, however anonymous its individual observations.

Over the past decade or so, systematic indicators have been developed by EU-level working groups to "monitor" member states, a terminology reminiscent of the work done by other supranational organizations like the Organisation for Economic Co-operation and Development (OECD) or the World Health Organization (WHO). The principles that underlie this practice, which can be routinely observed in bureaucratic environments, are deeply political: not only do data empower its agents with "hard facts" and "objective evidence," they also open up the possibility of measuring macro-level performance in the form of cross-sectional rankings or time-varying indicators. These, in turn, can be used as argumentative weaponry in discussions over the state of public health in individual member states or at the abstract level of the European region. The myriad symbolic tokens that are mobilized in the process of data reporting, such as in the calculation of an "average level" of mortality in European countries, are then turned into powerful cognitive cues in the speeches and writings of bureaucrats, politicians and interest groups alike.

This chapter specifically aims to describe the transformative effects of EU-level public health data on health policymaking. At the more general level, it also aims to show how a more precise understanding of the processes at play in public health data, namely quantification and standardization, might feed into current understandings of Europeanization. "Europeanization" is still what semiotics refer to as a floating signifier, that is, a notion that does not point to any agreed upon meaning.[2] Yet, in its most fundamental incantation, Europeanization does entail the idea of a collective space of reference that is shared by individual member states, and within which interactions are perceived to produce significant effects at the European and domestic levels. Public health data directly contribute to materializing this space of reference when such things as "Europe-wide data" or even "European data" start making sense to academics and to their human subjects of inquiry. In that sense, and several others, the matter of understanding how public health data has become a topic of interest for European political actors is closely linked to the scientific challenge of analyzing the Europeanization of public health policy in both practical as well as theoretical terms.

The empirical research question that sustains this inquiry has to do with how European institutions think, or rather, how participants in the EU policy process make sense of what they advocate, claim and discuss among each other. The puzzle takes particular importance for us at the level of the European Commission, because the object under examination, public health data, is produced and/or analyzed in part by Commission services. Specifically, the health statistics around which much of the analysis will revolve are often born out of joint ventures of the Directorate-General Eurostat (DG Eurostat) and Directorate-General for Health and Consumers (DG Sanco), the departments respectively responsible for statistics and for health issues within the administrative bodies of the Commission. The Directorate-General for Research and Innovation (DG Research) has also provided funding for a lot of the public health data that eventually gets spread through the EU statistical apparatus and well beyond it. Given the source of the data for this analysis, it likely expresses a strong "Commission bias" that understates and fails to document appropriately the diffusion and discussion of public health data in other EU institutions. Nonetheless, parliamentary debates or Council meetings do show that public health data is actively mobilized in these venues as well.[3]

Finally, the theoretical framework used in the present inquiry draws on what has been termed "common knowledge" in a different political setting (Culpepper 2008). Schematically, the notion of common knowledge designates an intersubjective configuration of human cognition where actors are mutually confronted to "a social fact that cannot be individually wished away"

(Wendt 1999, p. 161, cited in Culpepper 2008, p. 4). The essential property of common knowledge lies in the impossibility for political actors to discard its informational content. Specifically, once this form of knowledge has been shared between them, "its invulnerability to unilateral change" then allows it to produce "an independent impact on the bargaining power of actors" (Culpepper 2008, pp. 4–5).[4] Common knowledge requires a form of "convergent diagnosis" won through persuasion and "crossover appeal" among political actors (Culpepper 2008, pp. 5–7). As this diagnosis erodes past conceptions and delegitimizes their institutional settings, it coerces actors into experimenting with new mental sets under a high degree of cognitive uncertainty. The result of that process is the consolidation of a new ideational model to which political actors are eventually led to adjust their future strategies.

The following sections apply this analytical framework to the production and diffusion of public health data among European policymakers. The second section describes the most salient characteristics of the EU-level consensus that has gradually emerged and partially overridden former visions of public health. The third section then turns to EU powers over public health data and how even a constrained mandate over health policy can translate into substantial EU-driven activity in the field of public health. The final section concludes on not-so-future challenges for public health policy in Europe.

Technical characteristics of the issue

European public health data and government by numbers

Public health data are a compound of systematic observations that aim at measuring the state of health of selected populations. Since the inception of public health policy, these data have frequently taken the form of statistical reports commissioned by political authorities, including the European Commission, which mobilizes its own staff, national representatives from member states, other international organizations and private interests.[5] With regards to public health, the Commission has established particularly tight collaborative links with the WHO Regional Office of Europe, which works with European as well as Central Asian countries.

The keywords of the aforementioned institutions frequently refer to the lexical universe of quantification: in each of them, "data and evidence"—or simply "databases"—support the development of cross-country reports, geographical atlases and other communication tools such as Web platforms to explore tables and graphs built out of international health data. Some of the most detailed data series echo the origins of statistical integration in nation-states and focus on mortality and causes of death, using the successive versions of the International Classification of Diseases (ICD) as well as age-standardized death rates tailored specifically for European demographics.[6]

The history of modern state formation in Western countries indicates that the quantification of a territory is a precious power resource that political authorities have struggled to extract from the populations they rule over, in order to turn collective and discrete social entities into administrable labor or warfare power (Foucault 2004). By analogy, European politics is often conceptualized in the form of a conflict-ridden relationship between the supranational authority of EU institutions and the domestic preferences for national sovereignty of national governments accountable to their populations. The precise amount of statistical knowledge that the European Union has secured over nation-state territories is then not just an analogy: it measures the degree of precision with which the EU scrutinizes its member states.[7] That enterprise of turning populations into legible entities is in itself a practice intrinsic to modern statecraft (Scott 1998).

These general observations resonate significantly in public health, which has virtually always belonged to the core mandate of state power. When urbanization made it a pressing concern to maintain the health of the workforce, "vital" statistics rose to feature prominently along census data in the history of state-driven quantification (Desrosières 2008, 2010). The political history of disease control, however, features frequent acts of resistance to state surveillance, as in the decades since the AIDS epidemic and the emergence of claims to "democratic privacy" (Fairchild *et al.* 2007). As EU institutions successfully invest in the assemblage of public health data at their own territorial level, some of these conflicts are bound to gain a European dimension, gradually shifting the political space of public health towards supranational venues of decision making.[8] This new configuration is likely to change the rules of the game for member states when the legitimacy of a "European level" for the government of and by numbers becomes virtually unchallenged.

Evidence-based medicine and policy

The other language that European public health policy speaks rather fluently is that of evidence-based policymaking, although the arcane language of European bureaucracy sounds very modestly engaged on that path as compared to the "what works" lyricism of national bureaucracies in regulatory states.[9] At present, a striking aspect of the nexus of interests that binds medicine to politics concerns the shared legitimacy of evidence-based decision making in clinical as well as in policy circles, as seen in the wealth of literature on the topic that has blossomed in the past two decades.

Evidence-based medicine designates the scientific practice that aims at "generat[ing] objective knowledge of effective interventions based, where possible, on the results of unbiased experiments" (Daly 2005, p. 1; Timmermans and Kolker 2004). In the mid-nineteenth century, Edwin Chadwick, a pioneer of public health policy, formulated the oldest definition that one might accept for evidence-based policy, though today the randomization component central to "high-quality" clinical trials is still not applicable to policymaking (Klein 2003). Despite this difference, data-driven practices characterize high modernism and professional competition within both clinical medicine and public affairs. In these areas, establishing an evidence base has been simultaneously controversial and appealing to policymakers (Harrison *et al.* 2002).[10]

Regulatory reforms in European states are not limited to injecting evidence-based instructions into the machinery of government: other processes such as standardization play an increasing role in defining actual state capacity (Borraz 2007). Similarly, the various tokens of New Public Management have become deeply embedded into the principles of public service reform, inducing an epistemic shift for political and bureaucratic elites towards quantifiable policy performance measured by benchmarks, rankings, indicators of cost efficiency and other forms of public delivery targets (Bruno *et al.* 2006; Bruno 2008; Ogien 2010). The use of measurement, whether passive or active, has affected virtually all European health care systems in the past two decades, in a more or less gradual fashion and with mitigated success.[11]

The overarching logic couched in the deployment of quantification processes and evidence-based discourse at the EU-level is, in the end, fundamentally dependent upon its most immediate clientele, namely, the audience of public and private actors involved in reorganizing health care and public health in the shadow of European governance. To that audience, the investment of European resources into assembling "EU-level" public health data under the banner of informing policy by evidence has probably looked, and rightly so, like the first step toward a future of shared governance over public health issues. The current state of EU powers and initiatives further confirms that policymakers have adjusted their behavior to the existence of a political space of European public health, where data is carried by a diversity of stakeholders as a strategic symbolic resource.

EU powers and initiatives

Public health data and the "chaordic" dynamics of EU health policy

Having considered some of the cognitive properties of public health data, we turn to its institutional and political foundations, starting with the apparent paradox that EU powers over health matters are prima facie residual. At its origins, the European Union considered the possibility of supranational health authority through a "European Health Community" but briskly discarded that alternative, as it also discarded several other policy initiatives that tried to pool national resources under a European heading (Guigner 2008). Concordantly, the EU treaty base has always explicitly rejected the possibility that health care would fall under the remit of European rule-setters, as illustrated today in the unambiguous wording of Article 168 TFEU.[12] The political legacy and legal framework of European health policymaking hence seems oriented *against* the principle of European intervention.

However, a model of policymaking that pays attention to spillover dynamics effectively shows that, during the past two decades, policy arbitrages over health care have become increasingly Europeanized through both political and social learning, as shown by the contingencies of European court rulings (Greer 2006b), the adaptation of member states to European directives in the health care sector

(Greer 2009a), and the parallel formation of advocacy coalitions and interest groups around health issues in the Brussels beltway (Greer 2009b). Additionally, strategic interactions between the European Commission and the WHO Regional Office of Europe have led EU institutions to strike a series of ideational bargains over multilateral issues such as pharmaceutical market expansion or tobacco control (Guigner 2009). The overall public health policy arena has thus become increasingly Europeanized, through "vertically" binding regulatory measures and through "horizontally" diffused incentive measures (Guigner 2011a).

For more than 30 years, European public health policy has also been shaped by exogenous shocks that have opened policy windows for public health advocates to extend European powers to new areas of public health concern (McKee *et al*. 2010). The cumulative sum of EU responses to issues like nuclear radiation, food safety or organ donation has spun into a perhaps "spineless and toothless" but still identifiable European public health system, currently headed by DG Sanco and populated by three regulatory agencies, a federally inspired health surveillance unit,[13] and an executive branch responsible for EU programs in health promotion, consumer protection and food safety.[14] This trend has been progressively matched by explicit mandate adjustments in the EU treaty base, which today prominently asks for the European "mainstreaming" of health protection at Article 9 TFUE.[15]

While this state of affairs is explained largely by accidental logics and spillover effects, the expansion of public health data collection also contributes purposively to structuring the politics of European public health. EU cross-national comparative data provides a salient and shared argumentative resource on which to sustain policy initiatives and build evaluative judgments about the performance of domestic health systems. Steps taken by EU institutions that engage data reinforce the path of European integration of public health policy. This interplay of institutional and ideational factors has been insightfully coined the "chaordic" dynamics of European integration in health policy. On the one hand, the European health policy field has been formed through unpredictable spillovers and shocks. On the other hand, the accretion of deliberate European strategies aimed at governing over health issues form an "issue-specific, fragmented, and incremental process, necessarily technocratic and patchy, but quite consistent" (Lamping and Steffen 2009, p. 1375, emphasis removed).

The possibility for EU actors to be more involved—and more influential—in health policy relies on successful statistical integration, which requires organizational development and widespread trust in the reliability of the data. The history of EU statistical integration shows that producing reliable statistics that are available to market agents, policymakers and the general public has so far been a largely successful initiative for the European Commission and specifically its "Eurostat" directorate-general (Sverdrup 2006).[16] EU statistical services can furthermore count on the cognitive and institutional support of other members in the epistemic community of transnational data purveyors, such as the OECD or the World Bank, which also actively develop standardized health indicators and many other cognitive assets for global governance (Davis *et al*. 2011). Over the years, the EU has produced several collections of such indicators against which health system performance assessments can be elaborated in domestic policy environments.

The measurement of EU health system performance

Health performance indicators have been adopted rapidly by international organizations like the WHO, which ratified the principle and then published performance targets in its Health for All strategy in the early 1980s.[17] The recent history of EU public health, however, tends to show that EU decision makers expressed more measured ambitions in that regard. Calls to monitor domestic health systems at the EU-level appeared regularly in decisions from the European Parliament and the Council since at least the Community Action Programme on Health Monitoring of 1997, though they were implemented within narrower bounds than those recommended by the Commission. In reference to the first EU public health program, published in 2002,[18] Hervey and Vanhercke (2010, p. 89) note that limitations were applied to the instrumentation of EU public health data into what would have otherwise read like the formation of a supranational framework of comparative health system performance assessment:

> the Commission's proposals 'to stimulate EU-level action on comparing and assessing health care systems' through the program were removed during the first reading in the co-decision procedure in 2001, highlighting great reluctance by the Member States to accept interference in this domain, even if it 'merely' implied comparisons of performance.

Similarly, when another pledge to monitor public health progress in member states came out of Parliament and Council in 2007,[19] several member states requested that the budget of the proposed program be axed to thwart any significant advance in that direction (Baggott 2011, p. 96). Soft law instruments that encourage cross-national comparison within member states in order to identify "best practices" for policymaking, like the Open Method of Coordination (OMC), have also had to tread very carefully over health care, partly due to data limitations but primarily because some member states have expressed their outright hostility to specifically *supranational* target-setting and performance indicators for health services (Greer and Vanhercke 2010, pp. 209–12).[20] Even in the case of a policy instrument like Structural Funds, which can be allocated under a "what works" performance objective, the possibility of running comparative assessment that would concern "the running of the healthcare system" has been prudently ruled out so far (Hervey and Vanhercke 2010, p. 91).

In 2008, the ratification of the Lisbon Treaty provided another opportunity to further the case of EU-level public health monitoring. The Commission indicated in its draft that it would seek to support, "initiatives aiming at the establishment of guidelines and indicators, the organization of exchange of best practice, and the preparation of the necessary elements for periodic monitoring and evaluation."[21]

This text now appears verbatim in Article 168-1 TFEU. In a similar fashion, and in line with successive EU and WHO commitments to tackle health inequalities in European countries, an elaborate list of health determinants has now been published under the form of European Community Health Indicators (ECHI), ranging from infant mortality to waiting times for elective surgery.[22] It seems, then, that the defusing of EU-level health system comparison by understandably concerned domestic political elites has come to existence through the parallel policy pathway of EU public health programs.

EU health system performance monitoring still bears the marks of opposition from several member states. Its current state of development is that of an advanced battery of precise and systematic indicators that closely mirror national initiatives in that domain. At the same time, many national governments have invested in priority setting through targets in the past decade. In mapping out the strengths and weaknesses of public health in Europe, the EU has found close allies in other international organizations, as well as in more discrete, but nevertheless active and vocal, members of its epistemic community, such as the European Public Health Alliance and countless collectives of transnational medical elites. As of today, the joint work of EU services are not only inside rather than outside of the political space of European public health, as underlined in the previous section. They have also built a robust frameset of quantitative measurements that bring together various forms of accountability indicators, ranging from expenditure levels to health system inputs and outputs.

Cancer survival rankings and EU health policy

Cancer control provides an interesting illustration of the logic outlined so far. Using this example helps understand how the emergence of performance measures can affect future policymaking, but also reveals the still largely accidental ways in which the politics of European public health data unfold over time. The history of EU activity in cancer control indeed pre-dates and surpasses its involvement with the tackling of other diseases, as cancer, along with AIDS and drug use, has been a privileged target of EU programs and regulations. Since the inception of the "Europe Against Cancer" program (Trubek *et al.* 2008a) in the aftermath of the Chernobyl nuclear accident of 1986, several other EU policies have affected all aspects of cancer control, including clinical trials, screening recommendations, biomedical funding, and most visibly tobacco control, where comparative public health data has played an interesting role in the identification of well-disciplined and less-disciplined member states (Guigner 2011b).

One aspect of cancer control involves measuring cancer survival. Domestic governments are confronted with geographical inequalities in cancer epidemiology that make them aware of regional leaders and laggards within their territory. However, cross-national comparative data in cancer survival rates is a more recent element of common knowledge, which has been crafted by a small epistemic community of European epidemiologists over the past two decades. The EUROCARE research project, which received EU funding from the BIOMED and FP4 programs, was at the origin of cross-national cancer survival rankings that played an important role in shaping British health policy in the years 1999–2001; at the outset of its reform episode, the British decision created a policy point of reference for the "European average" of health expenditure, therefore injecting European criteria into national health care reform (Briatte 2010).

There is now a significant amount of consensus in reference to EU levels of conformity, in the form of either passive or active promotion of EU average measurements. These express the same logic of appropriateness and conformance as the "average American" did when surveys began having an impact on models of the mass public in the United States (Igo 2007). The political substance of European average levels also intermeshed domestic and supranational interests through the passive uploading of measurements and indicators, leading to a situation where they express crossover appeal to all actors. From 2001 onwards, as McHale (2010, p. 291) recalls, EU discourse started to act as a bandwagon on health issues as domestic interests had previously defined them, largely through the derivation of institutional health system characteristics:

> the European Committee of Social Rights expressed concern that there were increased waiting list times in the United Kingdom and they stated that, in light of the data, they considered that 'the organization of health care in the United Kingdom is manifestly not adapted to ensure the right to health for everyone.'

The referential and disciplinary properties of European public health data are only one instance of their political character. This section only scratches the surface of EU initiatives that revolve around public health data: other EU-level projects exist addressing biobanks of genetic information and tissue, as well as clinical trials. Some cross-national initiatives have also been suggested for the regulation of pharmaceutical markets, where domestic interests limit efforts at regulatory harmonization and comparative effectiveness assessments (Hancher 2010, p. 681). These initiatives follow a different but perhaps more predictable pattern of EU-level interests, strongly associated with market harmonization principles and standardization strategies.[23] They also operate jointly to mass information programs that advertise, for instance, patient information on public-private partnerships, as well as many other programs that assume a highly educated population capable of (responsible for) making its own health-promoting choices.

Overall, these policy developments have brought market concerns to weave together health, safety and public health concerns. They have affected the mental models and interest structures of states, markets and societies, reminiscent of what Michel Foucault tentatively captured in his theorization of biopolitics.[24] The politics of European public health data, which eventually revolve around the definition of health system performance issues across European states, match this general characterization, which carries its own risks, as currently reflected under radical austerity and financial crisis.

Future issues

In this analysis, the origins and politics of European public health data can be explained by the success of cross-national public health data becoming common knowledge that is shared by virtually all policy stakeholders in the emergent field of European public health policy. The cognitive properties of EU public health data have been gradually matched by institutional opportunities at the EU level, and finally by a structure of interests where member states tacitly compete to demonstrate high levels of comparative health performance. Every reference to EU benchmarks—such as the "European average" value of a given health indicator—adds to the cognitive harmonization and statistical "creep" of European public health data, leading in some cases to significant reform initiatives by domestic political elites in member states.

While every policy decision may produce positive feedback effects from which emerge path dependence and institutional "stickiness," it is possible that a macroeconomic decision, for instance, to some extent "reverses" or even "cancels out" practical policy effects. In contrast, public health policy and the statistical integration of European public health data are hardly concerned by radical reversals that would lower the policy sustainability of the public health field.[25] Harsher privacy rights, for instance, might thwart but very rarely *decrease* the precision of disease surveillance. Furthermore, the hypothetical policy decision to axe a public health agency like the European Centre for Disease Control would require many efforts not to look like a completely irresponsible move from a public relations perspective, given the critical context in which such agencies have often emerged in the first place. Finally, as research programs and quantitative information progress incrementally, their cumulative sum clearly pushes public health data towards more legibility rather than less, with ever-larger amounts of information becoming available through increasingly sophisticated instruments.

The future of public health is likely a trend toward more integration in the form of data streams under favorable political and technological circumstances. The internationalization of scientific activity is probably also a major contributor in assuring that public health practitioners look forward to a more collaborative epistemic culture. The future of public health looks quite similar to its past, which has also been a history of gradual expansion if one considers the *longue durée* of public health data. Additional innovations in computer and network infrastructures as well as in statistical and data science, helped by recent initiatives in favor of democratizing access to "open data," are likely to push that trend forward.

There is a bleak side to this rather optimistic narrative. Permanent fiscal austerity, now topped by financial crisis and dubious democratic politics in several European countries, both inside and outside the European Union, are important causes for concern to anyone with a professional interest in health. The universalization of health systems is a reversible trend: it might progress spectacularly somewhere and gradually retrench on a different subcontinent. European countries are not at all immune to the health effects of austerity on welfare, as Stuckler *et al.* (2009) have shown using the most recent Eurostat data. A country like

Greece, which is currently among the most stricken, is at serious risk of bearing higher death rates under radical austerity, whether due to suicide, drug use or lack of access to medical facilities as affordability collapses for large fractions of the population (Kentikelenis *et al.* 2011).

A cruel irony, of course, might be that the same institutions that are actively supporting these austerity shocks are also providing scientists with the means to analyze their effects on the health of societies. As McKee and Stuckler (2011, pp. 2–3) recently put it in their correspondence to the *European Journal of Public Health*:

> As researchers, the least we can do is to document the human costs of the crisis, to tell the stories of ordinary people throughout Europe whose lives are being blighted by radical austerity and risky bank maneuvers. There will be more unintended consequences, albeit difficult to predict, calling for a close monitoring of the situation. Our initial studies, recently published in the *Lancet*, were very simple to do and cost only our time as researchers.

However close the "monitoring," though, the body politic is the locus where the political economy of life and death unfolds (Foucault 2004). Modern states are hardly the sole site of these biopolitics anymore. The macroeconomic agenda of the European Union is, in itself, a public health policy that might enhance or forestall future public health efforts. The data will tell us.

Notes

1 The term "data" is used hereinafter as an analogue for statistical series made of standardized, quantified measurements, even if a narrative is technically a form of datum. The focus is hence set on numerical rather than literal information.

2 For a more formal introduction to the conceptual issues that come with the notion of Europeanization, see, inter alia, Radaelli and Pasquier (2007).

3 Some quantitative studies of health issues in the European Parliament do exist, however; for a full-fledged approach and comparison to environmental issues, see Princen (2009).

4 This perspective has the intrinsic merit of reconciling the long-established opposition between rationalist and constructionist views, as it grants causal power to "ideas" deemed appropriate by actors within a scheme of action that otherwise draws on strategic bargaining and consequentialist reasoning from actors who follow their individual "interests." The main background assumption of this analytical framework consists in translating the opposition between rationalist and constructionist arguments, initially exposed in the area of international relations (Risse 2000), to the study of European politics. That is arguably not a huge step to take. Common knowledge does indeed seem to be a very suitable candidate for a study of European politics that aims at avoiding the theoretical clash between intergovernmental and constructionist views of the European Union.

5 There is no reason to believe that this pattern of production is fundamentally different in other families of statistical data, and the observations made here might therefore carry implications for other sectors of European policymaking.

6 On the origins of population-level quantification by national governments, see Desrosières (2008, 2010) and Porter (1995) for two well-known historical works.

The ICD itself has its origins in the efforts of British and French medical statisticians commissioned by international congresses held in Brussels and Vienna (WHO, n.d.).

7 A different wording closer to the works of Michel Foucault would speak of the EU "gazing" at its member states as other dominant groups, like nation states or clinicians, "gaze" at society. For an elaborate account of the state as an assemblage of such technologies, see Márquez (2007), who draws on Foucault and Weber.

8 This pattern is neither unique nor universal. For a similar pattern between states, European institutions and geographic information, see Branch (2011) and Sibille (2010); For a different form of spatial politics expressed through the boundaries of welfare, see Ferrera (2005).

9 On the characteristics of regulatory states in relation to evidence-based policy and other instruments of impact assessment, see Humpherson (2010).

10 The most illustrative example of that trend probably still lies with the successive Blair and Brown governments (Faucher-King and Le Galès 2010, pp. 42–61).

11 On the general degree of state involvement in health care system development, management and reform, see Schmid and Wendt (2010) and other chapters in Rothgang *et al.* (2010).

12 Specifically, Article 168-1 TFEU specifies that EU action "shall complement national policies," and Article 168-7 TFEU that it should "respect the responsibilities of the Member States for the definition of their health policy and for the organization and delivery of health services and medical care."

13 On the European Centre for Disease Prevention and Control and its relationship to European health governance, see Greer (2012).

14 All measures are documented in the annual reports of the Executive Agency for Health and Consumers (EAHC). European public health programs operate under the conditions of Article 168-5 TFEU, that is, at the exclusion of "any harmonization of the laws and regulations of the Member States."

15 "In defining and implementing its policies and activities, the Union shall take into account requirements linked to the [. . .] protection of human health."

16 In addition to the institutional trajectory of Eurostat, other efforts at integrating European public health data have underlined the practical imperfections of comparative data collection and analysis over EU countries (McKee and Ryan 2003).

17 The WHO Regional Office for Europe published specific European targets in the same years. It should probably be reminded that the WHO has relatively little impact on domestic policies.

18 Decision 1786/2002/EC of the European Parliament and of the Council of 23 September 2002 adopting a program of Community action in the field of public health (2003–2008).

19 Decision No 1350/2007/EC of the European Parliament and of the Council of 23 October 2007 establishing a second program of Community action in the field of health (2008–2013).

20 The relevant policy documentation, such as the *Draft Joint Report on Social Protection and Social Inclusion* 2010, read like succedanea to the otherwise prolific research on national health accounts and comparative health outcomes developed by the OECD or the World Bank.

21 Similar objectives can also be found in the White Paper *Together for Health*, published by the Commission in 2007.

22 A shortlist of 88 ECHI indicators was initially conceived by national public health representatives, DG "Eurostat," DG "Sanco" (now DG "Health & Consumers"), WHO and OECD. For further details, see the ECHI Web pages accessible at http://ec.europa. eu/health/indicators/echi/list/ (last accessed February 13, 2012).

23 On the mix of public health and market interests that govern over the work of the European Food Safety Agency (EFSA) and the European Medicines Agency (EMA), see Demortain (2008). The third European regulatory public health agency, the

Community Plant Variety Office (CPVO), which enforces EU intellectual property rights over genotypes, also fits that pattern.

24 In a nutshell, biopolitics designate the balance of power established over the lifestyle of populations, in a dual process that both compels governments to rule over the vital signs of their citizenry and confronts individuals to their own responsibility in maintaining a state of health (Bossy and Briatte 2011). While originally studied in West European nation-states, biopolitics is currently understood to have potential empirical applications at all levels of government.

25 On policy sustainability, see Patashnik (2008).

5 European regulation and harmonization of clinical practice guidelines

Loes Knaapen

Countless standards do nothing. Some, however, obtain majestic results.
(Timmermans and Epstein 2010, p. 81)

European governance and clinical practice guidelines

The European Union (EU) has few legal tools and administrative institutions at their disposition to regulate health care systems in Europe, as this domain primarily remains the legal mandate of national governments. Instead of a traditional command-and-control-type government, the EU has developed policies to encourage various actors (non-state, public, private, international, NGOs) to form "networks" that establish their own standards and diffuse best practice (Hervey 2008). The term "new governance" is often used to refer to the broad range of regulatory tools, models and techniques to describe the focus away from the EU as an administrative institution that uses legislation to govern, towards "practices of governance," or "multi-level" governance (Delanty and Rumford 2005, p. 139; Scott and Trubek 2002). New governance is expected to expand the EU's regulatory impact "by utilizing new forms of knowledge and making use of global networking," instead of legal enforcement by a central authority (Rumford 2002, p. 72). The specifics of such "voluntary" mechanisms vary, but "policy learning" and the production and exchange of comparative information (e.g., benchmarking, name and shame) are considered viable strategies. EU officials and scholars alike have high hopes for such new governance structures to tackle the challenges of contemporary health care systems (Trubek *et al.* 2008b). The EU increasingly invests time, money and hopes into the development of standards, data and networks to regulate health care professionals and promote better health care practices in Europe (Greer 2006a), but few studies have empirically investigated the impact of specific European quality or safety standards in the health domain (Hoeyer 2010). Without traditional and centralized modes to impose changes on actors many scholars and EU policymakers remain skeptical about the mechanisms by which voluntary standards, knowledge and networks can achieve effective regulatory impact (see Greer, chapter 1). This chapter will present an empirical study of the establishment of the Guidelines International Network (GIN) to demonstrate how EU funding was successful in establishing a trans-national governance structure that regulates through knowledge and voluntary standards, yet did not succeed in a harmonization of European health care practices.

Clinical practice guidelines (CPGs) are a particular type of medical standard that aims to regulate physicians' behavior through knowledge. Based on a synthesis of evidence from medical research (ideally randomized clinical trials) CPGs provide clinicians with recommendations how best to treat a particular clinical condition. By providing a Gold Standard for clinicians to "live up to," such evidence-based guidelines carry the promise of simultaneously rationalizing and standardizing medical practices (Timmermans and Berg 2003). Since the late 1990s the European Union has invested in the development and harmonization of clinical practice guidelines by funding several closely connected research projects in this domain (Table 5.1). These projects have resulted in a quality standard for guidelines (AGREE; Appraisal of Guidelines Research and Evaluation in Europe), a formal recommendation on guideline methodology by the European Health Committee (Council of Europe 2002) and the establishment of the GIN. This chapter will chronicle how these EU-funded projects have been successful in establishing a sociotechnical network whose voluntary standards have worldwide regulatory influence in the domain of clinical practice guidelines. These projects were successful by realizing a change in regulatory structure, moving from centralized European guidelines to a distributed knowledge network. This structural change also meant transforming *what* was being regulated: from standardization of guidelines (products) to standardization of methodology (process). The result was a network that rejects the production of centralized European guidelines with which to harmonize health care practices in Europe. If EU policies pursue the establishment of networks as a policy goal in itself, with little attempt to coordinate harmonization policy with networks, European new governance may be highly effective, but the EU will have little control over *what* it is effective at.

The regulatory power of standards, knowledge and networks

To better understand the technical and knowledge practices that are central to giving voluntary standards regulatory impact, this chapter draws upon the field of Science and Technology Studies (STS). While "new governance" may be relatively new as an explicit and formal EU policy, STS scholars have repeatedly highlighted the importance of standards and standardization to regulate almost all aspects of modern life (Timmermans and Epstein 2010; Busch 2011). STS work provides myriad examples of successful and transformative (voluntary) standardization driven by practices of knowledge production. Scientific methods and classifications are not "naturally" and automatically universal, but are "a triumph of human organization—of regulation, education, manufacturing, and method" (Porter 1995, p. 29). For "universal" facts and artifacts to travel across boundaries of time, space, professional groups or languages myriad standardization processes are required (O'Connell 1993; Collins [1985]1992). By emphasizing the "leaky borders" between scientific categories, technical infrastructure, social norms and

Table 5.1 The AGREE collaboration led to many other international guideline projects (co-)funded by the EU

Founding year Nationality	1998 AGREE	1998 GRADE	2001 European Council Recom	2002 GIN	2005 ADAPTE	2006 CoCanCPG
Canada	Brouwers Browman				Brouwers Browman	
Finland	Mäkelä		Mäkelä	Mäkelä		
France	Fervers			Fervers	Fervers	Fervers
Germany	Ollenschläger	Ollenschläger	Ollenschläger	Ollenschläger		
Netherlands	Burgers Grol			Burgers	Burgers	
Scotland	Qureshi			Qureshi		Qureshi
Switzerland	Burnand	Burnand		Burnand	Burnand	
UK	Cluzeau Feder	Cluzeau		Cluzeau		
US	Littlejohns Slutsky			Littlejohns Slutsky		Littlejohns

institutional routines or personal habits (Lampland and Star 2009) scholars also emphasize the normative nature and political consequences of standards, classifications and knowledge (Bowker and Star 1999). The co-production of standards and knowledge takes place within a sociotechnical network in which both technical infrastructure (databases, standardized terminology, calibrated apparatus) and "social" connections (personal contacts between colleagues, peer review and peer pressure, tacit knowledge and face-to-face learning) are indispensable. In order to capture the mechanisms that give such sociotechnical networks regulatory "power," requires a departure from traditional conceptions of agency. Rather than including only humans as agents of change, STS has generally come to accept that all the interacting elements that constitute sociotechnical networks are "actors." Neither humans nor objects by themselves effect change. It is the strength of the connections between all constitutive elements that give a network regulatory and normative power (Latour 1983; Callon 1986). Objects and tools are not "merely passive objects of human manipulation" but as constitutive elements in a network they (co-)produce effects, they *do, perform* and *change* things (Barry 2001, p. 11). Although people (such as those listed in Table 5.1) are indispensable to this story, this chapter is not only about their ambitions, interests, beliefs and intentions, but objects (quality standards, evaluative instruments, comparative data) are equally important vectors of action.

This chapter draws on empirical material that was collected by studying international collaborations concerned with guideline development that received EU funding (Table 5.1). Besides document analysis, I conducted semi-structured interviews with five founding members of these projects; conducted participant observation (as user and evaluator of the AGREE instrument); attended international working group meetings (ADAPTE, G-I-N PUBLIC) and the annual conferences of the Guidelines International Network (2007–2011). Drawing on this empirical material, the chapter chronicles the emergence of a new sociotechnical network concerned with international regulation of clinical practice guidelines. I first introduce clinical practice guidelines and the promises and challenges they posed to the standardization of medical practices, setting the stage for the European Union's interest in funding collaborations to harmonize such guidelines. These efforts reject the standardization of guidelines on a European or international level, instead proposing the harmonization of the *methodology* to develop guidelines. It was the AGREE instrument, which, by defining the quality of guidelines in terms of its methodological process, transformed international guideline development. This chapter will discuss three different aspects of this transformation. First, it modified the notions of standardization and rationalization of evidence-based medicine. Second, by producing comparative knowledge the emergent network standardized guideline development practices around the world. Third, by founding the GIN it established a regulatory infrastructure that seeks to establish experts in guideline methodology as a new self-regulating profession. The chapter concludes with the claim that EU funding has been successful in establishing a "new governance" structure whose distributed regulatory impact has simultaneously reached beyond the EU, and is more localized than a nation state. The standardization of guideline methodology has professionalized this domain, establishing a novel meta-regulatory arrangement in medicine. Nevertheless, far from Europeanizing guidelines, this international network entrenches the development of guidelines further in national organizations.

The promise of guidelines as gold standards

Clinical practice guidelines are a specific kind of medical standard which are most commonly defined as: "systematically developed statements to assist practitioner and patient decisions about appropriate health care for specific clinical circumstances" (Field and Lohr 1990, p. 8). They first emerged in the 1970s, when widespread concern about the efficacy and cost of medical practice was heightened after analysis of treatment patterns in the USA showed that patients with the same condition were treated differently depending on geographical region. The production of guidelines was offered as one of the solutions to end unwarranted variation. They could function as "gold standards" that recommend and disseminate best practices to physicians in the clinic (Weisz *et al.* 2007). In 1990s the evidence-based medicine (EBM) paradigm emerged with the aim to "use the literature more effectively in guiding medical practice" (Evidence Based Medicine Working Group 1992, p. 2024). They emphasized that the fallibility of "intuition and unsystematic clinical experience" applied not only to local practitioners but also to national experts. They emphasize guidelines are "only worth following" when based on evidence from medical literature, especially randomized clinical trials (RCTs) (Sackett and Rosenberg 1995). By shifting the determination of "best practice" from individual clinicians, to national experts, to quantitative evidence, guidelines followed a more general shift in the "scientific" basis of medicine: "from a regime of trust in expertise and experts to a regime based on the mechanical generation of data, the elimination of human judgement and the adoption of a 'view from nowhere'" (Keating and Cambrosio 2009). Cronje and Fullan see EBM as an attempt to model medicine on the "classical rationality" of mathematics and logic: "The appeal of the classical model of rationality in medicine, operationalized by EBM, is clear: it promises a rule-governed procedure that, if followed faithfully, will necessarily result in improved health outcomes for all patients" (2003, p. 355). In this regime rationalization is identical with standardization: "any rational person, if s/he begins with the same information, will arrive at the same conclusions" (2003, p. 355). The appeal of guidelines is clear. By providing the evidence and rules to follow, they promise to automatically result in better medicine. With such high hopes, thousands of "evidence-based" guidelines for clinical practice are produced by private, professional, public and governmental organizations. For the European Union, guidelines are a way to harmonize European medical practices without recourse to health care legislation or regulation that is the legal competence of national states. In the late 1990s the EU started funding international collaborations of guideline developers to harmonize guideline development in Europe (Table 5.1).

European regulation of guidelines

The first survey of clinical practice guidelines in Europe found that the success and proliferation of guidelines posed a new challenge. It stated that the diversity in guideline-setting initiatives in Europe presented a "danger that in some years healthcare providers will drown in a guideline morass" (Grol *et al.* 1998, p. 65). The "overdose" of conflicting guidelines of varying quality questions the vision of guidelines as rational Gold Standards. Guidelines appear to reflect the practice variation they were meant to reduce, and are themselves in need of standardization and rationalization. In 1998 a consortium of guideline researchers was funded by the EU to develop the AGREE instrument, an evaluative instrument to address "the number of guidelines in specific clinical areas that contain conflicting recommendations" (Cluzeau 1998). Two of AGREE's members contributed to the European Health Committee's recommendation on guideline development addressing similar concerns (Council of Europe 2002, p. 12). AGREE members continue to establish or participate in a range of international collaborations that are supported by EU funding such as ADAPTE, GRADE and GIN (Table 5.1). The AGREE instrument comes to underpin international regulation of guidelines by sharing a distinct vision of international collaboration.

The official vision for international collaboration on guidelines articulated by the self-acclaimed "father" (Jako Burgers) and "mother" (Françoise Cluzeau) of the AGREE instrument rejects the discourse of guidelines as Gold Standards based on quantitative evidence that will standardize medical practices. They emphasize that in addition to evidence, "expert opinions, practitioners' and patients' preferences as well as societal priorities" play a role in standard setting and conclude that "each country has its own norms and values that influence the content and presentation of guidelines. Therefore, the aim should not be to develop international guidelines" (Grol *et al.* 2003, p. 6). The European Health Committee's Recommendation on guidelines reflects the same concerns. Instead of proposing a single "best" Gold Standard for Europe, it emphasizes the necessity of national and local diversity in guidelines in order to "suit the practical circumstances of the organisation applying [them] to accommodate the specific needs of guideline users," and to "enhance implementation " (Council of Europe 2002). As the EU subsequently funds other projects that reject international standardization of clinical practice guidelines (Table 5.1), the promise of guidelines to regulate physicians directly with "universal evidence"—avoiding national legislation or regulation—does not materialize and guidelines remain national documents.

From European guidelines to European guideline development

The rejection of guidelines as universal (or European) documents that can standardize medical practices is not simply a resistance to standardization or globalization. International collaboration on guidelines does not end, but shifts towards reaching "international agreement about the requirements for methodology and reporting of guidelines" (Grol *et al*, 2003, p. 6). Harmonization of the *process* of guideline development becomes the focus of European policy as expressed in recommendation Rec(201)13 "on developing a methodology for drawing up guidelines on best medical practices" (Council of Europe, 2002). Increased international networking between "organisations, research institutions, clearing-houses and other agencies that are producing evidence-based medical information" was also recommended (2002, p. 15), and in 2002 the GIN was established with EU funds. GIN now includes guideline development organizations from 46 countries, and around 400 guideline developers attend its annual meeting to exchange information, learn methodology and collectively define, defend, disseminate and enforce "good" guideline development. By establishing GIN, EU funding contributed to the creation of a network that creates, promotes and disseminates *the* international methodological standards for guideline development to which hundreds of guideline developers submit voluntarily. Significantly, not only the regulatory structure changed (from centralized European standards to the distributed regulatory power of a network), but *what* was being regulated had also changed: from standardization of guidelines (products) to standardization of methodology (process). It was the AGREE collaboration that was instrumental in achieving this shift.

AGREE: Guideline for guideline development

In 1998 an international collaboration of guideline developers from predominantly European countries was funded under the BIOMED2 program of the European Commission to develop the *European Union Critical Appraisal Instrument for Guidelines* (EUCAIG), a self-described "appraisal instrument to compare the different approaches to guideline development in Europe." It was renamed the catchier AGREE, and, aspiring to be the worldwide standard, eventually dropped "Europe" from its name. The AGREE instrument consists of a checklist of 23 items in six domains to assess whether "rigorous" guideline development methodology has been followed in the production of the guideline being appraised. It asks questions such as whether a systematic literature search has been done, if various "stakeholders" are included, and if the guideline will be updated regularly. AGREE thus evaluates guidelines based on the quality (reporting) of the methodological process, and "does not assess the clinical content of the guideline nor the quality of evidence that underpins the recommendations" (AGREE Collaborative Group 2003). Some consider this a serious limitation of AGREE (Vlayen *et al.* 2005; Hannes *et al.* 2005), as methodological quality only loosely correlates to measures of the quality, acceptability or validity of the content of the guideline (Watine *et al.* 2006; Nuckols *et al.* 2008). The founding members of AGREE, such as Jako Burgers, acknowledge that an AGREE score cannot *guarantee* the clinical validity of a guideline, but find it reasonable to assume "rigorous" methodology makes a good guideline more "probable." By jokingly adding, "I think it has an odds ratio of 2 out of 3," Burgers acknowledges but gently mocks the need to confirm assumptions with formal statistics, as the evidence-based medicine paradigm customarily requires (Burgers, interview

August 24, 2010, Chicago). In practice, AGREE scores are treated as a pragmatic shorthand for, or a straightforward representation of, the quality and validity of a guideline (Burgers *et al.* 2003; MacDermid *et al.* 2005). The AGREE collaboration has thus positioned "rigorous guideline methodology"—not the quality of evidence or the clinical content of guidelines—as the primary ground for evaluating the validity of guidelines. Disconnecting the quality improvement of guidelines from the standardization of guidelines allows them to vary from country to country, yet be legitimate if the process of arriving at the guideline is "up to" standard.

Transforming the debates of evidence-based guidelines

Rejecting global standards based on their failure to capture the complexities of (local) culture, values and environment is not new. It is a typical narrative that contests standardization for bringing about a dehumanizing uniformity that fails to capture the complexities that matter "on the ground" (Timmermans and Epstein 2010, p. 71). Guidelines have been at the center of similar contestations over whether evidence-based medicine brings about rationalization or standardization. Medical professionals have criticized clinical practice guidelines for creating "cookbook" medicine that ignores the expertise of physicians and values of patients (Berg 1997; Lambert 2006). The limitations of "universal" quantified evidence to properly capture the complexity of decision-making in clinical practice have also repeatedly been pointed out (Goldenberg, 2009). Many critics suggest a stark divide between "EBM advocates" who strive for "rational medicine" (which is universal) and those who resist EBM and strive for a "humane medicine" by preserving the "clinical art" (Timmermans and Mauk 2005; Mykhalovski and Weir 2004).

The international regulation of guidelines is remarkable as it fits neither side of such a polarized debate. Advocates of guidelines acknowledge the limitations of quantified evidence and problems of standardized medicine, but instead of rejecting guidelines and EBM they offer "systematic" guideline methodology as a solution to this problem. This new justification for guidelines proposes a new rationality for guidelines that cuts across both sides of the debate. It allows guideline developers to defend evidence-based guidelines while avoiding the unrealistic (and inaccurate) ideal of guidelines as one-size-fits-all Gold Standards.

We have already seen guideline developers collaborating in AGREE reject "classical rationality" as variation in guidelines is legitimized. Quantitative evidence such as RCTs and systematic reviews are important, but evidence does not *automatically* rationalize medical practice, and still requires guideline developers to consider processes in which evidence is found, translated, interpreted and implemented for the specific context (Grol *et al.* 2003, pp. 5–6). Instead of simply trusting individual guideline developers to perform this evidence translation, international guideline collaborations propose "rigorous" and "systematic" guideline development procedures to ensure the rationality of evidence contextualization. AGREE's 23 items provide requirements for assessing quantitative evidence as well as ensuring the presence and "objectivity" of "local" experts and stakeholders. The outcome of the process is neither universal nor based on the opinion of *individual* clinicians or experts, but specific to the practice in which the guideline will be used.[1]

The GRADE working group is one such international guideline collaboration that receives EU funding to rationalize the translation of evidence (Guyatt *et al.* 2008). GRADE is led by Gordon Guyatt of McMaster University who coined the term evidence-based medicine, and includes three AGREE founding members. It attempts to standardize the quintessential (and much criticized) EBM tool that assigns quality to evidence: the "evidence hierarchy." Despite terminological standardization and the use of the same software around the world, GRADE has not been able to establish universal rules for how to translate evidence. GRADE developers consider it a success because by revealing (rather than eliminating) judgments, guideline users can scrutinize (rather than simply trust) expert judgments. Standardized reporting of the guideline developmental process:

> Allows somebody else, who is taking the guideline and is applying it, to say: "Oohhh here is the basis on which they made the recommendation." If you follow their logic, I agree with their logic, therefore it is reasonable for me to follow the recommendation.
>
> (Guyatt, interview, October 7, 2009, Hamilton)

Instead of a mechanical view of guidelines in which evidence determines "correct judgments" and single outcomes, international guideline developers claim the evidence-based approach is defined by a methodological process that can "explicitly represent the issues for competing arguments and foster critical thinking by insisting on accountability to evidence" (Brouwers *et al.* 2008, p. 1026).

Redefining EBM's rationality based on a "rigorous" and transparent methodological process cuts across the polarized debates that surround EBM. This new legitimacy allows guideline developers to respond to the critiques that Evidence Based Guidelines encounter. The legitimacy of diverse guidelines and judgments reduces fears that "universal" guidelines erase distinct cultures, human values and clinical expertise necessary for high quality medicine. The insistence on the "contextualization" of evidence reduces concerns of EBM's over-reliance on quantification and reductionism. By promoting universal methodological procedures and evidence as well as local guidelines and contextual judgments, developers can claim their guidelines are universal *and* local, objective *and* inclusive of values. As Lambert (2006) has noted for evidence-based medicine in general, the limitations and critiques launched at EBM are not overcome by rejection or contestation but become incorporated. By focusing on process standardization instead of product standardization, AGREE has turned the variation in guidelines into a resource for more legitimate guideline development.

AGREE standardizes guideline development

AGREE not only provides an abstract ideal for guideline developers, it is a socio-technical instrument whose normative impact transforms and regulates the work of guideline developers around the world. While AGREE was not the first to formulate methodological standards for guideline developers (the highly regarded Institute of Medicine in the USA outlined similar ideals a few years earlier (Lohr and Field 1992)), it has had significant influence on standardization around the world. AGREE's regulatory impact is not the result of a more authoritative institutional origin, or the imposition of sanctions. Rather, AGREE distinguishes itself because it not only expresses an ideal to live up to, but provides a *test* of that ideal (Busch 2011, p. 52). Unlike other methodological standards, AGREE provides an evaluative checklist that produces a numerical, quantified score of guideline quality (Vlayen *et al.* 2005).

Many guidelines assessed by AGREE receive what seem to be rather low quality scores; for example, 85 percent of a collection of Canadian guidelines scored less than 5 out of 10 for "rigor of guideline development" (Graham *et al.* 2001). For fear of "misuse" of their instrument, AGREE never set a formal quantified norm or cutoff point (Cluzeau, interview November 3, 2009, Lisbon), so AGREE's numerical scores *alone* do not provide a basis to reject or approve guidelines. But by quantifying quality, AGREE's quality measurement is no longer "alone," but easily embedded, transferred, circulated and compared. The numerical score makes possible comparison and ranking of guidelines with entirely different content, format, clinical topic, or institutional, national, or linguistic origin. By ranking scores, over time or between guidelines, a relative norm is created. The act of quantifying produces comparative knowledge with normative effects (Espeland and Stevens 2008). In the medical literature guidelines and guideline programs receive negative publicity because they scored "low" on the AGREE scale, that is to say, lower than others (Brouwers and Charette 2001). Guideline development organizations are encouraged to reform their developmental programs to increase their AGREE scores in the future (Hurdowar *et al.* 2007, p. 657), and in the US, AGREE scores have been used to discredit guidelines that insurance companies relied upon to deny coverage (Manchikanti *et al.* 2008).

The normative pressures provided by AGREE are amplified by requirements that EU-funded projects use AGREE (Cluzeau, interview November 3, 2009, Lisbon). For example, the Coordination of Cancer Clinical Practice Guidelines (CoCanCPG), a EU-funded project that has established cooperation between 17 cancer guideline programs in and beyond Europe (Fervers *et al.* 2008), evaluated whether cancer guideline developers comply with the AGREE criteria. And, although the comparative knowledge created by this project is "descriptive," it creates a normative picture showing cancer guideline programs "where they stand" on the world ranking, creating normative pressure for "non-compliant" programs to adjust to the international gold standard set by AGREE (Figure 5.1).

AGREE's status as the Gold Standard of guideline development has become uncontested around the world. Its founding article has been cited 324 times

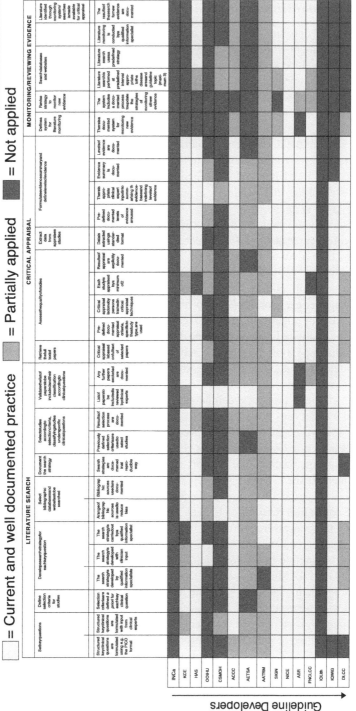

Figure 5.1 B. Benchmarking guideline development programs (vertical axis) along AGREE criteria (horizontal axis).

Source: Modified from Fervers, B. on behalf of CoCanCPG (2007) Benchmarking guideline development programs, presentation at DLCC, Montreal, October 9, 2007 (slide 1). Reproduced with permission.

(22-02-2012 Web of Science) and has been evaluated as the most useful of 24 guideline appraisal instruments (Vlayen *et al.* 2005). More than 1,100 oncology guidelines, including those from the UK, the Netherlands and European medical societies, have been evaluated with AGREE, the scores easily available in an online database, making comparison of AGREE scores very easy for physicians, policymakers and the public (www.cancerguidelines.ca, accessed September 7, 2012). As guideline developers anticipate their guidelines may be evaluated with AGREE in the future, the AGREE checklist is not only used to evaluate guidelines, but has become a "manual" on how to develop a guideline (e.g., Bloem *et al.* 2010, B2), and how to set up a guideline program (Van der Wees *et al.* 2007).

The AGREE instrument is a "voluntary" quality standard that simultaneously is an ideal to live up to, an *evaluative* instrument measuring the state of guideline methodology, and a normative standard that transforms and performs guideline methodology. It expresses and measures the ideal of guideline development, and by providing numerical scores that allow easy comparison of guidelines and guideline programs, it makes (relative) quality or its lack thereof visible, persuading guideline developers to modify their programs towards the ideal embedded in the AGREE instrument. AGREE has not only "*demonstrated*" an increasing harmonization of the methodologies used by guideline agencies and programs around the world" (Ollenschläger *et al.* 2004, p. 456, emphasis added), it has also been instrumental in *producing* this standardization.

The Guidelines International Network

The AGREE collaboration solidified its standardization impact through the establishment of the Guidelines International Network, which has become a single platform to promote, connect and embed the standards and knowledge produced by projects such as AGREE, CoCanCPG and GRADE. GIN was founded as a result of the AGREE collaboration's renewed funding under the 5th Framework, whose objective was to promote AGREE and establish "an international network of guideline agencies and related organizations." Previous research conducted by AGREE members had shown large divergence in guideline development initiatives throughout Europe, both in the content of guidelines (Burgers *et al.* 2002) and in the methods of guideline development (AGREE Collaborative Group 2000).

Much guideline development takes place at organizations for which guideline development is only a minor activity, such as medical specialty organizations, regional health care networks, academic institutions or health care financers. Individual guideline developers may be information specialists, librarians, epidemiologists or medical professionals and do not share national professional associations, educational trajectories or even job titles. So while the AGREE collaboration brought together a dozen guideline developers from large national organizations exclusively dedicated to guideline development such as NICE (UK), CBO (Netherlands) and AZQ (Germany), GIN does more than provide an international platform for guideline developers previously organized on a national level.[2] GIN brings together "professional" guideline developers that previously did not share any identity or community on a national, regional or even local level.

Knowledge about the diversity in guideline development in Europe served to make the contours of a distinct (albeit diverse) "guideline world" visible for the first time, providing a picture of who is participating, in what way, and what might be improved. The results of one such survey were presented at an international workshop on guideline development to advertise the need and desirability of an international guideline network (Figure 5.2). In November 2002 the Guidelines International Network officially registered as a not-for-profit "international network of excellence for the research and implementation of guidelines" (Ollenschläger *et al.* 2004, p. 456), with 22 founding committee members from 12 countries. Since then, GIN's membership has grown to "93 organisations and 89 individual members representing 46 countries from all continents," and its website has put guideline development quite literally "on the map," by providing hyperlinks to all its members.[3]

GIN's founding documents explicitly state an opposition to the standardization of guidelines, and instead see diversity as a resource for "building partnerships" and "to promote information sharing and cooperation in guideline development" (Guidelines International Network 2002). GIN promotes its methodological standards (AGREE, GRADE, ADAPTE) as "ideals" for all guideline developers

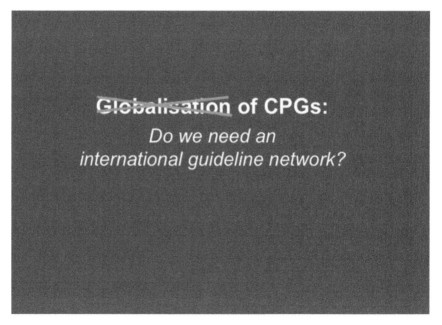

Figure 5.2 J. Miller and G. Ollenschläger, slide 17 from presentation: "Globalisation of CPGs: Do we need an international guidelines network?" Berlin, June 2002.

Source: Available at: http://www.aezq.de/mdb/edocs/pdf/azq-veranstaltungen/cpg/miller.pdf

to live up to, but they are voluntary standards: GIN accepts members regardless of whether they comply with GIN's standards, and no sanctions or enforcement are in place. The development of formal certification has been discussed at GIN meetings, but remains controversial. Jako Burgers, founding member and former chair of GIN, opposes certification and sees the role of the network to "connect organizations like a kind of highway, a kind of infrastructure, and in that way tries to improve communication and exchange" (interview August 24, 2010, Chicago). This echoes the EU's policy to establish networks of excellence as *social connections* between people to advance research. This model considers diversity a resource for innovation, and is uncoordinated with the broader policy of harmonization, which is associated with an alternate model of networks as *shared infrastructure of technical standards* aimed at facilitating harmonization (Barry 2001, pp. 89–93). Despite GIN's opposition to standardization as a formal and explicit policy, its standards and knowledge practices do standardize guideline development.

GIN standardizes guideline development

The Guidelines International Network creates voluntary standards and comparative knowledge with which guideline developers self-regulate their practices. GIN standardizes based on the same normative pressures of emulating what is considered best practice, as described above. GIN's annual conference provides an important forum for guideline developers to measure, compare, and rank their own and other's guideline development practices along methodological Gold Standards such as AGREE. But it is not only the exchange of knowledge that *results* in standardization. Standardization is also *required* to establish knowledge exchange in the first place. A session at GIN's 2011 annual conference illustrates this. The speaker compared several approaches to grading evidence, without finding any of them superior. But instead of concluding that diversity in grading systems was legitimate and harmless, attendees preferred having a uniform approach in order to understand and learn from one another, to interpret and judge each other's evidence summaries, and to reduce efforts by using each others' evidence summaries (fieldnotes, GIN conference 2011, Oral Session 3.10). Since variation itself is considered an obstacle to improve (and reduce) guideline developers' work, attendees preferred the GRADE system simply because many guideline developers around the world already use it. Since standardization is required for establishing knowledge and collaboration, GIN's goals of "improved communication and exchange" result in standardization. Such shared standards may not represent "the cheapest, most efficient, safest, scientifically most reliable, or technically most advanced outcome" but may be established by repeating "how things are already done by most parties" (Timmermans and Epstein 2010, p. 79).

Adherence to methodological standards may be cumbersome, time consuming and expensive, but GIN's growing membership suggests members expect such constraints to be overshadowed by its benefits. As Timmermans and Berg have shown, shared standards can be appealing because they increase the legitimacy of criticized or unrecognized work. For weak professional groups "the process of standardization forms an attractive strategy to rally members and claim expertise" (2003, p. 93). Standardization is particularly attractive when standards are developed and monitored from *within* the professional group, and they display enough flexibility to allow for professional judgment and discretion.

GIN aims to transform guideline developers from a heterogeneous, unorganized group whose work is criticized by medical professionals (who denounce standardization) and policymakers (who demand more standardization), to an emergent profession that claims its own domain of expertise. Following AGREE helps defend guidelines against criticism (and globalization) because the process of arriving at the guideline is "up to" standard. According to the subtitle of its logo, AGREE advances "the science of guideline development," allowing guideline developers to lay claim to *scientific* procedures. GIN makes experts in guideline methodology visible as a distinct group of "guideline methodologists" and provides a platform to learn and display their skills, expertise and procedures. The standards do not provide universal rules that can be mechanically followed, and judgment and discretion of guideline developers remains necessary. And since there are no fixed norms or sanctions, standards may be endorsed as ideals without (fully) living up to them. Failure to do so may be grounds for petitioning guideline financers for more resources to bring guidelines "up to standard."

The extensive (and expensive) proposed methodological requirements explicitly encourage guideline production to take place within centrally organized and well-funded organizations dedicated solely to the "guideline business" (Grol *et al.* 1998, p. 265). The standards process excludes local groups of medical professionals— disapprovingly referred to as "GOBSAT" or "Good Old Boys Sat Around a Table" (Guyatt, interview 7 October, Hamilton)—from developing guidelines without "professional" guideline methodological experts (Hirsch and Guyatt 2009). By encouraging the standardization of "professional" and "systematic" guideline development, GIN's methodological standards thus result in a rejection of both global and local guidelines and a strengthening of the development of national guidelines.

Conclusion

By developing quality standards for guidelines and establishing the Guidelines International Network, EU funding created a new governance structure wherein the voluntary nature of standards has not limited its regulatory success, but made it successful. By connecting people, practices, technologies, standards and knowledge across disciplinary and national borders this sociotechnical network is neither "bottom-up" nor "top-down" standardization, but is a coordination of social, organizational and technical elements across local, national, and international levels. GIN's regulatory impact is distributed along these dimensions. It is both more "localized" than EU regulatory structures by affecting the daily practices of individual guideline methodologists, and also by operating far beyond the EU, shaping guideline development in South Korea, North America and the WHO.

Yet, despite initial hope and promise of universal Gold Standards for health care, this new governance structure has not resulted in increased Europeanization of health care. Not because it lacked the "power" to regulate and standardize across Europe, but by changing *what* was being regulated and standardized. The vision of guidelines that regulate physicians directly with "universal evidence" is rejected, insisting "norms and values" co-determine guidelines. By measuring the quality of guidelines in terms of methodological process, guidelines do not require uniformity of clinical content. The rationalization of guidelines, then, is disconnected from the standardization of guidelines. Experts in guideline methodology have emerged as a new (self-regulated) profession indispensable for ensuring the "objectivity" of medical regulation. This new governance structure can be considered a new type of meta-regulation in medicine, distinct from medical professionals' self-regulation and from governmental legislative powers (Cambrosio *et al.* 2006). Methodologists pursue meta-regulation by aiming to improve quality improvement instruments, while rejecting meta-standardization and legitimizing variation in guidelines. This meta-regulation of guidelines further entrenches guideline development at the national level because it rejects global guidelines, and its extensive quality standards discourage local guideline development.

Since GIN does not consider clinical practice guidelines to be universal objects, it rejects the establishment of European guidelines as a "technical" infrastructure to standardize health care practices. Instead, GIN is supported by, and supportive of, EU policies that aim to establish "social" networks in which diversity is considered a resource for learning and knowledge production. However, collaboration amongst diverse stakeholders both produces and requires shared infrastructure and objects, therefore the notion of a sociotechnical network is more productive in capturing these dynamics than are models of strictly technical or social networks. The case of GIN illustrates how a sociotechnical network can transform local practices around the world with voluntary standards. Without an EU institution (or other central actor) determining who will enroll in such networks, and how standards are going to be used (if at all), the EU has little control over the kind of standardization that a network will produce. Since standardization is not always the emulation of a Gold Standard, but may be established by the lowest common denominator or a consolidation of existing practices, there is no guarantee that standardization will result in rationalization or Europeanization. If the EU pursues the establishment of networks as a policy goal in itself, with little attempt to coordinate harmonization policy with networks, European new governance may be highly effective, but the EU will have little control over *what* it is effective at.

Notes

1 The validity of "universal" evidence or standards for "local" settings is a familiar and contested issue in most standardization processes. The "contextualization" of evidence during standard development is only one of many possible solutions to bridge the radically different environments of "context-free" RCTs and clinical practice. Timmermans and Berg (1997) describe how "universal" standards require informal

work-arounds and local adjustments to be workable in practice. To avoid this "implementation gap," Zuiderent-Jerak (2007) suggests standards to be produced *within* the practice where they are to be used, which he calls situated standardization. Carl May (2006) describes how "universal" quantified evidence was rejected outright in favor of what he calls "practice-based evidence" (local experimentation and qualitative evidence). Others advocate for prioritization of evidence from observational studies (Black 1996), which would rely on entirely different kinds European networks, such as EUROCARE (see Briatte, this volume). Attempts to "contextualize" or localize the production of randomized clinical trials include what Epstein (2007) calls "niche standardization," as well as comparative effectiveness research (Keating and Cambrosio 2012, pp. 376–81).

2 In the Netherlands a similar informal network of guideline developers call "EBRO platform" did exist. As neither organization nor individual, the EBRO Platform did not become a GIN member, but several of EBRO's members did.

3 See http://www.g-i-n.net/about-g-i-n, accessed February 9, 2012.

6   The European regulation of medicines

Boris Hauray

Medicines play a key role in public health. The twentieth century has seen the advent of many new and efficient drugs (from penicillin to tritherapy HIV treatments, as well as cortisone or antidepressants, for example) and these have become the main tools of modern medicine. They have therefore become an important part of our daily lives; on average each French person consumes one box of pharmaceutical products every week. However, crises such as cerivastatin (Baycol, Lipobay)[1] in 2001, hormone replacement treatments for menopause in 2002, rofecoxib (Vioxx)[2] in 2004, and benfluorex (Mediator)[3] in 2009, regularly remind us that medicines also constitute a threat to populations and that their adverse effects are one of the foremost causes of mortality. Given the high stakes for health care and the weakness of the European Union's competence in health-related issues (Greer 2009a), as well as the importance of medication in national economies and public finance, one could expect the EU's involvement in this domain to be relatively low. Yet, pharmaceutical policies are very firmly implanted within a common European framework. Not only has the EU become involved in pharmaceutical economic policies (regulating the length of patents and the procedures for fixing prices and reimbursements), but also drug safety control now largely takes place on a European scale. Since 1995, the European Medicines Agency (EMA, formerly EMEA) has coordinated the assessment and monitoring of medicinal products sold in Europe and has become a key figure in defining world standards in this domain. This chapter will focus upon these later health policies, analyzing the history of, and current issues at stake within, what I call a "Europe of Medicines."

The regulation of pharmaceuticals

The public health issues involved in drug safety control

> There are no therapeutic roses without their thorns.
>
> (Dunlop 1962)

Medicines are amongst the products subject to the most regulation from public authorities. In Europe, the latter supervise the tests carried out on new drugs, authorize or prohibit their sale, specify their conditions of use and monitor their adverse effects. They also define intellectual property rules applicable to pharmaceutical products, and regulate prices, rates of reimbursement and even how they can be advertised. This considerable involvement can be explained by a number of factors: the importance of medicines in public health; the atypical consumer relationship that they induce (unlike a normal good, neither the prescribing doctor nor the patient pays directly for the product, nor can either make a precise judgment about the actual characteristics of the product); the cost they represent for health insurance systems (approximately 15 percent of health expenditure in Germany and nearly 20 percent in Spain and Italy); and the strategic nature of the pharmaceutical industry, which is a lucrative knowledge-based sector many governments are keen to promote (Permanand 2006).

Regulating the safety of pharmaceuticals, which will be the main focus of this chapter, is an age-old phenomenon that can be dated back to antiquity (Dunlop 1962). Initially, the quality of medicinal preparations, measured in terms such as how accurately they reflected the declared composition, or by the presence of impurities, was at the heart of drug regulation, which took the form of the inspection of apothecaries' dispensaries. From the fifteenth century onwards, pharmacopoeias began to be drawn up in Europe thus providing inventories of medicinal products, their fabrication, and their conservation. That a public authority ought to scientifically evaluate the effects of a given therapy, and formally approve it prior to sale, was a notion that only came into existence much later. It is only in the twentieth century that public authorities progressively began to develop real policies in this matter.

Beyond the general increase in state intervention in the well-being of populations—the responsibility for "fostering life" (*faire-vivre*) to use Foucault's expression—several other elements were instrumental in the establishment of pharmaceutical regulation. The first is the shift in the production of medicines from the dispensary to an industrial context, thus allowing regulation to be centralized. The second is that advances in chemistry and biology led to the elaboration of more numerous and more concentrated products. The third, which is linked to the latter (Marks 1997), is the development, from the second half of the twentieth century onwards, of new knowledge tools such as clinical pharmacology and randomized clinical trials,[4] supplementing laboratory tests and research on animals. Finally, the fourth is the advent of health crises that catalyzed the emergence of more stringent control measures. The most infamous of these is the case of thalidomide, a drug that was prescribed as a sedative and to treat morning sickness for pregnant women and that later claimed thousands of victims in the 1960s due to its teratogenic effects (toxicity to the fetus). It was presented as completely harmless according to the tests in place when it was put on the market, and therefore later became emblematic of the risks inherent in the use of any medication. This scandal also encouraged public authorities to require manufacturers to prove the efficacy of their products: while all medicines can be harmful, they should all provide treatment.

Despite the rise in public authority regulatory practice, the impact on public health of the adverse effects of medicines remains high. One study has shown, for example, that over 6.5 percent of hospital admissions in the UK are linked to adverse drug reactions (Pirmohamed *et al.* 2004). Another has indicated that such reactions were responsible for more than 100,000 deaths each year in the United States (Lazarou *et al.* 1998).

Until the 1960s, drug regulatory systems were weak in Europe and largely determined by the respective histories of the nations in question (Abraham and Lewis 2000; Daemmrich 2004; Hancher 1990). From this period onwards, however, countries progressively put in place national, public structures to evaluate the properties of medicines via the assessment of marketing authorization (MA) applications that collated the results of tests and trials carried out by manufacturers while developing their products (Hauray and Urfalino 2009). The Western world became increasingly demanding regarding the data required from manufacturers, making the process of developing a new product both time consuming—from five to ten years—and costly, even if the sums involved—sometimes claimed to reach over one billion dollars—are probably largely overestimated (Light and Warburton 2011). In order to evaluate these data, states usually have recourse to a combination of internal experts, employed by the administration, and external experts, for example academics and practitioners, who are called upon in committees to provide specific and clinical knowledge.

Decisions regarding MAs have become more refined. Today it is no longer simply a question of approval/rejection: a drug will only be authorized for strictly defined uses and decisions also mention contraindications, posology, precautions for use, adverse effects, and the like. Systems of pharmaceutical oversight (i.e., "pharmacovigilance") have also been implemented to monitor medicines in their actual conditions of use: these systems work mainly on the basis of declarations made by health professionals or pharmaceutical companies regarding the side effects of treatment, and by carrying out epidemiological surveys. The analysis of these data can lead to the reevaluation of products, to changes in the marketing authorization and even to withdrawal from the market.

The foundations of European intervention in the pharmaceutical sector

The EU has become involved in most areas of public action regarding medicines (Permanand 2006). However, given how vigorously member states defend their competence in health care (Greer 2009a), "positive" integration has been much more limited on the economic side of pharmaceutical policies (Hancher 2004).

Conversely, despite the speed with which the idea of creating a unified "Europe of health" was abandoned (Guigner 2008), the European Union has become the main player in drug safety regulation in Europe. Much as in other domains, this role has been founded on competences relating not to health but rather to the single market (art. 100 and 235 of the EEC Treaty, then art. 95 of the EC Treaty, and art. 114 of Treaty on the Functioning of the European Union—TFEU). Defining unified health standards became a necessity after the Treaty of Rome when the EC member states united to implement a common market for pharmaceutical products. This endeavor initially took the shape of establishing a European pharmacopeia, carried out within the Council of Europe in order to include Switzerland and Great Britain.

EU intervention in the economic regulation of medicines

The EU "Transparency" directive 89/105 established a specific timeframe for pricing and reimbursement decisions regarding medicinal products and required them to be individually justified by presentations grounded in "objective and verifiable" criteria in order to avoid national bias. A revision of this directive was launched in 2010.

The EU also developed a specific framework for intellectual property related to medicines and the data produced during their development. In particular, regulation 1768/92 (replaced by regulation 469/2009) implemented the right for manufacturers to request a supplementary protection certificate that would extend the duration of a patent up to five years.

The EU also negotiates in the World Trade Organization on behalf of member states regarding intellectual property rights in the pharmaceutical sector (ADPIC Agreement).

Efforts were then made to reach agreements regarding the nature of public-authority control and to implement European procedures for marketing authorizations, allowing national expertise and decisions to result in "Europeanized" approval. In contrast to other health sectors, this led to an extremely substantial body of regulations regarding the properties of medicines and the organization of product assessment, as well as, for example, the promotion of the development and marketing of "orphan medicinal products"[5] or of pediatric medicines.

It was only in 2007, more than ten years after centralized authorizations were implemented on a European scale, that the Treaty of Lisbon formally ratified this long-standing and deep involvement of the EU in controlling medicines. In the article concerning public health, the Treaty includes "measures setting high standards of quality and safety for medicinal products and devices for medical use" amongst the rare domains in which the EU can take restrictive action in order to bring national policies in line with common safety concerns (article 168 of the TFEU, paragraph 4). Despite this recognition, when the new directive concerning pharmacovigilance was adopted in 2010, it was not only on this more recent legal basis, but also on the "traditional" internal market provision of article 114 (ex-article 95 EC).

The progressive institutionalization of regulation by network

Dynamics of European integration in the pharmaceutical sector

Several phases can be distinguished in the development of EU policies on medicines. Until 1975, national measures remained underdeveloped and the community was mainly working toward defining common ground for drug safety control. In 1965, a framework directive was adopted giving a European definition of a medicine, imposing mandatory marketing authorization for any medicine, contingent on demonstrating efficacy, safety and quality. In 1975, after a ten-year deadlock largely attributable to Germany's objections (Hauray 2006), two directives emerged that defined the content of tests that had to be carried out by the manufacturer (directive 75/318) and the basic procedures through which experts' evaluation was to be carried out (directive 75/319).

The year 1975 also saw the start of a second period in which the first EC bodies and licensing procedures were created. Directive 75/319 allowed manufacturers to request the recognition of marketing authorizations obtained in one member state by other states. In theory, the latter were supposed to accept. In cases of refusal, a committee composed of different state representatives then provided a non-binding opinion on the MA. This process of mutual recognition, reformed in 1983, did not work well: it was rarely used by manufacturers, states usually refused to recognize the decisions made by their partners, agreement within the European committee was often minimal (Hankin 1996) and the opinions provided had no important bearing on national decisions. However, after 1978, working groups brought together experts on specific issues. Among the first issues to be addressed were acute and long-term toxicity, carcinogenicity studies, and anti-inflammatory products and their efficacy. This paved the way for the formalization of a great number of European standards regarding the development and control of medicines (Hauray and Urfalino 2009).

The 1985 *White Paper on the Completion of the Internal Market* made provisions for the reform of European procedures for issuing marketing authorizations. After long negotiations, a new system was finally adopted in 1993. Three pathways were laid out: 1) a national procedure, reserved for medicines only marketed in one state; 2) a centralized European procedure (only mandatory for biotechnological products and optional for innovative ones) within which assessment is carried out by the European Medicines Agency (EMA)—which incorporates the European committee created in 1975 that then became the CHMP (Committee for Medicinal Products for Human Use)—and the marketing authorization is delivered by the Commission; and 3) a procedure for mutual recognition between states based on national marketing authorizations and restrictive arbitration by the EMA in cases of persistent disagreement. The centralization of the control of medicines and the EMA's expertise have been bolstered on several occasions since 2000. In 2000, the EU adopted a policy for promoting orphan medicines that the EMA implemented. In 2004, revised legislation extended the list of medicines that had to be authorized by the centralized procedure (regulation 726/2004)[6] and changed the procedure for mutual recognition (directive 2004/27). In 2010, the pharmacovigilance reform led notably to recording all adverse drug effects in a single European database (Eudravigilance) run by the EMA.

Regulation by network

The EMA is not a European version of the US Food and Drug Administration (FDA) (Abraham and Lewis 2000) and relies strongly upon national authorities

(Gehring and Krapohl 2007). These national authorities make up the majority of the agency's management board (27/35 members).[7] The management board appoints the Executive Director, and approves the budget as well as the annual reports and work programs. In order for the EMA's opinions to be transformed into decisions by the Commission, they must first go through a complex system of "comitology" allowing further control by the states afterwards.

Above all, members of the CHMP are appointed by their home states and continue to represent national authorities. In the centralized procedure, two *rapporteurs* are appointed from members of the CHMP to conduct the initial evaluation of every application dossier. Several deliberations take place within the committee in order to reach a common verdict, which is ratified by a vote. Although *rapporteurs* work independently and are free to choose their teams from amongst EMA-recognized experts (approximately 5,000 for the whole agency), in reality they work with their national agencies. Incidentally, the latter receive a quarter of the fee paid by the manufacturer to the EMA.

However, the EMA does represent real European pharmaceutical expertise. Within the CHMP, it is no longer seen as legitimate to invoke national specificities and it is the ability to convince others on the basis of technical arguments that is decisive (Hauray 2006). Neither the states nor the European Commission contest the opinions of the agency, which are made public the very day they are adopted and considered as decisions by the pharmaceutical sector's stakeholders. When controversies about medicines develop in Europe outside of the centralized procedure, as occurred recently in considerations of medication for obesity or depression, a common, European-level position is defined through several referral procedures. In cases where a member state has suspended or withdrawn a medicine from the market, the CHMP is required to provide a European opinion.

The "external" legitimacy of this "regulation by network" is strong. Not only is it rare for pharmaceutical companies to take any legal action against the EMA's decisions (Groenleer 2011), but the agency is also considered to be the FDA's main partner/competitor. Interactions between the two agencies, protected under a confidentiality agreement, are frequent and they often consult each other on application dossiers that they are assessing in parallel (Kermani 2009). Whether in terms of timeframe or content, the decisions of the two agencies are also compared by administrative and political leaders, by non-governmental organizations (NGOs) and by companies or specialists in the sector. The affirmation of the EMA's role has gone hand-in-hand with a substantial increase in its in-house staff (the secretariat has gone from 50 to nearly 500 employees) and in their influence upon the EMA's work.

Steering and mutual transformation

The Commission's competence in implementing the necessary measures to build the Single Market and the process set in motion by the White Paper have obviously played a key role in the processes described (Permanand 2006). However, how can we explain and account for the very successful centralization of regulations in the pharmaceutical sector? In keeping with the main theories regarding European integration (Grossman 2004), the decisive influence of the pharmaceutical industry has been put forward as one explanation. Gehring and Krapohl underline the fact that "most contributions focus on the origins of the authorization system and correctly point out that it has been promoted by industry within the Single Market project, rather than by stakeholders with public health interests" (Gehring and Krapohl 2007, p. 209).

Industry is either viewed as initiating and steering the processes analyzed (Abraham and Lewis 2000; Greenwood 1997) or—in approaches that consider the EU's intervention in the health sector to be biased towards economic interests—as being the main influence and preoccupation of the Commission in drawing up its proposals (Permanand and Mossialos 2005). Explanations for the decisive role of industry are corroborated by a number of elements: the fact that the Directorate General Enterprise and Industry has taken on pharmaceutical policy; the highly successful organization of the industry on a European level; the overall satisfaction of industry stakeholders with the European system; and, the extent to which pharmaceutical companies' requests about procedures have been taken into account (e.g., reducing the timeframe for assessments, or allowing preference to be expressed regarding the *rapporteur*). For several years now, proposals by the Commission have also been severely criticized as being too pro-business. Examples include proposals concerning the promotion of patient access to information on medicines, which was seen as a disguised manner of allowing prescription drug advertising to the public, and the proposed withdrawal of the need to revise marketing authorizations every five years (which was not adopted in the end).

The strong consideration given to industry interests is undeniable. However, its role in creating the European system itself should not be considered self-evident or over-estimated for four reasons. First, from the 1960s until the early 1990s the Commission met with considerable opposition from the majority of businesses regarding centralizing assessments on a European scale (Hauray 2007; Permanand 2006). Therefore, although these corporations might be relatively satisfied now, it is difficult to claim that they initiated the system that was adopted.

Second, it is problematic to reduce the Commission's motives simply to the promotion of industrial interests. This does not account for the priority given to integration as an aim within the "practical identity" of the Commission—which can be pursued in ways that both are and are not amenable to business interests. The reductionist approach also does not account for the specificity of the pharmaceuticals unit within the DG Enterprise and Industry. The Commission's pharmaceuticals unit grew out of the secretariat of a committee on health issues—the ancestor of the CHMP—and its main state partners—as concerns drug safety regulation—are the different state health authorities. F. Sauer, the director of this unit between 1986 and 1994, and main leader for the reform adopted in 1993, was a pharmacist, member of the French health administration and, after having been the first director of the EMA, was appointed head of public health within the DG Health and Consumers, with great expectations (Guigner 2008).

   Third, unlike the pharmaceutical companies, patient and consumer associations consistently supported the centralization of control (Orzack *et al*. 1992). However, for a long time they were unable to counterbalance the strong lobbying carried out by companies to influence the precise definition of legislative content. This imbalance seems to have been somewhat redressed by the creation, in March 2002, of the "Medicines in Europe" Forum bringing together patient associations, family and consumer organizations, health care insurance providers and organizations of health care professionals.

   Fourth, reducing the creation of the European regulation of medicines to a purely economic project fails to situate this process within its historical context and to trace the progressive manner in which a European policy space for medicines has taken shape (Hauray and Urfalino 2009). The creation of the EMA and the integrated system is grounded in more than 30 years of interactions between European and national levels and of progressive alignment of state practices. Even though the regulatory mechanisms created prior to 1993 were of limited efficiency, they nonetheless played an essential role in the Europeanization of the sector. After the late 1970s, formal common European standards for product development and assessment began to be implemented through guidelines. Later, European committee meetings of national experts and leaders initiated the existence of a "European medicine evaluation" and developed cooperative methods and even interpersonal links. Furthermore, the initial European procedures encouraged comparisons and competition between member states as health authorities could now verify their work. This comparison encouraged member states to align safety controls, assessment modes, and organization through, for example, the replacement of central administration by semi-independent agencies beginning at the end of the 1980s. The implementation of the EMA and new European procedures after 1995 augmented the combined effects of the definition of common standards, socialization (Checkel 2005) and comparison/competition between nations in institutionalizing European regulation.

Issues at stake

The implementation of a new system for the regulation of medicines, and in particular of the EMA, has generally been seen as a success and as a potential model for other sectors (Demortain 2008; Groenleer 2009). This system is nonetheless repeatedly called into question by stakeholders in the sector like S. Garattini (former member of the CHMP), medical journals, NGOs and members of the *Medicines in Europe Forum* collective (HAI Europe, ISDB, and MiEF 2010). Three main issues seem to be discernable regarding its workings, although they are strongly intertwined.

Autonomy and accountability

An essential dimension to the political accountability of regulatory authorities is their transparency, which determines to what extent third parties can reach independent judgments about the decisions they make and how they function. The creation of the EMA was presented as a step forward in this regard due to the agency's decision to publish on its website summarized meeting minutes of its committees and management board, as well as public assessment reports containing the CHMP's opinions and a summary of the scientific data and expert assessment upon which these opinions are based. Since March 2011, the EMA also holds a public register of ongoing clinical trials in the European Union. Initially, the same efforts were not made regarding national procedures or mutual recognition procedures (the committees that work as forums for arbitration between states did not even have any legal existence before 2004). A 2005 directive extended the principles adopted at the EMA level to national authorities and established new rules for the committee responsible for mutual recognition.

However, European practice remains behind that of its American counterpart (Garattini and Bertele 2010).[8] Not only are the FDA's advisory committees public, but full transcriptions are also available online. The EMA also takes a very comprehensive view of what consists of confidential trade information that cannot be made available to third parties. Faced with the EMA's refusal to make available certain documents justifying their decisions, stakeholders have turned to the European Ombudsman on several occasions. In cases involving results of clinical trials for an anti-acne medicine and two anti-obesity medicines, as well as the adverse effects of an anti-bacterial medicine, the Ombudsman's verdict required the EMA to provide the information requested.

The great autonomy enjoyed by the EMA has also led to questions concerning the quality of the controls to which it is subject. To use the terms of the principal–agent model, have the principals (the states and European institutions) lost control of the agency? Although the EMA does make marketing authorization decisions de facto without actually having the legal competence to do so, it has generally been underscored that it still reserves an important role for the "principals" in question (Gehring and Krapohl 2007; Groenleer 2011). The states are able to weigh in on the decisions that are made via their members of the CHMP and the management board. The European Parliament also has two members on the management board, but above all it supervises the agency's activities through the annual budgetary discharge vote that must be obtained by the director of the EMA (see *infra* the question of conflicts of interest). As for the Commission, it keeps a permanent watch on the legal implications of the EMA's work, for example by attending CHMP meetings. These mechanisms of multiple controls (Dehousse 2008) allow tensions to be expressed, thus tempering any overly consensual view of the workings of the EMA. Recurrent sources of conflict between the EMA and the states include how the licensing fees paid by pharmaceutical companies should be divided between the EMA and the member states (Groenleer 2011), the precise definition of the size and responsibilities of the EMA "secretariat" (Hauray 2006) and the composition of the CHMP. Behind these issues lie deeper questions regarding the future of national authorities and the emergence—or not—of a form of "European FDA."

The relationships between pharmaceutical companies and the
European regulation of medicines

European policies and the EMA are criticized for the links between the pharmaceutical industry and the regulatory authorities. The fact that EU pharmaceutical policies were placed under the responsibility of the DG Enterprise and Industry encouraged the idea that economic aims prevail over those of public health. When the Commission was renewed in 2009, these policies were eventually handed over to the DG Health and Consumers and the Health Commissioner. Within the routine working of the European system, certain mechanisms adopted since the 1990s have proved more specifically problematic. For example, pharmaceutical companies have been given the right to indicate their choices for *rapporteurs* in the centralized process, introducing possible bias in the assessment relationship. Also, the fact that European law and its strict enforcement by the EMA impose stringent assessment deadlines that seem to favor industry interests in rapid approval, despite well-documented links between deadline pressure and lower quality of assessments (Carpenter *et al.* 2012). What is more, the licensing fees paid by pharmaceutical companies represent 73 percent of the EMA's budget. Although not a problem per se, it contributes to spreading the idea of a structure that is in fact at the service of industry.

The scientific advice offered by the EMA, which consists in offering help to manufacturers in developing their products—in exchange for remuneration—has also been a point of contention (Hauray 2005a). While this is a way to improve regulatory activity, it can also create a form of prior engagement on the agency's part and lead to increased financial dependence upon industry. The mechanisms for the mutual recognition procedure—which generates strong competition between national authorities to serve as point of entry to the EU, has long-remained untransparent, and favors industry's influence—have been criticized (Abraham and Lewis 2000).

Due to the pharmaceutical industry's extensive funding of medical research and the links established between scientific experts and companies, the question of conflicts of interest is also extremely important. Although this was always handled far less rigorously in Europe than in the United States, it has been subject to increasing control since the early 1990s. The EMA traditionally put in place a system of annual declarations of interest for its experts and the members of its committees, which was augmented in 1999 by a *Code of Conduct* (that has since been revised) in order to oversee EMA employees' actions. In practice, however, regulation of these declarations proves difficult due to the substantial number of experts who work for the agency.

Several affairs have recently rocked the European system calling for improvements in addressing conflicts of interest. First, the EMA's former director, who served from 2001 to 2010, began advising pharmaceutical companies immediately after leaving his post with the EMA, thus providing a tangible illustration of the proximity between the EMA and the pharmaceutical industry. Second, a NGO (Corporate Europe Observatory) brought to light the fact that certain patient associations, who were not only members of the EMA management board but also sat on several expert committees, had not declared the substantial funding they received from the pharmaceutical industry (Corporate Europe Observatory 2010). Finally, the Mediator (benfluorex) scandal revealed the extent of Servier Laboratories' influence upon both experts and political powers in France. The incident had repercussions on a European scale because the medicine had been the subject of debate and arbitration on a European level. These different controversies were significant factors in the May 2011 Parliament decision to postpone its vote until October on the budgetary discharge for the EMA's director in order to encourage the agency to reform and improve its handling of conflicts of interest. In response, the agency reinforced its policy in this domain and created a public database containing the declaration of interests of all of its experts. Following the request of French Eurodeputies, the European Anti-Fraud Office (OLAF) opened an investigation into possible conflicts of interest within the EMA concerning Mediator.

Although the question of conflicts of interest is important, it should not subsume reflection about the interplay of private and public interests. The pharmaceutical industry's key influence is present both before and after the public assessment of products. It can be seen in the definition of research protocols, and therefore in the information provided about products, and in the lobbying of doctors (thanks to journals and pharmaceutical sales representatives). Above all, the way in which private and public interests intersect is deeply embedded in the content of medicine policies that shape the framework for scientific expertise.

The politics of expertise

The strong integration that exists in the pharmaceutical sector has been obtained as a result of a highly technocratic approach to drug control (Gehring and Krapohl 2007; Hauray and Urfalino 2009). The goal of reaching common decisions despite different medical cultures, public health policies and sometimes even sanitary conditions, was based upon the view that harmonized criteria and technical standards would lead to identical judgments. In actuality, European procedures—and the coordination that they entail—work by setting aside the involvement of political officials, separating discrete aspects of policies regarding medication (though questions of price remain largely national), and concentrating on regulatory science as both a-national and apolitical. As one member of the CHMP stated (Hauray 2006): "Regarding the other issues, issues of a political nature, the impact of decisions . . . that isn't science so it has no place here."

However, the observation of agency deliberations reveals political dimensions of some of the committee debates (Hauray 2005b), which have policymaking consequences. Furthermore, the architecture of European medicine policies and the criteria used in the evaluation process are called into question. The European system of drug control, for example, has focused on the initial assessment phase at the expense of post-authorization regulations, which have developed in a less complete and systematic fashion (Bauschke 2012; Demortain 2011). Only over the last few years, since the cerivastatine and rofecoxib crises, has there been a real increase in European investment in questions of pharmacovigilance, of which directive 2010/84/EU offers a concrete illustration. Another recent trend, aiming to improve links between the pre- and post-marketing phases, is the rise of pharmacovigilance planning, which requires pharmaceutical companies to better anticipate—beginning at the authorization phase—the monitoring of adverse effects and the possible response measures (Demortain 2011). The effects of this change have yet to be evaluated (Frau *et al*. 2010), but many fear that it will lead to more relaxed pre-marketing controls with an increased use of conditional marketing authorizations[9] or of fast-track procedures.

Another central political issue in the European regulation of medicines is that of defining criteria for registration. Many observers lament the fact that insufficient demands are made upon pharmaceutical companies to provide comparative studies that would evaluate their products in relation to the best medication currently available. The use of placebo studies as well as "non-inferiority" trials (which simply establish that the new medicine is not significantly less effective than the comparator treatment) are also criticized. While agencies do request explicit product comparisons depending on the situation and pathology in question, this is not considered enough. Further demands are being made to either amend European medicine law to require demonstrating the relative efficacy of medication (Sorenson *et al*. 2011) or to add a fourth criterion for approval: "therapeutic advance." A medicine could only be marketed if it makes a proven contribution in terms of public health when compared with existing products.

Conclusion

The European Union has taken on a central role in policies regulating medicines since the 1960s. A positive outlook on the development of these European policies would highlight the way in which the obvious logic involved in creating common assessments in Europe progressively took shape through an interplay of cooperation and socialization processes, through the comparison of expertise and the steering of the European Commission, and ultimately through the cross-effects of European integration and Europeanization. Pharmaceutical policymaking has led to the implementation of an innovative institutional framework—an agency— able to organize efficiently the coordination of national expertise and to embody an emergent European identity in matters of medication.

A more critical analysis of these European developments would rather underscore the negative implications of defining health policies through market aims, the cumbersome nature of inter-state communication and, above all, the extremely technocratic aspects of the process, that is to say, the rise in pharmaceutical policies within the "secret garden" of European health policies (Greer 2009b). From this perspective, rather than undermining the legitimacy of European regulations, the ways in which both the European Agency and the content of Community policies have been called into question recently seem to constitute a new stage in the development of a real European policy space in this field.

Notes

1 Cerivastatin (Baycol, Lipobay, Staltor) was marketed in the late 1990s to treat hypercholesterolemia. It was the fifth molecule of the highly lucrative statin class. Bayer voluntarily withdrew it from the market worldwide in 2001, after almost 100 reported deaths.

2 Rofecoxib (Vioxx) is a non-steroidal anti-inflammatory drug marketed by Merck & Co. in the late 1990s. This arthritis and acute pain medication was withdrawn from the world market in 2004, due to safety concerns of an increased risk of cardiovascular events.

3 Mediator was first marketed in the mid-1970s as an anti-diabetic drug, but was mostly prescribed by doctors as a weight-loss pill. It was only withdrawn from the French market in 2009, years after being forced off other markets (in 1997 in the US), amidst scandal, and appears to have caused more than 500 avoidable deaths in France.

4 Patients are randomly allocated to an "experimental group" (they receive the drug) or to a control group (they receive a placebo or a comparator drug) and the results of the two groups are compared.

5 A medicine can be qualified as orphan if it treats a serious illness that affects no more than five in ten thousand people in the EU or if it is unlikely to generate sufficient profit, without incentives, to justify the necessary investment for its production.

6 This now also includes orphan medicines and medicines for the treatment of AIDS, cancer, neuro-degenerative disease, diabetes, auto-immune and viral diseases.

7 The other members are two representatives from the Commission, two representatives from the European Parliament, two representatives from patient organizations, one representative from doctors' organizations and one representative from veterinarian organizations.

8 For a recent evaluation of the European agencies' internet sites, see Bauschke 2012.

9 A conditional marketing authorization—valid for one year but renewable—can be given to a medicine in cases where the application dossier did not provide the data usually required, providing that the drug provides treatment for *unmet medical needs* and that the benefits to public health outweigh the risks inherent to the fact that the assessment of the medicine is incomplete.

Part II

The EU and global health governance

7 The EU as a global health actor

Myth or reality?

Sébastien Guigner

Almost two-thirds of the population die of infectious diseases in developing countries, while these diseases kill only 1 percent of the people living in developed countries (Zacher and Keefe 2011). Such disparity does not suggest that infectious diseases affect only a limited part of the world. The recent global spread of SARS (Severe Acute Respiratory Syndrome) and influenza A (H1N1) are dramatic reminders that "microbes ignore borders." Such events put the global nature of health in the spotlight and serve as a reminder that, more generally, "*health issues* ignore borders." In a globalized world, global health is not confined to communicable diseases and health-related challenges increasingly transcend national boundaries. Chronic diseases and health issues linked to individual behavior have also become global. Diet, tobacco, and alcohol, for example, are strongly influenced by marketing strategies of multinational food companies (see Chapter 11 by Kurzer).

In light of the global spread of a wide range of threats to public health, a landmark event took place in New York in September, 2011. The United Nations (UN) general assembly convened to set a global agenda on the prevention and control of *non*-communicable diseases. It was only the second time in history—after AIDS in 2001—that the general assembly of the UN met on a health issue. Three key issues spurred this UN action. First, the global chronic disease burden currently places seemingly endless and often excessive demands on health care that jeopardize the sustainability of health systems worldwide (Blank and Burau 2010). Second, many developing countries do not have access to essential medicines produced in developed countries. Drugs are protected by intellectual property international regulations that preserve high prices often unsustainable for individuals and health care systems. This situation encourages smuggling and counterfeiting, which may endanger the health of individuals. Third, the worldwide flow of patients and health professionals is another major global health concern. Competition for patients and poor distribution of health professionals can lead to medical desertification in some countries or hyper specialization in areas that do not serve the health care needs of local populations.

In this chapter we will define global health as encompassing "those issues which transcend national boundaries and governments and call for actions to influence the global forces that determine the health of the people" (Kickbusch and Lister

2006, p. 7). Nonetheless, the meaning of global health is extensively debated, as shown by the increased attention paid by national and European authorities to global health (Koplan *et al.* 2009; Harman 2012). In the last decade, health has increasingly been recognized to directly impact economic development, security and trade, and, as a result global health, has become a key policy issue and a fast-growing field of research.

The European Union (EU) hopes to be a major actor on the global health scene. In a recent communication on "The EU role in global health," the European Commission called for the expansion of its role (2010c). To date, think tanks and committed scholars have been the main sources to analyze the EU's contributions to global health (Kickbusch and Lister 2006; Silberschmidt 2009). Conceptual approaches to the EU's international role (Bretherton and Vogler 1999; Elgström and Smith 2006) offer several frameworks with which to appreciate the EU's role in global health.

In this chapter, we build on the concept of "actorness" (Sjöstedt 1977; Jupille and Caporaso 1998), which can be understood in terms of the EU's "ability to function actively and deliberately" (Sjöstedt 1977, p. 16) in global health politics. Rather than determining the specific nature of the role the EU—which poses significant methodological problems and can easily drift into normativity—the investigation of actorness takes "one step back" (Groen and Niemann 2010, p. 4). It is about the EU's *capacity* to act. Starting from the premise that being present[1] (i.e., positioned) within the global health field does not necessarily imply being an active player in this domain, this chapter begins by describing the EU's global health activities and confirms the presence of the EU on the global health stage. We then assess the EU's global health actorness through three criteria: authority, cohesion and recognition.[2]

EU's global health policy: Action all-fronts

The European Commission defines global health as the: "worldwide improve-ment of health, reduction of disparities, and protection against health threats" (European Commission 2010c, p. 2). This broad understanding has justified the EU's presence on all fronts of global health from infectious diseases[3] to non-communicable diseases (NCDs) to health care/health services challenges. Furthermore, in dealing with these diverse issues, the EU deploys its full range of usual policy instruments such as regulation, funding or knowledge gathering and dissemination. Many of the EU global health policies are not new per se, but they have recently become integrated in a common EU framework.

The framework of the EU's role in global health

The EU has recently multiplied initiatives to address global health more compre-hensively and efficiently. In October 2009, the Commission's Directorates General for International Development (DG DEV), Research (DG RTD) and Health (DG SANCO) launched a public consultation to gather opinions "regarding the rationale, scope and strategic objectives for an EU role in global health" (European Commission 2009a). Following this initiative, the European Commission issued a communication on the EU's role in global health that is now the cornerstone of EU's activities (European Commission 2010c).[4] This document, the first of its kind, points to four challenges facing global health:

- governance, which consists of coordinating diverse actors and initiatives engaged in global health;
- universal coverage, which consists of ensuring access to health services for all and addressing health problems, including non-communicable diseases;
- policy coherence, which consists of consistently addressing the main factors that influence global health (trade, climate change, migration, etc.) across policy domains; and
- knowledge, which consists of two things: first, translating research findings into evidence-based decisions and policies; and second, addressing access and innovation so as to make new interventions and pharmaceuticals effective, safe, acceptable, affordable, and accessible.

The document identifies several action areas to improve the EU response to these challenges, including development of:

- Democratic and inclusive governance. This involves EU support of the participation of all stakeholders in national health policies and, at global level, the support to a stronger leadership by the WHO and an effort to cut duplication and fragmentation. In the international context, this also requires the EU to speak with one voice. To accomplish unity in communications, the Commission proposes the designation of global health coordinators appointed by the Commission and the member states.
- Universal health care coverage. The EU proposes to support the strengthening of health systems to ensure that they are able to deliver basic health care for all and that they are based on fair financing mechanisms. The European Commission will propose a list of priority countries to concentrate its health Official Development Assistance over a period of at least three years.
- Coherence. To ensure that all relevant internal or external policies contribute to improving global health more effectively, the communication proposes creation of an impact assessment mechanism to analyze the effects on global health of EU policies.
- Evidence-based intervention. The communication calls for incentivizing the collection of comparable data and statistics to allow benchmarking, to promote mechanisms for partner countries to build and sustain their national research capacity, and to promote the dissemination of information on hazards in areas where global normative action is required (e.g., food, feed, medical devices).

The fact that the EU has adopted such an inclusive strategy confirms its ambition regarding its role in global health. This new framework is evident in three main fields of global health: infectious diseases, non-communicable diseases, and health care.

Infectious diseases

The EU has invested particularly extensively and intensively in the field of infectious diseases at global level. The European and Developing Countries Clinical Trials Partnership (EDCTP), created in 2003, provides a first illustration. The goal of the EDCTP is to develop new or improved drugs, vaccines, microbicides and diagnostics against HIV/AIDS, malaria and tuberculosis to address the needs of sub-Saharan Africa. Its specific aim is to focus on the translation of medical research into clinical applications adapted to the needs of developing countries.

The EDCTP was the first EU program to use a very specific article of the Lisbon Treaty to provide a legal basis for EU support of an integrated set of research programs undertaken by several EU member states and that promoted partnership with sub-Saharan countries. The EDCTP had a projected budget of €600 million for the period 2003–2007, one-third of which came from EU funding, one-third from member states, and one-third from industry, charities and private organizations. The EDCTP, in turn, has contributed more than €4 million to tuberculosis (TB) prevention and treatment projects that strive to shorten, simplify, improve adherence to, and reduce costs of treatment regimens. Since 2011 the EDCTP has provided significant funding to a study evaluating a new tuberculosis vaccine. The study tests the vaccine in approximately 1,400 adults age 18–50 in Senegal and South Africa and involves the University of Oxford and the Institute of Infectious Disease and Molecular Medicine in Khayelitsha, South Africa.

The European Commission has also been a founding member of the Global Fund to fight HIV/AIDS, tuberculosis and malaria in developing countries. Set up in May 2001, the Fund is now the main financier of programs to fight these diseases. The Global Fund allocates money raised from public authorities and private donors to local structures best suited to manage efficient use of funds. The European Commission is a voting member of the Global Fund's Board, which is responsible for overall governance and the approval of grants. The EU is also a major participant in financial terms: the European Commission has pledged €790 million for the period 2001–2007 and the European Commission plus EU member states are the largest donor. To date, they have delivered over 50 percent of total pledges (€2.8 billion, up to 2007) (Global Fund to fight AIDS, tuberculosis and malaria 2011).

EU action on infectious diseases does not only concentrate on these three poverty-related diseases.[5] For example, the European Centre for Disease Prevention and Control (ECDC) focuses on EU countries, but also works daily with the World Health Organization (WHO) and participates in WHO's Global Outbreak Alert and Response Network (GOARN) (see Greer in Chapter 10).

Non-communicable diseases

Non-communicable diseases are a second field of EU activity in global health. In his opening remarks of the September 2011 Special Meeting of the UN

General Assembly on NCDs, the Secretary General stressed that, worldwide, three out of five people die from NCDs and that the trend is on the rise. Deaths from non-communicable diseases—principally cardiovascular diseases, cancers, chronic respiratory diseases and diabetes—are expected to increase by 17 percent in the next decade and in Africa, that number could rise to 24 percent (United Nations 2011a).

NCDs are a global heath issue for three reasons. First, they cause great health and socioeconomic harms to residents in all countries in the world. Second, there is a vicious cycle by which poverty, chronic diseases, infectious diseases and fragile health care systems feed off each other. Third, risk factors form a chain at the world scale. The example of tobacco illustrates the complex linkage of risk factors for NCDs. Since the mid-1980s most industrialized countries have developed wide-range tobacco control policy. In response, the tobacco industry shifted its business strategies to focus on developing countries and/or to countries where tobacco control policy is weak or non-existent (World Bank 2003; WHO 2003). Contraband coming from developing countries now impairs developed countries' ability to regulate and control price and content. Governments have recently adopted, by consensus, a "Political Declaration on the Prevention and Control of Non-communicable Diseases" that recognizes the need for measures at global, regional and national levels that cut smoking. The consensus statement also prioritizes the reduction of harmful consumption of alcohol, and high salt, sugar and fat foods (United Nations 2011b).

Following the lead of global health figures such as Ban Ki-moon, Secretary General of the UN, and Margaret Chan, Director General of the WHO, John Dalli, European Commissioner for Health and Consumer Policy, took the floor on the UN General Assembly stage to outline EU initiatives at the EU and global levels. EU's scope of action is less expansive in the area of NCD prevention and control at global scale than it is in infectious diseases. One exception is that the EU assumes a central role in the issue of tobacco control as evidenced by Dr Gro Harlem Brundtland, the former WHO Director General, presenting a special award for leadership in global tobacco control to David Byrne, the former EU Health and Consumer Commissioner on June 16, 2003. This event acknowledged the EU's role in adopting the WHO Framework Convention on Tobacco Control (FCTC). The World Health Assembly adopted the FCTC, negotiated under the auspices of WHO, in May 2003.

The FCTC outlines seven actions of its sponsors. Specifically, it requires parties to: First, adopt measures to regulate tobacco advertising, promotion and sponsorship; second, regulate packaging and labeling of tobacco products; third, regulate the content of tobacco products; fourth, control illicit trade in tobacco products; fifth, protect from exposure to tobacco smoke; sixth, promote public awareness on the risks of tobacco use; and seventh, establish tobacco cessation programs. The EU has clearly inspired some of the major articles of this treaty and facilitated its adoption through its negotiating strategies and tools (Guigner 2009). EU's commitment to this treaty has turned out to be vital to its implementation. In July 2011 one-quarter of countries had not remitted any payments of their so-called voluntary contributions to the implementation process, while all EU member states (except Slovenia) have paid all their contributions for the period 2006–2009 and the EU has contributed nearly $600,000 (WHO 2011).[6]

Health care

In addition to infectious and non-communicable diseases, the EU also addresses the global implications of health care issues such as access to essential medicines and workforce development. The EU regularly praises its efforts to widen access to vital medicines in developing countries in accordance with the 2001 World Trade Organization (WTO) Doha Declaration. The 2003 Council regulation to avoid trade diversion of certain key medicines (European Community 2003) is consistent with the Doha objective to improve access to essential medicines. The Council regulation aims to encourage European pharmaceutical companies to make medicines available at heavily reduced prices (so-called "tiered-priced medicines") in developing countries, while ensuring that these products are not to be sold back into European markets, thus threatening profits in European countries. In order to avoid the development of parallel markets, the regulation mandates a logo to be affixed on packaging or products and documents used in connection with the products sold at tiered prices. This provides a system for spotting tiered-priced products and facilitates inspections by customs authorities.

The EU uses licensure as an additional mechanism to improve access to essential medicines. The Trade Commissioner Pascal Lamy once declared that "the EU leads the way in ensuring access to affordable medicines for poor countries" (European Commission 2004a). The EU further played a decisive role in introducing the public health provision in the WTO agreement on Trade-Related Aspects of Intellectual Property Rights (TRIPS) (Wiechoczek 2006). This agreement establishes minimum standards for protecting and enforcing all forms of intellectual property rights, including those for patents. These rights help patent-holding firms by facilitating a return on their investment in research and development, incentivizing the development of new products, notably innovative medicines. The consequence of the patent system is that is keeps prices high and limits access to medicines, especially in developing countries. To limit this effect, WTO members adopted an agreement during the Doha Round of negotiations in 2001 (Abbott 2002; WTO 2001).

The Doha agreement includes the possibility of compulsory licensing, which is "the practice under which a foreign government insists that a company wishing to sell an intellectual property product in that market license the use of its technology to a firm within the foreign country or to the foreign government itself" (Mastel 1996, p. 64). In theory, compulsory licensing allows countries to manufacture pharmaceuticals that they could not otherwise afford in the global marketplace. However, policy has turned out to be counterproductive. The same countries that cannot afford high-cost medications are the same as those that have no or limited capacities in their pharmaceutical sector.

To address the unintended consequences of the original compulsory licensing agreement, WTO members introduced—and actively pushed by the EU—an amendment to the TRIPS Agreement in 2005 that allowed medicines produced under compulsory licensing to be exported to developing countries with limited manufacturing capacity. This amendment was integrated into EU law in 2006 (European Community 2006) and in 2007 the EU formally accepted the amendment to the WTO. The EU's acceptance spurred 28 additional ratifications— the 27 member states, plus the EU. This highly motivated the endorsement of the amendment. Indeed, before the EU's formal agreement only 13 countries had accepted the change, while two-thirds of the WTO's 151 members are required to ratify a decision before it takes effect.

A competent health workforce is of vital importance to health systems as well as for global control of communicable diseases. Developing countries have always faced a shortage of health workers but in recent years this shortage has become critical, especially in sub-Saharan countries (WHO 2006). This trend is partly due to actual and/or perceived health workforce shortages in developed countries, including those in the EU. The differential in living and working conditions between developed and developing countries has led to a brain drain from poor to rich countries (Marchal and Kegels 2003). All EU institutions have issued documents conceding the problem and the European Commission (2006a) has adopted the "European programme for action to tackle the critical shortage of health workers in developing countries." This resolution defines actions that the EU ought to pursue to reduce harm due to brain drain. For example, it proposes supporting the expansion of country-level training capacity and supporting the development of a regional observatory on human resources for Africa.

While the EU's position promises to be effective, the problem is not limited to the health care sector. Brain drain cannot be solved without reducing the broader "suction effect" engendered by developed countries. The EU's response has since evolved to include internal policies aimed at producing and retaining sufficient numbers of European health workers (European Commission 2008b). The EU has also made a commitment to develop a Code of Conduct for the Ethical Recruitment of International Health Workers, and has collaborated with the WHO's work to develop a "Global Code of Practice on the International Recruitment of Health Personnel" (WHO 2010). This Code asserts that recruitment of health personnel from developing countries facing critical shortages of health workers should be discouraged. Endorsing the Code is voluntary, but EU member states are encouraged to incorporate it into applicable laws. The Council of the EU (2010a) acted quickly on the issue and in December 2010 invited member states to adhere to this Code.

EU's fragile ability to act in global health

The EU is vocal in the global health arena, but what is its ability to act and to what effect? Based on Jupille and Caporaso's (1998) work, we will consider three aspects of the EU's global health actorness and its ability to act in global health affairs: authority, cohesion and recognition. These criteria are not absolute; actorness and its attributes are matters of degree. Moreover, they interact with each other and can be evaluated empirically in terms of legitimacy. For example, if a significant number of credible actors broadly recognize the EU's legitimacy to act in global health, the EU consequently expands its authority. Cohesion and authority, in turn, improve legitimacy with other actors and thus augments recognition. Though all dimensions of actorness are more or less addressed, the EU's ability to act in global health is, as yet, not firmly established.

The EU's authority in global health

Authority in the context of Jupille and Caporaso's actorness (1998, p. 216), refers to the "EU's legal competence in a given subject matter." The EU's legal competence to act in global health comes from two sources. First, it derives from explicit treaty provisions. Health competencies are laid down in article 168 of the Treaty on the Functioning of the European Union (TFEU), commonly known as the Treaty of Lisbon. Ever since the first version of this article—dating back to the Treaty of Maastricht, 1992—the Union has been invited to act at the international level. Indeed the EU shall "foster cooperation with third countries and the competent international organizations in the sphere of public health" (article 168.3 TFEE). Other provisions in the treaty support this objective and competence as in Article 168.1, repeated in Article 9 of the TFEU, stating that "a high level of human health protection shall be ensured in the definition and implementation of all Union policies and activities." This addresses the EU's capacity for external action and foreign policy development such as the EU's humanitarian aid and development cooperation.

When it comes to assessing the EU's authority in global health, *implied* power is at least as important as actual power given the international aspects of global health. During the 1970s, for example, the European Court of Justice (ECJ) stated that the EU can conduct external relations and become a party in international agreements in a given domain—even when there are no explicit provisions in the treaty—when the EU has already legislated internally in this domain or when external activities are necessary to attain the internal objectives mentioned in the treaty. This implied power is also referred to as the parallelism doctrine between internal and external competencies. In the case of health, the doctrine of parallelism's impact can appear rather limited since the EU's internal health competencies are still relatively narrow and allow minimal space for legislation. However, the EU has adopted a significant amount of secondary legislation directly targeting health goals on the basis of legal competencies in relation to the common market (i.e., EU legislation on tobacco control, on pharmaceuticals, on free movement of patients and health professionals, etc.). The Lisbon Treaty further sets out the protection of health as one of the objectives of a broad range of EU policies (consumer protection, environment and social policy).

There is thus sufficient legal basis for the EU to be involved in global health, suggesting the EU has the capacity to act in global health. However, the EU's degree of actorness in global health depends on *how* these legal tools are used. We now turn to other facets of the EU's actorness to understand its actions in the global health arena.

Recognition of the EU in global health

External recognition is another important component of actor capacity in global politics. Recognition means being registered on the "analytical radar" (Jupille and Caporaso 1998, p. 215) of other players. The more a third party interacts with the EU, the more it can be said to be recognized. With increased interactions "a process of socialization occurs according to which EU activity comes to be accepted and expected" (Jupille and Caporaso 1998, p. 216). The EU comes to influence the way third parties think and act, because the EU is a recognizable actor. It is not possible here to discuss the interactions of the EU with all the global health actors; instead, we focus on the WHO's recognition of the EU given the considerable and growing agreement that the WHO remains one of the pivotal actors in global health (Harman 2012), and that the WHO is on the analytical radar of all other global health players. When the EU interacts with the WHO, then it also indirectly interacts with all other actors.

The EU benefits from limited *de jure* recognition from the WHO. The EU formally holds observer status, which means that the EU is a second-class player and that the WHO does not interact with EU institutions as it does with other member nations. The practical implication of observer status is that it limits the EU's ability to participate fully in the politics of the WHO arena. EU representatives participate in the World Health Assembly, WHO Executive Board meetings, and various WHO committees only if invited. When the EU is present, it cannot vote, and EU representatives can only take the floor after WHO full members, and cannot raise point of order (Guigner 2009). In May 2011, the UN granted the EU *enhanced* observer status thereby reducing, in the short term, some of these limitations.

Prior to granting elevated status to the EU, the WHO and European Commission formally exchanged letters (December 2000) to formalize cooperation. The agreement notably states that the Commission will be systematically invited to WHO, Executive Board and WHO Regional Committee meetings, and that the WHO shall encourage the Commission's participation in the work of its diverse bodies by sharing reports and soliciting input. Formal membership of the EU in several international negotiations that took place under the WHO auspices is another sign of *de jure* recognition (Van Schaik 2009). We previously discussed the participation of the EU to the FCTC negotiations. The EU's involvement in the revision process of the International Health Regulations (IHR) is another example.[7]

These two international agreements (the FCTC and IHR) also provide symbolic proof of de facto recognition of the EU by the WHO. We already mentioned the WHO award for leadership in global tobacco control given to David Byrne, then European Commissioner for Health and Consumer Protection. Significantly, at the end of his mandate David Byrne also became WHO special envoy to revise the IHR, and was charged with building political consensus. De facto recognition is also evident in the creation of a WHO office in Brussels in 1999 to manage WHO–EU cooperation. The EU–WHO projects cited in the first part of this chapter represent a small sample of examples of de facto recognition, as do the countless informal and formal meetings that take place between European Commission and WHO officials (Guigner 2009).

But this expanding recognition (Eggers and Hoffmeister 2006) should be interpreted cautiously. Recognition does not always imply legitimacy, which ultimately determines the nature and credibility of recognition as criterion of actorness.[8] WHO cooperation with the EU may be largely motivated by self-interest than by the recognition of the merits of the EU's contribution on the substance of global health issues (Guigner 2009). Nevertheless, even if the recognition is minimal, it is significant and amplified by interactions. Recognition ultimately plays an attributive role in EU's actorness in global health.

The EU's cohesion in global health

The cohesion criterion evaluates the consistency of the EU's behavior within a given field. For the present analysis, we will distinguish between two types of cohesion: goals and strategy. A low level of cohesion on these two points would challenge EU credibility, power and, as a result, actorness.

The EU's goal in global health seems clear when reading the European Commission's communications on the EU's role in global health, and is largely consistent with the EU's definition of global health as the "worldwide improvement of health, reduction of disparities, and protection against global health threats" (European Commission 2010c, p. 2). The EU is not, however, the sole purveyor of services and support in this international arena. Notably, the Commission also states that "the Union shall uphold and promote its values" (European Commission 2010c, p. 3). In other words, the EU does not summarily support the best solution for global health, but the best solution for global health *that fits its values and norms*. For example, the EU was an ardent supporter of the FCTC insofar as it advocated adoption at the international level of norms already adopted at the EU level. As soon as the proposed regulation moved away from the *acquis communautaire*, the EU strongly opposed it, despite the added efficacy in the fight against tobacco use. The EU fought the abolition of tax and duty-free sales (Guigner 2009).

For similar reasons, in its comments and proposals on the draft Global Code of Practice on the International Recruitment of Health Personnel, the EU systematically replaced strong, binding language with weaker commitments (Spanish presidency of the EU 2010). Achieving better health worldwide may oppose some vested EU interests, but the compelling, positive economic, security and diplomatic effects that investment in global health can produce partly explain the growing attention to global health. As noted by the American Institute of Medicine (1997), healthier populations mean more markets for goods and services, and less money spent on disease outbreaks. In this spirit, the EU strongly supported the public health amendment to the TRIPS Agreement, which ultimately protects the European pharmaceutical industry and appears less philanthropic than at first blush (Abbott 2002; Guigner 2009) (see Chapter 9 by Massard da Fonseca).

Considering global health as a tool of "soft power" (Kickbusch 2011) leads to an understanding of why the EU launched the EDCTP program, despite its obvious drawback, corroborated by the ECDTP 2007 independent external review report, of further fragmenting global health policies and governance (Garrett 2007).

In summary, sometimes EU's goals favor the global improvement of health, sometimes they do not. The EU's activities in global health are guided by its values, norms and interests. As a fragmented and low coordinated organization pursuing several and sometimes competitive objectives (Smith 2004), the EU does not always behave consistently in global health and does not behave only in a completely disinterested and neutral way.

The EU acts with varying degree of strategic cohesion when participating in global health governance. The EU is much more efficient in international negotiations in areas of exclusive competence (Bretherton and Vogler 1999), such as trade. In these areas, the Commission develops an EU position and represents the EU in negotiations, under the supervision of member states. This process does not always prevent conflicts between EU member states, between EU member states and the European Commission, or between different Directorates General of the Commission. However, tensions usually remain confined in-house. This allowed the EU to speak with one voice and play a decisive role in the global arena, as illustrated by the WTO TRIPS agreement (Wiechoczek 2006). In the case of health, however, most EU competencies are shared or complementary. When it comes to negotiations at the international level, the EU's external representation is more complex. The EU is habitually represented both by the member state holding the presidency of the Council and by the European Commission. Despite a plethora of procedural mechanisms intended to adopt and defend a common EU position, conflicts between member states and the European Commission are inevitable.

In the field of health, the Commission fails to broker consensus among member states, nor do they trust the Commission to negotiate on their behalf (Van Schaik 2009). The reasons are manifold, but often linked to the limitations and the recency of the EU's involvement in the health. The general feeling is still that the EU is motivated by purely economic goals and has low expertise in the area of health (Guigner 2006). This leads EU units to express clashing opinions and adopt disparate strategies, as they did during the negotiations on the WHO global strategy on diet, physical activity and health (Van Schaik 2009). In cases where the EU has already proven its value internally to its members, it has reduced discrepancies between national arrangements and demonstrated that it is capable of cohesion, as during most of the negotiations of the FCTC (Guigner 2009; Mamudu and Studlar 2009; Studlar in Chapter 13). In a similar vein to the EU's authority and recognition, the EU's external strategic cohesion is deeply linked to the EU's internal competencies, policies and intra-EU institutions power relationships.

Conclusion

The EU has made many and strong declarations in support of global health and has expressed its intention to play a role in this area. The EU implements this commitment and, in practice, the EU is present on all fronts of global health. It is involved in the control of communicable and non-communicable diseases, in issues of global health care. In geographical terms, the EU informs and acts on global health policies not only in Europe or in developing countries, but world-wide, mostly through its participation in WHO programs and regulations. Despite all this apparent activity, the EU is at times simply a "decorative element" on the global health stage. The examination of actorness criteria in terms of authority, recognition, and cohesion shows that the EU's ability to act in global health is fragile. Health is neither a strong EU competence nor an objective that takes prec-edence over other EU objectives and policies. Furthermore, the European Commission often confuses legality and legitimacy as exemplified in communi-cations on the EUs role in global health. Invoking legal authority to act is neces-sary, but is not sufficient to be recognized by other actors. The EU nevertheless fulfills actorness criteria. It is able to, and does, act in global health. To continue with the theatrical metaphor, the fact remains that the EU is not merely a margin-alized agitator delegated to a corner of a stage where nobody pays attention. Rather, the EU plays a main role on the global health stage, but whether as antag-onist or protagonist remains an open question.

Notes

1   In this text the term "presence" is employed in the usual meaning, not in the conceptual sense used in some studies on EU's role in international affairs (Allen and Smith 1990).

2   According to Jupille and Caporaso (1998) the EU's capacity to act is a function of four criteria: recognition, "understood as acceptance of and interaction with the entity by others"; authority, that is to say "authority delegated to EU institutions by nation states"; autonomy, "conceived as institutional disctinctiveness and independence from other actors," namely EU member states; and cohesion, which is the ability "to formulate and articulate internally consistent policy preferences" (Jupille and Caporaso 1998, pp. 214, 216). While obviously drawing on Jupille and Caporaso's proposals, we do not fully replicate these criteria. Some criteria, like cohesion and autonomy, as designed by their authors, can be inconsistent (Groen and Niemann 2010). Furthermore, these criteria are essentially relevant to assess the EU's behavior in the negotiations of international agreements. To cover the whole scope of the EU's global (health) activities—including funding programs, for instance—they shall be interpreted very broadly.

3   Literally, « infectious diseases are defined as diseases cause by the actions of a living organism » (Zacher and Keefe 2011, p. 197). Consequently infectious diseases can be communicable or non-communicable. However, here when we use the term non-communicable diseases we refer only to non-infectious diseases or health problems.

4   See European Commission (2010d) for a detailed presentation of the Commission's views on EU's role in global health.

5   For an overview of EU strategic plans on these issues, see also European Commission (2002, 2005).

6   The implementation of the FCTC is mainly financed through voluntary assessed contributions (VAC) made by the Parties to the treaty. These assessments are based on national income.

7   The IHR, adopted in 2005, is an international binding agreement aimed at containing the spread of infectious diseases. Concretely, it contains detailed public health measures, to be implemented in ports and airports for instance, and obliges 194 states

Parties to develop certain minimum capacities to detect, notify and report events that may constitute a public health emergency of international concern. Such events shall be notified to the WHO, which will issue recommendations, coordinate the responses and provide assistance to the countries. In doing so, the IHR "greatly expanded WHO's authorities in global governance" (Katz and Fischer 2010, p. 3).

8 Massard da Fonsesca's work on intellectual property enforcement demonstrates this particularly well (see Chapter 9 in this volume). The EU became a central actor in this global health issue because the EU itself and member states generated the issue, which in turn obliged them to interact with the EU. This case thus reminds us that the actorness capacity cannot be simply associated with the impact in a given field.

8 Trade in services and the public's health

A "Fortress Europe" for health?

Holly Jarman

Introduction

In the current economic climate, considerable tension exists between states' economic policies and their stated social goals. Many EU member states have made decisions to drastically cut public spending, including health budgets. These cuts, as well as Europe-wide measures to instill "fiscal discipline," have been justified in many countries on the grounds that they are essential if states are to bring down government debt and end economic uncertainty (European Member States 2012).

At the same time, EU officials have focused their attention on strategies designed to bring back economic growth via innovation, increased economic competition, and free trade. These strategies support the liberalization of some areas of the economy, particularly services and some public utilities, while defining those services which should be protected from the market (Commission 2010b, 2011e).

The latest budget cuts and innovation strategies come amidst ongoing, broader trends towards the commodification and globalization of health care. Since the 1970s, deregulation and privatization in some EU health care systems has led to increased roles for private companies in providing health care (Feigenbaum *et al*. 1998; Pierson 1994). Beginning in the 1980s, states, as members of the World Trade Organization (WTO) or as bilateral or regional trading partners, have debated the creation of global service markets, including health service markets (Blouin *et al*. 2006). And from the 1990s, a series of European Court of Justice (ECJ) decisions have applied internal market rules and principles to the area of health (Greer 2008, 2009a; Hervey and McHale 2004; Hervey 2011; Mossialos *et al*. 2010).

These trends have had several important effects. First, health has been defined as a service, both informally, in political debate, and in formal law. In EU law, health services were treated like other commercial services in several key ECJ decisions. This implied that health services can and should be traded—causing political aftershocks through the EU system which led member states and the European Commission to attempt to circumscribe, and define exceptions to, this idea (Greer 2008, 2009a).

Second, the ability of constituencies—both private companies, and individual patients—to demand trade in health services has been strengthened (Greer 2009b). If corporate actors are active in some elements of EU health care, then it makes sense that they would use EU-level and national political institutions to lobby for wider market access. If patients see successful cases under EU law that support the ability of individuals to attain care abroad and be reimbursed by their home state, then they are more likely to consider their own claims. In 2011, EU institutions supported such claims by consolidating ECJ case law in the patient mobility directive (see Lamping in Chapter 2).

Third, health care is increasingly being talked about less as a drain on public finances than a potential contributor to national GDP. From an economic policy perspective, health services form a huge part of the EU's economy. Europe's highly skilled population of medical professionals, advanced medical and information technology, and specialized facilities could enable the EU to export health services to other countries (Commission 2007, 2011b). This concept of health services as profitable commodities is a popular one that can be seen in policy debates in many industrialized countries from the United States to New Zealand, often inspired by the development of "medical tourism" sectors in countries such as Singapore, India, or Thailand (Jarman and Greer 2010; Glinos *et al.* 2010; Laugesen and Vargas-Bustamante 2010).

But health services are also *public health* services: outside of the benefits attained by treating each individual, they play a vital role in attaining good population health, controlling the spread of communicable disease, and preventing and treating non-communicable disease. Many of the "goods" produced by health services are public goods, meaning that they are both non-excludable (no one can be excluded from the positive effects of controlling the spread of communicable disease, for example) and non-rival (freedom from disease enjoyed by one individual does not reduce the availability of that good for consumption by others). In a broader sense, European states have an individual and collective interest in building and maintaining reliable and effective public health services (Michalos 2008). As the perceptions and the realities of what health care is and how it is provided change, so too do the challenges for achieving and maintaining good public health within the EU and around the world.

This chapter examines the links between the external and internal aspects of EU health policy, and between the role of EU institutions as promoters of a large global market for health services, and their role as promoters of European public health. I explore the idea that the EU is creating a "Fortress Europe" for health—a liberalized internal health market combined with external barriers to trade in health care.

The next section explains the EU's formal powers supporting action on trade in health services. I then detail the EU's current policy in relation to the cross-border movement of health professionals and patients, commercial presence for foreign health providers, and cross-border health services where there is no commercial presence. Finally, I discuss future trajectories for EU policy on trade in health services.

What power does the EU have to construct or constrain cross-border health markets?

Trade in health services is an issue spanning two areas of activity—the economic and the social—and two jurisdictions—the internal and external faces of EU policymaking.[1] At one extreme, health care services can be viewed as just another form of economic exchange. At the other, they can be seen as a distinct form of social activity that should be protected from market forces. Likewise, health services form part of an internal market where patients, professionals, and providers move between EU member states, but they are also part of a global debate on how these actors can and should move. The EU's formal power to act, as well as the strength of consensus around policy norms and principles, varies a great deal along these dimensions (see Table 8.1).

EU treaties have historically granted the Union little power to act in health policy. This may seem surprising, given the longstanding coordination of social security rules between EU member states. Although elements of the TFEU allow the Union to act collectively on some public health issues,[2] health services are part of territorially based, distinct welfare states, often funded and managed by governments, and so remain a member state competency. The TFEU commits EU institutions to encourage cooperation between member states on health services in "cross-border areas,"[3] but states clearly that member states are responsible for both defining health policy, and for managing and financing health services.[4]

In contrast, the EU has long held strong internal market and external trade competencies. In the internal market, member states and the Union formally share competence while the Union has exclusive power to set important rules, such as those for competition, which shape the market. The ECJ has played an important role in supporting a free internal market, and applying internal market law to other policy areas. In multiple decisions, the ECJ has rejected arguments that health services, which form part of social security systems, should be considered "non-economic" in nature, and excluded from the application of EU commercial law (Hervey 2011).

Table 8.1 Dimensions of EU power in trade and health services

	Internal to EU	*External to EU*
Economic Dimensions	Shared competence for the internal market, but exclusive Union competence to establish competition rules.	Exclusive Union competence to negotiate almost all trade matters, but mixed agreements still needed where member state competence exists, including health. Ordinary legislative procedure, but unanimity requirement in some sensitive areas, including health.
Social Dimensions	Member state competence to define health policy, and to manage and finance health services and medical care.	Union and the member states will "foster cooperation" on public health issues with international organizations.

In terms of external trade, the Union has almost[5] exclusive jurisdiction to conduct external negotiations under the TFEU through the EU's common commercial policy. This includes the ability to negotiate agreements on trade in goods, trade in services, the commercial aspects of intellectual property, and foreign direct investment. A body of Court doctrine has partially supported the Union's competence on trade in the past,[6] placing important limits on the Community's ability to negotiate on services and intellectual property. The TFEU goes further in making trade in services entirely a Community competence, in theory reducing the need for mixed agreements requiring national parliamentary ratification (Eeckhout 2011, pp. 60–68).

On paper, therefore, the TFEU gives European institutions considerable power and autonomy to negotiate and conclude external trade agreements as compared to their ability to influence directly the internal configuration of member state health systems (as we can see from Table 8.1). But there are some important limitations to this power that demonstrate the difficulty of regulating trade in health services and the need for messy compromises.

The EU has not yet made many commitments to liberalize health-related services through international trade agreements, but it has made some (see Table 8.2), including some important bilateral arrangements with states interested in cross-border health services, such as India. In these agreements, states commit to provide market access to foreign companies, and to treat those companies on an equal footing with their domestic firms.

Trade agreements that touch on member state competences, including issues such as health and social policy, require mixed agreements, which member states must ratify. Art. 207(6) of the TFEU states that the "exercise of competences over common commercial policy shall not affect the delimitation of competences between Union and member states" and shall "not lead to harmonization of legislative or regulatory provisions of the Member States insofar as the Treaties exclude such harmonization." Furthermore, actions affecting trade in health services (along with those in education, cultural, and social services) require unanimity within the Council (Eeckhout 2011).

In practice, it is still unclear how the relationship between the EU's external trade in services commitments and its attempts to build an internal health market will unfold, but there is some evidence that the EU institutions have made promises that they cannot keep.[7] In *Commission v. Council*,[8] Advocate-General Juliane Kokott gave a detailed opinion on this relationship. In detailing their commitments under the General Agreement on Trade in Services (GATS), states must indicate the limitations they will place on foreign trade for each sector. Under the part of the agreement that deals with hospital services, certain EU member states list limitations on the ability of foreign health providers to establish a commercial presence within their borders. Belgium, for example, states that the number of beds in the Belgian health system is limited by a national health plan, and that the number of hospitals in Belgium is subject to an economic needs test. Kokott concluded that limitations such as these needs tests fall under national competency, supporting the argument that the Community acting alone should not

Table 8.2 EU health-related commitments under the GATS

	Cross-border Supply (Mode 1)	Patient Mobility (Mode 2)	Commercial Presence (Mode 3)	Professional Mobility (Mode 4)
Horizontal Commitments (applying to all sectors)			Market Access: National or local public utilities may be subject to public monopolies or exclusive rights granted to private operators. Some country-specific restrictions on investment and subsidies (France, Spain, Ireland, Portugal). National Treatment: subsidiaries of third country companies do not have to be treated as well as their parent companies, some limitations on land purchases. Subsidies to firms may be limited to those established in an EU state or region, with no commitments on subsidies for R&D. "The supply of a service, or its subsidisation, within the public sector is not in breach of this commitment."	Market Access: No commitments, except for some measures concerning temporary stays. National Treatment: Subsidies for investment may be limited to EU nationals. Union directives on mutual recognition of diplomas do not apply to third-country nationals. recognition of diplomas is a member state competence unless Union law says otherwise, and the right to practice in one ms does not grant the right to practice in another.
Hospital Services	No commitments made.	No limitations on trade.	Market Access: limitations based on health service plans, economic needs tests for numbers of beds. National Treatment: No limitations on trade.	Market Access: No commitments, except horizontal commitments, which are subject to limitations on access to management functions (France) and nationality for public hospitals (Greece). National Treatment: No commitments, except horizontal commitments.
Social Services	No commitments made.	No limitations on trade.	Market Access: limitations based on local authorization (France). National Treatment: No limitations on trade.	Market Access: No commitments, except horizontal commitments, which are subject to limitations on access to management functions (France). National Treatment: No commitments except horizontal commitments.

Source: WTO services database, accessed November 14, 2011.

be able to make amendments to the GATS—in this case, to allow the accession of Vietnam to the WTO (Kokott 2009).

This example illustrates how difficult it is to unravel the relationship between the internal and external faces of EU health policy. Limitations on the EU institutions' power to conclude trade agreements without member state involvement may seem favorable at first glance for those who oppose the liberalization of health services markets. But this may not be a sustainable compromise over the long term. Preventing regulatory harmonization between member states is not the same as maintaining the status quo—and the global policy debate around cross-border health services is rapidly moving. Governments around the world with expensive health care systems are interested in the potential for trade in health to decrease costs, and those with profitable health sectors are keen that international laws should support their global health ambitions. The following section addresses the EU's policy responses to these ongoing trends.

How does the EU currently construct or constrain cross-border health markets?

Trade in health services can be thought of as a policy problem with four different aspects: the provision of a health care service across a national border where neither the provider nor the patient nor the professionals move (such as telemedicine or outsourced medical transcription), the movement of patients across national borders to seek treatment, the establishment of foreign providers and foreign direct investment, and the movement of medical professionals across national borders to give treatment. In the GATS, these aspects are described as "modes of supply": mode 1 refers to cross-border supply of a service, mode 2 refers to consumption abroad, mode 3 relates to commercial presence, and mode 4 to the presence of natural persons (see Table 8.2). As with the EU's internal health policy, there is no coherent policy on trade in health services, but several smaller policies that collectively address these key aspects.

Cross-border supply of health services

The first form of cross-border health services relates to the provision of a health care service across a national border where no commercial presence is established in the host state. Perhaps the most often cited health example of this is telemedicine, although other examples include outsourced administrative services, insurance processing, or medical transcription.

Telemedicine (or in some cases, telehealth) refers to the use of telecommunications or information technology to facilitate health care, health education, or health research (Oh *et al.* 2005). It can include many different aspects of health care such as sending patient information electronically, or using technology to manage chronic conditions, to facilitate remote consultations with patients, or for medical education. Interest in telemedicine and telehealth among policymakers and providers has grown considerably in the last decade. The virtual provision of some cross-border health care exists in many countries around the world, but remains fragmented and underdeveloped (McLean 2007). Nevertheless, a legal framework already exists in trade law that could govern the future of global telemedicine markets.

In the context of new technologies, policymakers in developed and developing countries have turned their attention to encouraging the development of "eHealth" systems, in which cross-border health services such as telemedicine would exist as part of a broader network of electronic health information. Despite sustained interest in the cost savings and increased access to care that telemedicine may provide, most of the resulting policies remain weak (Mars and Scott 2010).

The EU is invested in promoting a European eHealth system (a "European eHealth Area") despite the many problems in developing such a system, and the weakness of its relevant policy tools. Research in various aspects of telemedicine is supported through the EU's Research and Development Framework, while assistance for implementing new systems is provided through the Competitiveness and Innovation program and the cohesion and structural funds (Palmer *et al.* 2009).

At this stage, telemedicine policy consists of much talk and much less action. The European Commission has been active in raising the issue of eHealth, producing an eHealth Action Plan in 2004,[9] adopting a Communication supporting telemedicine in 2008,[10] and addressing eHealth in the "Digital Agenda for Europe" in 2010.[11] The vast majority of the EU's member states now have a stated policy on eHealth, although implementation of these policies remains patchy and is largely dependent upon national political will (Lang and Mertes 2011).

In 2009, the Employment, Social Policy, Health and Consumer Affairs Council recognized the huge problems preventing the deployment of eHealth services, including market fragmentation, a lack of interoperability between systems, patient privacy concerns, and the need to improve legal clarity on the regulation, licensing and accreditation of eHealth services and called for greater cooperation between member states to remove these barriers.[12]

Responding to the Council's call, Art. 14 of the Directive on Patients' Rights in Cross-border Healthcare allows the Union to establish a "voluntary network connecting national authorities responsible for eHealth designated by the Member States" in order to "support and facilitate cooperation and the exchange of information" (Commission 2011a).

Undoubtedly, the supporters of a European eHealth Area hope that it would strengthen the economies of EU member states and give the EU a competitive edge in developing telemedicine markets. According to the Commission's ICT for Health Unit, the European market provides a "strong base" from which EU telemedicine providers can "tackle the global market" (Commission 2012a).

Indeed, EU telemedicine providers may face some tough international competition from providers in other states. A recent study found that providers in India, for example, see significant opportunities in the EU to sell services such as teleradiology, telediagnostics, telepathology, remote monitoring of patients in intensive care, remote diagnosis in areas such as ophthalmology and dermatology, telepsychiatry and continuous online remote monitoring. Indian companies and hospitals already provide some of these services in the United States, Singapore and countries in South and Central Asia. In relation to the EU, stakeholders view telemedicine services as less politically sensitive than other forms of cross-border care, with the UK's NHS seen as a strong potential client (Chanda 2011).

Patient mobility

The second aspect of trade in health services is cross-border patient mobility. At the present time, the number of EU patients traveling between member states to receive care abroad is fairly low, and mostly limited to regions where the best, closest, or most desirable care might be just across a national border or determined by expatriate populations. However, the EU's internal law supporting patients' rights to move is far ahead of that in any other region of the world.

The benefits and costs of increased patient mobility vary between sending and receiving states (see Table 8.3).[13] In sending states, patients with limited or no health care coverage may seek out cheap care abroad, or receive treatments or specialized care that is not available in their home state. By sending patients abroad, a state may be able to lower waiting times within its health care system. But sending patients abroad in higher volumes could have a detrimental effect on national health care capacity and planning.

Receiving states have the potential to grow their economies by receiving patients. In poorer states, growing their domestic health care sectors might seem like a much better policy option than losing medical professionals to better paid markets.

Hungarian interest in receiving foreign dental patients is largely driven by this phenomenon, for example. The fear that accompanies this argument, however, is

Table 8.3 The opportunities and costs of increased patient mobility

	Opportunities	*Costs*
Sending States	Lower waiting times. Access to specialized knowledge and treatments. Access to treatments not covered by home state. Potentially cheaper care for patients without coverage. Patients denied care on moral grounds can receive it abroad, e.g., abortion.	Potential spread of infection. Difficult continuity of care. Impact of sending patients in high volume on domestic health care capacity. Loss of ability to use cost containment measures such as waiting lists.
Receiving States	Health sector as a contributor to economic growth. Better alternative to sending medical staff abroad. Potential to use excess health capacity more efficiently.	Potential spread of infection. Difficult continuity of care. Impact of receiving patients in high volume on domestic health care capacity. Risk of establishing a parallel health system for local population.

that this will set up a parallel health system for the local population. Capacity is also a concern for states like Belgium, where a sudden influx of patients could potentially overwhelm local health care capacity.

Patient mobility became a very significant issue within the European Union after two important decisions made by the ECJ in 1998. The *Kohll* and *Decker*[14] decisions were significant in that they applied EU internal market law to health care much to the surprise of many national officials who believed that they were protected from such competition. A series of further decisions refined these initial judgments. The Court confirmed that health was part of the internal market, that patients should not be prevented from seeking care in another EU member state, and that states should, with some important limitations, pay for that care abroad. This jurisprudence and the policy debates which followed at the European level and in member state capitals culminated in the 2011 Directive on Patients' Rights to Cross-border Healthcare, which confirmed much of the Court's decision making but also went further in terms of outlining what member states may do to restrict cross-border patient movements (see Greer and Jarman 2012; Greer 2009; Lamping in Chapter 2).

In comparative terms, the EU's long history of social security coordination means that Europe is further advanced in terms of the portability of public health care insurance between states. But this internal patient mobility policy does not extend to states outside the EU. Member state health insurance is not portable beyond EU borders, although countries such as India would like this to be the case. Nevertheless, the EU does not mind receiving patients. The EU commitments under the GATS schedules on hospital and social services place no restrictions on inward patient mobility, but clearly limit government subsidies to third-country nationals.

Commercial presence for foreign health providers

The third form of cross-border health services refers to the establishment, including through foreign direct investment, of providers in a foreign state. Acting somewhat retrospectively, the Commission has put in a great deal of effort to frame the EU cross-border health care debate around patient mobility and patients' rights. But the original ECJ jurisprudence on health referred to above was based on Articles 49 and 56, which address the freedom of health *providers* to provide services across borders (Greer 2008). Article 49 and 56 decisions referred to the "freedom of establishment" for foreign undertakings (bodies offering goods or services in the internal market) wishing to move or establish a subsidiary in another EU member state (Hervey 2011).

In considering a future EU-wide Services Directive, the EU institutions and member states engaged in a messy and heated debate about how to apply to health both the right to freedom of establishment and the "country of origin" principle—the right of providers established in a foreign member state to be regulated by their home state. The controversial nature of these and related internal market principles and their lack of popularity among member state governments is illustrated by the fact that not only was health eventually stripped from the services directive, but that the country of origin principle was almost entirely stripped out too.

In this debate and subsequently, EU member states have shown little interest in (and have often been actively opposed to) changing the status quo regarding freedom of establishment in health care. Where foreign commercial presence does exist, it has been the result of member states choosing to invite in companies rather than systematic change (Greer and Rauscher 2011b). Companies in Germany's health and social services sector have a comparatively high number of foreign affiliates (Smith *et al*. 2009) as some German municipal governments have been selling off local health facilities to raise revenue. Central governments in the United Kingdom have shown interest in contracting with foreign firms to provide certain procedures through a system of day clinics, although this has not led to the wider liberalization of contracting in the National Health Service on the scale that foreign providers had hoped.

Under the GATS, the EU has made commitments that support the commercial presence of foreign health providers, with some important limitations. The EU states that national or local public utilities may be subject to public monopolies or exclusive rights, and that some of its members may apply restrictions on foreign investment or subsidies provided to foreign investors. Subsidiaries of third-country companies do not have to be treated on the same terms as those established within the EU. On hospital services specifically, the EU retains the right for its member states to apply an economic needs test or refer to a national health plan before allowing foreign providers to access their markets.

EU policy towards professional mobility

The fourth aspect of cross-border health services, professional mobility, refers to the ability of a medical professional who has been educated and trained in one state to register and work in another. While there are as yet only weak frameworks at the global level to manage professional mobility, the EU, along with several other regional trade blocs such as ASEAN, has more extensively attempted to harmonize professional accreditation among its member states, although not without some difficulties (Smith *et al*. 2009; Arunanondchai and Fink 2007). The Directive on the Recognition of Professional Qualifications consolidated EU rules on this subject in 2005, but as of 2012 is already being reviewed again as part of the push to rejuvenate the single market.

Again, we see a difference between sending and receiving states in terms of the costs and benefits of professional mobility (Table 8.4). Receiving states can benefit by hiring cheaper staff for a more flexible health labor market. Richer Western countries have been able to solve their own staffing crises by hiring doctors from poorer accession states, who come with fewer, or at least different, transaction costs than doctors from outside the EU. This can have an ongoing dampening effect on wages, as well as reducing the number of nationals who consider a medical career. This might be what governments want, but it is not in the interests of existing medical professionals, causing increased political conflict.

Table 8.4 The opportunities and costs of increased professional mobility

	Opportunities	Costs
Sending States	Benefits from remittances sent home. Could encourage greater capacity to train more medical staff.	Encourages experienced medical staff to leave. Encourages new medical staff to leave.
Receiving States	Flexible health workforce. Potentially cheaper health workforce.	Risks of different medical training and experience. Displacement of domestic workforce. Dampening effect on wages and numbers training as medical professionals.

The other risk that states take in recruiting from abroad is that the licensing and training of medical professionals varies a great deal between countries. These differences are not necessarily attributable to the quality of professional education across countries per se—but rather to differences in professional responsibilities, approaches to treatment, and expectations of staff that can vary a great deal between health systems. Some duties required by a nurse in a UK hospital, such as inserting an IV, are not required of nursing staff in Germany, for example.

The EU attempts to manage this problem through the principle of "mutual recognition." Under mutual recognition, member states come together to agree on a certain standard, such as a minimum number of hours of education, and then accept each others' credentials on that basis. This promotes professional mobility, but does take into account many of the distinctions between systems. In response to these persistent differences, receiving member states are allowed to test for certain skills, including language skills, and can apply their national regulations to foreign professionals working within their state (Nicolaïdis and Schmidt 2007).

Sending states face different issues. On the one hand, they may benefit from remittances sent back by their nationals when abroad. But those remittances may not make up for the serious shortages in staff numbers and experience faced by their state as medical professionals find work in higher-paid countries. Just after the Baltic states joined the European Union in 2004, the UK and Germany hired away large percentages of their medical workforces at salaries much higher than those available domestically. Some states at risk of professional out-migration might prefer to import patients than to export their professionals.

Both internal and external professional mobility is a significant challenge for EU member states. Western member states receive significant proportions of their medical professionals from abroad, while newer member states in Eastern Europe are sending doctors and nurses in large numbers. At the same time, there are examples of large professional mobility from third states—for example between the UK, India, and the Philippines (Glinos forthcoming; Wismar *et al.* 2011a). But while governments regulate external professional mobility, internal mobility falls under one of the EU's core principles: freedom of movement for people

(Glinos forthcoming). In the late 2000s, the UK government chose to choke off medical immigration from third countries at the same time as it ramped up incentives for domestic medical recruitment. But the ability for member states to control internal professional migration is somewhat more limited.

The EU's debate on professional mobility becomes still more important in the face of efforts to liberalize international labor markets. A number of international organizations, including the World Health Organization, World Trade Organization, and the UN Educational, Scientific, and Cultural Organization are attempting to set global standards on professional education and licensing, but with different end goals (Frenck *et al.* 2010, p. 1939). Some organizations, including the WHO, are highly engaged with promoting the "social accountability" of accreditation, where criteria for assessment reflect the health priorities of the relevant community (WHO 1995, 2010). Others, such as the WTO, are concerned with promoting the harmonization of professional licensing in order to streamline labor regulation and reduce barriers to trade (WTO 1994).

One might argue that these two goals—socially accountable accreditation and international harmonization—are mutually exclusive. For its part, the EU's policy on professional mobility fits much more closely with market promotion than social accountability. Perhaps if internal professional mobility continues its upward trend, the internal market principle of free movement will increasingly come up against complaints from member states struggling to manage their domestic health capacity. This is one of the many issues being tackled in debates surrounding reform of the Professional Qualifications Directive.

Current and future trends: EU 2020 and the single market

EU member states, taken as a group, have a grand vision: vibrant, innovative, high-technology health sectors, enough of an internal market in health services to drive down health costs and generate growth, but not enough to risk the integrity of their domestic health systems, and an external trade relationship which allows them to take advantage of cheaper foreign labor, without allowing "too much" migration or unintentionally opening up sectors to foreign competition. They want trade in health services—on their own terms. Unfortunately, the international and European legal systems seem to have already established key parameters.

This summary of member state policies skims over significant differences between member states, regional governments, and local authorities, and the political factions within them. Nevertheless, it does help explain why the EU's policies on the social and economic, internal and external aspects of cross-border health care often seem at odds with one another. The EU's big innovation and growth agenda, EU2020, addresses several issues pertinent to the future of health services policy. It is unclear at this point to what extent these policy proposals will be implemented, but their underlying ideas are likely to be much more persistent. Although the EU2020 strategy relates to the EU's future competitiveness in global markets, many of the individual policy proposals are the subject of "old wounds" inflicted by past debates.

In relation to the health workforce, these proposals include reviews of the Working Time Directive,[15] which stipulates maximum weekly working hours, as well as rest breaks and annual leave, and the Posting of Workers Directive,[16] which regulates minimum conditions of employment for workers who are temporarily sent by their employers to work in another EU member state.

The Working Time Directive, in particular, was heavily criticized on its initial implementation not just on economic grounds, but also for limiting the hours of junior doctors and nurses, with the resultant medical problems and mortalities from patient handovers proving to be worse than those resulting from overworked medical staff. Since that point, however, managers and officials in EU health systems have learned to work with the Directive, and special rules implemented for doctors in training, and so the resultant gains from revisiting this issue may not be as large as some expect. Nevertheless, the perception that the EU's labor market requires liberalization to compete internationally comes through clearly in this proposal.

Other proposals with a similar focus on cost-savings include the "Digital Agenda for Europe" discussed above, which includes funding for research on telemedicine and interoperability of medical data. The proposed pilot, the European Innovation Partnership on Active and Healthy Aging, rides in part on the assumption that a competitive social services market, and longer working lives for European citizens, will be necessary and desirable as governments struggle to fund future retirement.

The European Commission, for its part, has proposed an ambitious package of single market reforms. The "Single Market Act," adopted by the Commission in April 2011, and expanded in 2012 but mostly not passed by the other EU institutions, includes proposals to:[17]

- promote the liberalization of public procurement policies, and clarify the relationship between rules on state aid and public procurement that affect Services of General Economic Interest (which include Social Services of General Interest);
- simplify procedures for mutual recognition of mobile workers, and legislate on the posting of workers overseas to "clarify the exercise of freedom of establishment and the freedom to provide services alongside fundamental social rights";
- review the EU's standardization system for goods in order to apply it to services; and
- legislate to promote a "digital single market" which will, among other things, increase "the effectiveness of public services and procurement," and promote consumer empowerment through alternative dispute resolution mechanisms, particularly in relation to digital services.

One key question regarding these proposals is whether they will apply to health. Past disagreements between the EU institutions, member states, and European interest groups including businesses, NGOs, and professional associations have resulted in health being excluded from some important internal market legislation and policy such as the services directive. Health services are also sometimes regarded as distinct from Social Services of General Interest, although these services often have public and population health consequences (van de Gronden 2009; Jarman 2011b). But these categorizations are not permanent. They were hard won with considerable member state support, and there is no reason to assume that a further debate on the appropriate policy space for health services would have exactly the same outcome, given the current ideological standpoints and budgetary shortfalls in many member state capitals.

A second question is whether this ambitious agenda will gain any traction. Given the current economic climate, there may be little room on the EU's agenda for grand reforms, even pro-market reforms. It can be assumed, however, that this document gives a good indication of the Commission's strength of feeling on these issues, and that if there are ways for them to implement some of these proposals without needing the cooperation of the other institutions and the member states, they will pursue them.

At the same time as the Commission is pushing forward this innovation agenda, EU Member states are using "spot markets" in cross-border health care—informal, ad hoc transactions which allow them to supplement their domestic health care systems (Greer and Jarman 2012). By signing contracts for a certain number of procedures, or outsourcing one particular element of the system on a limited term basis, member states show that they are keen to gain the benefits from trade in health services, but cagey about broader free trade in health services. For this reason, the current system of spot markets is likely to continue, at least in the short term.

Internationally, the EU is not formally negotiating on health in WTO negotiations on trade in health services, but as the global market in health services grows, pressure from states outside the EU with expanding international health care sectors (and also perhaps from EU member states with stakes in exporting health care such as Germany or Hungary) to liberalize cross-border care is likely to grow.

The question framing the next decade of health services policy in the EU is whether the current status quo—a liberalized internal health market and protectionist external trade policy for health—can be maintained in the face of this pressure. The further that the EU moves down the path towards health services liberalization within its own market, the harder it might be for EU institutions to defend limitations on the participation of businesses from third-party countries within that market.

Conclusion: A "Fortress Europe" for health?

In a policy environment where the boundary between internal and external poli-cymaking is increasingly blurred, the EU is attempting to bridge the gap between perceived imperatives for innovation and economic growth and increasingly trans-border health care markets by making bets on future demands for care.

The result is, to some extent, a "Fortress Europe" for health. In trade policy, "Fortress Europe" refers to the argument, often made in the 1980s and early 1990s, that the creation of an internal market in the EU with few barriers between states would lead to increased protectionism between the EU as a trading bloc and the rest of the world (Hanson 1998).

While the EU's internal health market has been substantially liberalized, the EU has remained a relatively protected trading bloc in relation to global health markets. There remain some important formal and informal barriers preventing the EU's greater participation in these markets.

Formally, the EU has made relatively few commitments to liberalize trade in health services through the World Trade Organization, although it has made some in hospital services and related business services such as insurance. Informally, even if the EU were to expand its health sector commitments under the GATS, there is currently some constitutional uncertainty as to whether the Commission has the right to negotiate on health services liberalization without directly involving the member states.

Attempts to manage the EU's internal health market have been focused on the movement of people across national borders. Patient and professional mobility are sensitive topics where opinions vary considerably between EU member states. Some states such as Hungary see a clear advantage in receiving patients, others such as Sweden in sending them, while a further group of states have an interest in addressing their workforce shortages through professional mobility.

But the most likely avenue for increased liberalization is actually in electronic and other direct services where neither patients nor professionals nor companies move. It is in this sector that outsourcing seems most plausible, with a less visible impact on the receiving health system as a whole. Political visibility, as well as budget pressures and decentralized decision making, make it perhaps more likely that a hospital manager will outsource a particular service through tele-medicine than a government will rethink its immigration policy. We should not underestimate the power of such small internal changes to change both the EU's internal health market and its relationship with health providers in the rest of the world.

The often-prophesied "Fortress Europe" for goods did not materialize as some scholars expected. Overall, the EU member states did not block imports or systematically veto legislation that was not seen as protectionist enough as their economies integrated with one another. What did happen, in the EU as elsewhere, is that as tariff barriers to trade were removed, regulatory barriers to trade became much more important as targets for liberalization.

The key point here is that "Fortress Europe" was not seen as a viable, or desirable, long-term policy option in an increasingly open global market for goods. Nor was protectionism a viable strategy for member states wishing to protect their health systems from the development of an EU-wide health services policy. In much the same way, we should not expect "Fortress Europe" to be a viable long-term policy option for health services. Even if Europe remains a "fortress" that limits the migration of medical professionals, other aspects of health services, particularly services provided across borders like telemedicine, are likely to be liberalized. This is what many European and foreign policymakers want, and they have the tools to achieve it.

Notes

1 For an examination of health in internal market EU law, see Lamping, this volume.
2 TFEU Art. 4(k) grants shared competence in public health matters. Art. 6(a) allows the Union to take action to "support, coordinate or supplement" the actions of member states in the "protection and improvement of human health." Art. 168 mandates a "high level of human health protection" in the definition and implementation of Union policy.
3 Art. 168(2) states that the Union shall "encourage cooperation between the Member States to improve the complementarity of their health services in cross-border areas."
4 Art. 168(7) states that Union action shall "respect the responsibilities of the Member States for the definition of their health policy and for the organisation and delivery of health services and medical care. The responsibilities of the Member States shall include the management of health services and medical care and the allocation of the resources assigned to them."
5 The Union does not have exclusive competence to conduct external negotiations on transport matters.
6 This is an intricate history that is too detailed to be explained here. For discussions of this jurisprudence, see, among others, Meunier and Nicolaïdis (1998) and Eeckhout (2011).
7 The following section relies heavily on Eeckhout (2011), p. 61.
8 Case C-13/07 Commission v. Council. AG Kokott, opinion of March 26, 2009. Withdrawn following entry into force of Lisbon Treaty, paras 142–56.
9 See European Commission (2004b).
10 See European Commission (2008b).
11 See European Commission (2010a).
12 See Council of the European Union (2009).
13 For a full typology of patient mobility, see Glinos *et al.* (2010).
14 C-120/95, Decker v. Caisse de Maladie des Employés Privés, 1998 E.C.R. I-1831, Case C-158/96, Kohll v. Union des Caisses de Maladie, E.C.R. 1998I-1931.
15 Directive 2003/88/EC of the European Parliament and of the Council of 4 November 2003 concerning certain aspects of the organization of working time.
16 Directive 96/71/EC of the European Parliament and of the Council of 16 December 1996 concerning the posting of workers in the framework of the provision of services.
17 See European Commission (2011e) for updates, and the second Single Market Act of 2012, see http://ec.europa.eu/internal_market/smact/index_en.htm (accessed 21 October 2012).

9 Intellectual property enforcement in the European Union

Elize Massard da Fonseca

What are intellectual property rights?

Intellectual property (IP) rights and patent protection of medicines are controversial topics in public health. IP rights provide legal protection to intellectual activity in the industrial, scientific, literary and artistic areas. IP laws aim to safeguard creators and other producers of intellectual goods, such as research-based pharmaceutical industries, by granting them certain time-limited rights by which to control the use made of those products. In the pharmaceutical sector IP issues exist in delicate equilibrium. On the one hand, governments and decision makers sustain monopolies over the price and production of medicines, which motivate research and development; on the other hand, they want to guarantee affordable prices to life-saving medicines.

Since 1994, the World Trade Organization (WTO) has been responsible for coordinating the minimum standards for intellectual property protection in its member countries through the Agreement on Trade-Related Aspects of Intellectual Property Rights (TRIPS). As an important global economic and political player, the European Union has participated very closely in the debates drafting and implementing TRIPS. Several studies have analyzed the controversial decision to regulate intellectual property at the supranational level (cf. Weissman 1996), while others have explored the unyielding alliance between developing countries and non-governmental organizations (NGOs) to clarify the TRIPS safeguards to public health (cf. Abbott 2004; Sell 2007). However, as with other regulatory arenas, intellectual property rule–making is dynamic. While discussion in the 1990s focused on the content of what should be protected and to what extent, in the 2000s it centered on how to enforce these rights. This chapter discusses the latter of these debates analyzing IP enforcement policies in the European Union.

The remainder of this chapter explores the dynamics of the IP and public health debate. The first part documents the EU competencies and policies aimed at enforcing intellectual property rights through customs authorities. The second part examines the effects of these decisions on developing countries. The third section discusses the social phenomena underpinning the controversies of the IP enforcement agenda: definition of public interests and where to promote them. The key message of this chapter is that trade in medicine through European ports and airports has become a problem of global health governance.

The EU agenda on enforcing intellectual property and curbing counterfeit medical products

Resolutions on intellectual property enforcement in the European Union have gained importance over the past decade. In 2006, the European Commission issued a statement cautioning consumers about potentially unknown quality and origin of pharmaceutical products commercialized on the internet. The European Parliament echoed this concern (2006). Controversial decisions have subsequently been discussed to enforce intellectual property rules. Proposals have included the introduction of a common identification for online pharmacies, or use of an obligatory authenticity feature on packaging. Perhaps the most controversial are the stringency rules on customs and products in transit through the EU.

If member states take unilateral actions to address the problem of counterfeit medical products, it could lead to different standards of public health protection. Additionally, it could raise concerns about the compatibility of their actions with the internal market and encourage counterfeiters to focus on countries with lower levels of protection in the distribution chain (DG Enterprise and Industry 2008a). For these reasons, the European Commission has taken steps to promote the intellectual property enforcement at supranational level.

EU and the WHO

The European Community has worked closely with the International Medical Products Task Force (IMPACT). IMPACT is a voluntary initiative of WHO member states intended to curb counterfeit medical products. Currently, it consists of 40 member states, representatives from the Council of Europe, the European Commission, the International Criminal Police Organization (Interpol), as well as other international agencies, and non-governmental organizations (IMPACT 2011). In 2007, the Director-General of the DG Enterprise and Industry, Heinz Zourek, gave an enthusiastic speech at the First European Parliament Symposium on the EU and International Initiatives against Counterfeits (Zourek 2007). He publicly expressed strong support for the IMPACT and raised concerns about the quantity of fake medicines seized at the EU external border. A few months later at the IMPACT international conference, the DG Enterprise and Industry voiced strong warnings linking counterfeit products to low quality medicines: "counterfeit drugs kill," "counteract counterfeiters," "put an end to drug counterfeiting" (Lalis 2007).

With the financial support of the DG Enterprise and Industry and the Commission's Competitiveness and Innovation Framework Programme, the IMPACT presented a document proposing the principles and elements for legislation to minimize the risk of counterfeit. This highly controversial document (as discussed in the next section), proposes a set of principles to guide national legislation to counteract counterfeit medical products. The relationship between IMPACT and the EU has been mutually beneficial. While the EU has fostered the IMPACT initiative, IMPACT has served as a basis to justify and legitimize several decisions taken by the EU to enforce IP rules.

Internal activities to curb counterfeit

In 2008, the European Commission released the outcomes of a two-month intervention to inspect medicines entering and in transit through the EU, known as the Medi-Fake action program. A team of customs experts, a pharmaceutical specialist and the Commission developed key risk assessment indicators and named high-risk pharmaceutical products that should have reinforced controls. This first joint initiative between the 27 member states intercepted several medicines ranging from life-saving drugs, such as anti-cancer and anti-cholesterol medicines, to lifestyle drugs (such as drugs to treat impotence, wrinkles, or acne). Program records indicated that more than 34 million illegal medicines were seized (Europa Press Release 2008).

The Commission has also promoted the implementation of a pan-European resolution, enacted in 2001, to control the supply chain of pharmaceuticals and medical products for human use (Directive 2001/83/EC). The motivation for the Directive was the increasing sales of counterfeit medicines over the internet. Directive 2001/83/EC, along with Regulation 1383/2003 concerning customs actions against goods suspected of infringing IP rights, are the legal bases of the European Union's customs actions to protect and enforce intellectual property rights. Regulation 1891/2004 relates specifically to the submission by member states of information on the detentions made.

IP right-holders (the pharmaceutical companies) can request border officials inspect shipments in transit through the EU, or customs officials on their own initiative (*ex-officio*) can examine cargos if there is suspicion of IP rights violation. Nevertheless, very few cases are initiated *ex-officio*. The collaboration between private industries and customs has resulted in an increase in applications from 1,000 in the year 2000 to 18,000 in 2010 (European Commission—Taxation and customs union 2010). However, this collaboration has raised several concerns as it can be argued that public officials are acting in the interests of private actors (Cozendey 2009).

The increased volume of confiscated goods raises the question of the relationship between counterfeit and substandard products. While the former implies a violation of trademarks and IP, the latter refers to medicines with sub-standard active ingredients that can not only cause severe side effects, but also pose a risk of death. Fears of the latter led, in April 2008, the DG Enterprise and Industry to propose a public consultation seeking suggestions to amend the Directive 2001/83 (DG Enterprise and Industry 2008b).

Several stakeholders contributed to the consultation though among the 123 participants, 100 were from industry (DG Enterprise and Industry 2008b). This suggests an imbalance in the direction and content of the proposed amendments. There was a strong reaction of NGOs and developing countries against the EU seizures (as we shall see in the next section). There was little participation from civil society in this public hearing for reasons that are unclear.

Pharmaceutical industries have welcomed and supported the EU decisions at different levels. For instance, the European Federation of Pharmaceutical Industries and Associations (EFPIA), which represents the pharmaceutical industry operating in Europe, suggested that communication between customs and right-holders should be strengthened and speeded up to allow quick actions (European Federation of Pharmaceutical Industries and Associations 2010).

Together, the WHO-IMPACT initiative, the public consultation, and the impact assessment served as a basis for a new legislation on falsified medicines, approved in July 2011, Directive 2011/86/EC (European Parliament 2011). This new rule maintained previous responsibilities for pan-European IP enforcement and introduced more stringent measures for the trade of medicines (e.g., record-keeping requirements for wholesale distributors).

The flip side of IP enforcement: Impact on developing countries

Following the agenda in enforcing IP rules/counteracting fake medicines, in December 2008 Dutch customs authorities seized a cargo of 500 kilos of Losartan Potassium (Active Pharmaceutical Ingredient used in the production of generic medicines for arterial hypertension) (Bloomberg 2009; Reuters 2009; Valor Economico 2009). The seizure was motivated by a request from its patent-holder in the Netherlands. The product was in transit from India (Dr Reddy's Laboratories) to Brazil (EMS Pharmaceuticals) and off-patent in both countries. However, Losartan Potassium was protected by patent in the Netherlands (a supplementary protection until September 2009) under the brand name Cozaar, owned by Merck (McAviney 2009). The Indian government stated that as many as 16 shipments in 2008 were seized from India and China to Peru, Colombia, Ecuador, Mexico, Portugal, Spain and Nigeria and additional confiscations in 2009 took place in France, Holland and Germany (*Business Standard* 2009a,b; India 2009). In one case, UNITAID's[1] shipment of antiretroviral AIDS medications, certified by the World Health Organization, was intercepted under the misleading claim that it contained counterfeit goods (UNITAID 2009).

Due to fears of confiscation en route to destination countries, Indian generic makers have diverted shipments to transit hubs outside the EU through Singapore and Malaysia at great expense (*Wall Street Journal* 2009). Mobility of pharmaceutical products and enforcement of intellectual property law has rapidly become a problem for health diplomacy. Arguing against the European agenda, international non-governmental organizations (e.g., Oxfam, Doctors Without Borders and Health Action International) and developing countries such as India and Brazil have urged clear conceptual differentiation between generic drugs and counterfeit products, and have argued that the seizures and shipping delays affect their capacity to provide prompt access to affordable medicines. Seizures have been contested on the basis that the definition of counterfeit products is unclear and that there is dissonance between the EU and WTO regulations on transit of goods.

Definition of counterfeit medicines

One of the core objections to the seizures of pharmaceutical products and the EU regulatory standards is the definition of counterfeit products. Several international non-governmental organizations and developing countries have claimed that the term "counterfeit," according to the World Trade Organization, refers less to the quality of the product than to the infringement of trademarks (*Médicines Sans Frontières* 2009; Oxfam 2009). The TRIPS agreement defines counterfeit trademark products as those goods that use, without the permission of the right holder, a trademark that is identical or which cannot be distinguished in is essential aspects from the registered one (World Trade Organization 2010c). Importantly, products that infringe on intellectual property protection do not necessarily imply a poor-quality product (e.g., incorrect type of pharmaceutical ingredient or concentration). Thus, from a public health perspective, the relevance is not the illegal or fraudulent reproduction of a logo or brand name, but whether the pharmaceutical product has a toxic or incorrect quantity of active ingredients. This discussion has been transferred to the World Health Organization, under the IMPACT initiative.

The current IMPACT definition of counterfeit connects violation of trademarks with public health concerns (IMPACT 2007). This broad definition could be applicable even to legally available generic medicines, depending on its interpretation. Generic medicines can be commercialized by a non-proprietary name, for example making them potentially illicit under the proposed "Principles and Elements for National legislation against Counterfeit Medical Products" (ibid.). Whilst opponents of the IMPACT argue that it misleadingly uses intellectual property rather than public health objectives to address the poor quality of products, IMPACT representatives argue that certain measures aimed at counterfeit medicines are similar to the measures taken to reduce the rates of substandard medicines, such as monitoring the distribution chain (IMPACT 2011). Although IMPACT documents are not official recommendations of the WHO, they provide technical guidelines that can influence the agenda of the WHO and other member countries.[2] Much of the European Union decisions on this matter have been grounded on IMPACT suggestions (as previously discussed), while the IMPACT guidelines resemble, to a great extent, the initiatives proposed by the EU.

In 2009, a report on counterfeiting was scheduled to be presented at a WHO Executive Board meeting (Pharmabiz 2010). Brazil and India fiercely opposed the content of this document. The concern was that associating counterfeit drugs with concerns about drug quality would open the door for the WHO to get involved in IP enforcement and for generic producers vulnerable to IP challenges (IP Watch 2009). The Brazilian Ambassador for the WHO, Maria Nazareth Azevedo, declared:

> Brazil opposes the draft resolution on counterfeit medical products. Any definition related to the falsification of medical products cannot be used to undermine the access to legitimate generic medicines, especially in countries where they are part of national public health policies. As well as on branded medicines, any deviations of quality or non-compliance to Good Manufacturing Practices are infractions against public health, but should not be taken as examples of falsification.

(Farani-Azevedo 2009)

Brazil further stated that the WHO is the forum to discuss proposals to ensure the quality, safety and efficacy of medication, not the enforcement of IP rights (IP Watch 2009). The problem of substandard drugs has greater impact on public health than counterfeit medicines as suggested by a "Doctors without Borders" – MSF study (Ford *et al.* 2002; Caudron *et al.* 2008). This coalition of developing countries and international non-governmental organizations acknowledges the problem of substandard pharmaceutical products as a threat to health. However, they argue that the best way of dealing with poor-quality medicines is to strengthen national drug regulatory authorities than through the enforcement of intellectual property laws (Oxfam 2011a).

The UK Department for International Development conducted an assessment on drug registration and regulation in developing countries to shed light on this debate about drug quality. They found problems related to poor manufacturing capacity, lack of human resources and funding for drug regulatory activities, as well as inadequate knowledge of regulatory science in order to assess quality generic drugs locally. The findings suggested the presence of grave barriers to generics meeting the need for essential drugs (Hill and Johnson 2004). The issues were not related to IP infringements as much as the need for capacity building. Proposals to improve quality controls, then, should refer less to enforcement of IP rules than to bilateral capacity building to upgrade technical skills in low-income countries, such as the Promotion of Quality Medicines funded by USAID (Oxfam 2011a). International procurement agencies such as the Global Fund for TB, AIDS and Malaria rely on the WHO Pre-Qualification Programme (an international certification program for generic medicines) can contribute to improving quality by ensuring that medicines meet global standards of safety, quality and efficacy (*Médicines Sans Frontières* 2009). Advocacy can contribute to quality improvement efforts as well. To broadcast their disagreement with the EU's agenda on IP enforcement, Doctors Without Borders launched a campaign to pressure the European leaders to reformulate its position: "Europe! Hands off our medicine" (Figure 9.1) (*Médecins Sans Frontières* 2010b).

Violation of international trade rules

Generic drug seizure highlights a possible regulatory and power gap forming between the World Trade Organization (WTO) and European Union law (Seuba 2009). In 2009, Brazil, India and 15 other developing countries expressed their disagreement with the European generic drug seizures at the WTO General Council Meeting in February. These concerns were also reaffirmed at the WTO TRIPS Council meeting supported by Colombia, Ecuador, China, Cuba, Egypt, Argentina, Venezuela and South Africa (March 2009) (Azevedo 2009; Farani-Azevedo 2009; Valor Economico 2009; Brasil 2009).

Subsequently, both Brazil and India initiated a request for consultations with the European Union and the Netherlands at the World Trade Organization (World Trade Organization 2010a,b). (Consultation is the first step in the process of a formal trade dispute at the WTO.) Both Brazil and India were concerned with the

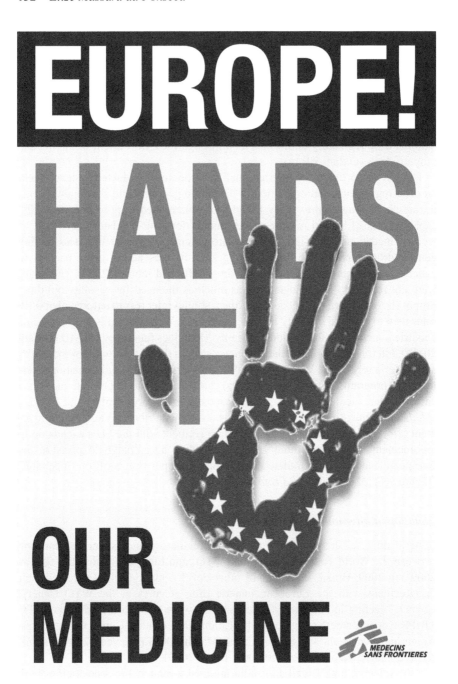

Figure 9.1 Médecins Sans Frontières' international campaign (access to medicines).

Source: Médecins Sans Frontières 2010a—Design by TaunusGrafik.

constant seizures of off-patent medicines originating in India and other third countries and transiting through ports and airports in Europe. Brazil and India claimed that various European Union and Dutch measures are inconsistent with the obligations of Articles V and X of GATT 1994 (which refer to transit of goods), various provisions of the TRIPS Agreement (e.g., definition of "trademark"), and Article XVI:4 of the WTO Agreement (see e.g., Seuba, 2009, for a detailed discussion of these international regulations). For the purpose of this chapter, it is important to understand that they refer to the freedom of goods in transit and the fact that confiscated medicines are not protected by patent in the country of exportation and importation. One of the key foundations of the TRIPS agreement is the principle of territoriality; that is, patents are territorial and their protection depends on the national regulation enacted by each member country of the WTO (article 28). Therefore, it would be irrelevant if the pharmaceutical product is patent protected in the country of transit, and would not justify the seizure.

The opposers of the EU generic drug seizures point to two additional considerations (Seuba 2009) beyond the legal. The first refers to the fact that customs authorities do not have jurisdiction over the validity of foreign patents. Even if they were qualified to evaluate patent infringement, doing so often requires laboratory examination or other complex procedures. Second, and perhaps more problematic, pharmaceutical products have acquired a special status in the WTO and other public international laws after the TRIPS and Public Health declaration. European regulations and seizures, then, could jeopardize the pro-public health interpretation of the TRIPS agreement. To resolve this concern, sixteen public health and consumer NGOs sent separate letters to the head of the World Trade Organization requesting him to resolve with the EU the conflict between their rules of goods in transit and the commitments made in 2001, and to encourage the EU to interpret TRIPS in a manner supportive of public health (Knowledge Ecology International 2009).

In response to the developing countries and NGOs concerns, EU Ambassador Eckart Guth declared at a WTO General Council that he would have liked Brazil and India to have first raised their concerns bilaterally to clarify the facts and figures, "before triggering a highly emotional debate" (Guth 2009). He assured the Council that "the EU has absolutely no intention to hamper any legitimate trade in generic medicines or to create legal barriers to prevent movement of drugs to developing countries, nor have our measures had this effect" (ibid., p. 1). It was not until 2011 that the EU and India reached an agreement on the WTO dispute. Nevertheless, the new legislation approved by the Parliament in July 2011 (Directive 2011/62/EC) did not solve this issue completely. The international NGO, Oxfam, released a statement that this legislation not only fails to ensure that generic medicines will not be detained in the future, but also creates more obstacles by requesting that trade partners of the EU should also comply with the Union regulations, including those related to IP (Oxfam 2011b).

The controversies of intellectual property enforcement

So far this chapter has presented different perspectives on intellectual property enforcement and the disparate interests involved in it. I now turn to two critical analytical reflections on this highly controversial regulatory policy arena. One hinges on the definition of public health interest, while the other refers to the choices regarding jurisdictional control over where and how IP policies are developed, enforced, and evaluated.

Definition of public health interest

The narratives presented in this chapter suggest that both the claims of the coalition of EU representatives and pharmaceutical firms on the one hand, and the alliance of developing countries and non-governmental organizations on the other, all make claims to acting based on social concern. They express relevant concerns for patient safety and public health. The rhetoric and identities of these stakeholders (i.e., the State, pharmaceutical firms or NGOs) express a fundamental social phenomena underpinning the controversy in the IP enforcement agenda that reveals similarities/differences of the coalitions' demands.

Some social scientists understand the political process as a game in which actors behave rationally as to maximize their preferences (whether it is profit or staying in power) (cf. Scharpf 1997). The contestation over intellectual property enforcement is explained by observing that powerful/resourceful research-based pharmaceutical industries, backed by their home countries (mainly developed nations), promote an agenda maximizing their economic preferences. The industry uses a clever strategy of portraying their issues such as "counterfeit kills" to graft decision makers' attention and public opinion to their demands. Developing countries and NGOs have social motivations for questioning how this agenda can prevent access to medicines by causing a shortage/delay of supply. Connecting a trade activity (brand name of products) to a public health issue (quality of medicines) becomes a phony discourse that fails to foster health protection. While the industry is motivated by material concerns, the NGO sector is motivated by principles and values. In both cases, participants of the policy process act rationally in order to maximize their stakes. Several studies examining European interventions resemble this perspective (cf. Abbott 2009).

Another set of social science scholars and analysts argue that the differences between North and South nations, businesses, and NGOs are less evident than their similarities (cf. Sell and Prakash 2004). Private actors can be guided by normative beliefs just as public or non-profit agents are; that is to say, the spread of counterfeit products is a legitimate social concern of pharmaceutical firms as it jeopardizes competition, employment opportunities and, ultimately, the safe distribution of medicines. By looking too narrowly into IP enforcement, it would appear that the EU is hampering global public health. However, by expanding the view into other decisions taken by the EU on global health matters, it is possible to observe several important actions that foster global health policy.

Examples include improving access to health services, the development of medical technologies and close monitoring of pharmaceutical regulatory practices (Oxfam 2009). For instance, in 2009, a partnership between the EU and the private sector (European Federation of Pharmaceutical Industries and Associations) committed €246 million for research projects on diabetes and severe asthma, and to training scientists and clinicians engaged in drug development (Community Research and Development Information Service 2011). Additionally, in 2008 the European Commission released a highly praised report on the competition inquiry into the pharmaceutical sector. This report evidenced for the first time that innovator pharmaceutical industries were promoting unfair practices to delay and limit the market entry of generic medicines (e.g., requesting multiple patent grants for the same medicine, and initiating disputes and litigation against generic companies) (European Commission 2008e). Therefore, it is not that the EU has a counterproductive or negative agenda on global health, as suggested in a publication by Oxfam (Oxfam 2009). Actors can have multiple, controversial interests and these are fluid rather than static. These preferences change over time in response to evolving experiences (cf. Hall 2005).[3]

Venue shopping: Where does IP enforcement belong?

Where does IP enforcement take place? Another political phenomenon that reveals the controversies of intellectual property enforcement is that of venue shopping (or forum shifting). This refers to the strategy of shifting the policy discussion to the most receptive institutional arena (Baumgartner and Jones 1993). Because the EU and right-holders have expressed their concern with intellectual property enforcement along a narrative that cites security and competitiveness, border control seems an adequate venue. Three examples illustrate this form of venue shopping.

First, the IP agenda has been promoted simultaneously and coordinately at various forums in relation to customs authorities, despite the fact that customs, for example the World Customs Organization (WCO), is not the traditional arena for discussing intellectual property. The Working Group Standards to be Employed by Customs for Uniform Rights Enforcement (SECURE) was an initiative at the WCO, motivated by the fact that the G8 (top industrialized countries) suggested that customs authorities should pay greater attention to IP violations. This initiative was highly supported by the EU. The Secure group faced strong opposition by South American countries, particularly Brazil and Ecuador, who claimed that the WCO was being used to set norms, standards and best practices and to put new obligations on the WCO Members beyond its purview (cf. South Centre 2008). After many disagreements, the group was discontinued in 2009. A new working group addressing Counterfeiting and Piracy (CAP) was created; as opposed to Secure, it did not make reference to IP enforcement in terms of health and safety.

Second, customs authority over IP enforcement has been added as a conditional clause of bilateral trade agreements and economic partnership agreements. For example, an operational document released in 2005 by DG Trade, *Intellectual Property Rights Enforcement Strategy in Third Countries*, suggests that future trade agreements emphasize improving enforcement at the highest-level possible (DG Trade 2005, p. 7). Agreements should include clauses on IP enforcement, clearly defining what the EU understands as highest standards in this area, and providing technical assistance to countries that normally lack resources and capacity to provide IP enforcement. This regulation was put into practice, in the Cariforum (15 Caribbean Community states and the Dominican Republic) economic partnership agreement. An independent evaluation of the 2005 DG Trade strategy found that the EU has been mostly successful in providing technical assistance projects on IP enforcement (DG Trade 2010).

A third venue of discussions of IP enforcement is the Anti-Counterfeiting Trade Agreement (ACTA), which is perhaps the most controversial one. This is a plurilateral trade agreement for promoting international standards of IP enforcement among participating countries. It was launched by the US and Japan in 2008, while the EU, Canada, Australia and other countries jointed later. The confidentiality of ACTA's negotiation procedures and leaks of the contents of parts of draft documents raised strong criticism from civil society (cf. *Médecins Sans Frontières* 2010a; Oxfam 2010). Oxfam suggests that ACTA is "proposing a new, expanded framework of intellectual property protections [. . .] which will be combined with border measures to stifle the trade in legitimate generic medicines. This will mean that poor people will be denied legitimate and life-saving generic medicines" (Oxfam 2010). The closed-door nature of negotiations makes it challenging to confirm or refute these claims.

The alliance of developing countries and NGOs criticize the strategy of spreading the authority for IP regulation beyond the WTO, arguing that these forums lack legitimacy to decide on this matter (Tellez 2009). International agencies such as the WHO and WCO would end up providing financial resources and coordination assistance without having an express mandate or consent from member states (including developing countries) to do so. Nevertheless, this coalition of developing countries and NGOs used a similar strategy years before by reframing the IP rights as a public health concern and promoting the agenda of access to medicines as a component of the human right to health (cf. Sell and Prakash 2004). This agenda was diffused through several health and trade forums such as the WTO, WHO and the United Nations General Assembly Special Section (UNGASS) (Sell and Prakash 2004; Nunn *et al.* 2009) and culminated in the "TRIPS and Public Health" declaration in 2001, which recognized the rights of governments to override patent protection in cases of public health emergencies and affirmed governments' rights to define what constitutes a national emergency.

Conclusion

This chapter has explored the evolving debates on intellectual property enforcement in the EU and its implications for developing countries. The core message of this chapter is that the shipping of medicine through European ports and airports, an ordinary trade procedure, became a problem of global health governance that is far from being resolved.

The EU supports the belief that counterfeit pharmaceutical products could hinder public health, particularly with the increasing illegal trade of substandard life saving drugs, such as medicines that treat chronic disease. On the other hand, a coalition of developing countries and NGOs has accused the EU of promoting stringent IP enforcement rules that confuse trade rules (violation of trade marks) with public health concerns (substandard products). This chapter did not intend to solve this disagreement. The intention was to highlight the recent dilemma in regulating pharmaceutical products: although there is a rising concern with intellectual property enforcement, less has been agreed on how to develop enforcement mechanisms that ensure public health interests.

Looking ahead, two key issues should be considered in the IP enforcement debate. First, pharmaceutical firms have had greater participation in the EU policymaking process of IP than other civil society members. The EU regulatory policy should respond more effectively to the preferences of non-governmental organizations and patient advocacy groups. The voice of these groups should be introduced carefully into the initiatives to enforce intellectual property. Not all groups have had the same capacity to participate in the decision-making process. Future studies should investigate why they have not been full participants, and the extent to which imbalanced participation promotes social/policy inequalities.

Second, modern pharmaceutical regulation has included not just multiple stakeholders but also many jurisdictions. As this chapter has demonstrated, there is an overbearing presence of a number of agencies and departments promoting IP enforcement, which provides a substantial challenge for regulators and the potential for fragmentation. International agencies with less traditional input in IP debates (such as the World Customs Organization) have taken leading roles while other institutions with a clear stake in this policy have been less vocal. For instance, the DG Sanco—whose mandate is to promote equitable access to health care services to patients and consumers across Europe—is yet to express its position in this debate. A more strategic approach to pluralism in IP regulation would promote effective collaborations geared to health improvement, avoiding arbitrary partnerships.

An estimated two billion people lack regular access to essential medicines globally (World Health Organization 2004). Pharmaceutical regulations (whether intellectual property or health surveillance) can have sweeping effects on public health, as they can limit or foster the supply of affordable drugs. Poorly regulated products can also lead to abortions, malformation or even death. Therefore, understanding the factors influencing the formulation and development of intellectual property can help EU policymakers make balanced and informed decisions on how to regulate and enforce these rules without hindering access to medicines.

Notes

1 UNTAID is an international procurement facility responsible for the purchase of drugs against HIV/AIDS, malaria and tuberculosis and distribution to less-developed countries (www.unitaid.eu, accessed September 11, 2012).

2 The IMPACT document did not refer to the WHO Guidelines for the Development of Measures to Combat Counterfeit Drugs, as elaborated in 1999 and a core guide for member states. Whilst the WHO Guidelines suggest that the high price of medicines contributes to the proliferation of counterfeits, the IMPACT document did not refer to drug prices but rather suggested that inadequate regulation/enforcement contributes to counterfeiting.

3 This division between rational and constructed preferences was simplified here for clarity. These are routed in philosophical discussions of human rationality (cf. Elster 1983) and some authors suggest that they are complementary approaches (cf. Katznelson and Weingast 2005).

Part III

The EU and population health

10 Catch me if you can

Communicable disease control

Scott L. Greer[1]

Communicable disease control has been a concern of states for as long as there have been states. Control of epidemic diseases, including legendary killers such as cholera, plague, and tuberculosis, is a coercive and expensive public good that can never be private and whose absence cannot be compensated by even the richest person's housing or flight.

Precisely because it has long been a concern of the state, communicable disease control is deeply entrenched. In fact, is it done so well that it is almost invisible to the outside observer, buried in primary care, or local government, or little-known agencies. While ignoring communicable disease control might not be so hard in the age of childhood vaccines and antibiotics, the option of ignorance is a luxury paid by generations of bureaucratic, legal and political investment.

But as viruses voyage and bacteria cross borders, there is increasing attention to communicable disease control as outbreaks of major infectious diseases seem to become more frequent while new security concerns, and new actors based in security rather than health organizations, reshape older structures (Fidler and Gostin 2008; Weir and Mykhalovskiy 2009). If there is any theme to European integration, it is increased border crossing and the breaking down of state borders and consequent reasons for integration in public health (Greer and Mätzke 2009). In public health, as a long-established part of the state, we see the development of new EU powers—European integration—and an effect on how communicable disease control works in Europe—Europeanization (Greer 2012c). European integration in communicable disease control means the development of new EU powers and actions including funding technical networks, engaging in research, and creating a new agency, the European Centre for Disease Prevention and Control. With each public health crisis, the increasingly well-organized and Commission-funded networks of European experts have an opportunity to suggest that member states might deepen integration. Europeanization, meanwhile, is always harder to study but shows in the empowerment of networks and experts who advocate for adherence to, or promotion of, "European" practices in field epidemiology, disease reporting, prevention campaigns or the other administrative and intellectual tasks of communicable disease control.

Integration through crisis and advocacy, and Europeanization through networks and low-profile agencies, is perhaps the most common kind of European Union politics today. This makes it a case study for a kind of Europeanization, and European integration, too often forgotten in the focus on high-level politics and the history of integration: *neofunctional political integration* (Greer 2006b).

Communicable disease politics matter for public health as well as for European integration. Vaccination demands an effort every day, across public bureaucracies and doctors' offices, as well as a constant plebiscite among the citizens who might not accept it. Enough citizens refuse them to worry the epidemiologists of the European Centre for Disease Control and Prevention's Annual Epidemiological Reports. Antibiotics, the other half of the health care system's contribution to the control of infectious diseases, give us cause to worry: the number of infections that resist antibiotic treatment, combined with practices in medicine and agriculture that increase antibiotic resistance, threaten us with a future in which antibiotics are less able to compensate for problems in prevention and infection control.

Communicable disease control policy in the EU

Communicable disease control is the identification and management of infectious diseases in the population. It comprises a variety of activities, whose form and substance takes remarkably different forms in different countries. These practices are described here non-technically, since every sentence in the next paragraph has enough content to sustain several entire disciplines.

One is identification of the disease. This involves surveillance, monitoring populations in various ways in order to identify the burden of disease and changes such as new outbreaks, and laboratory work to identify new agents (public health language is often unreconstructedly Benthamite). A second is management of an outbreak: the detective work to identify the source of infection, measures to control spread (such as destroying dangerous food or quarantining people with infections), and sometimes health care initiatives. A third is prevention: notably, vaccination, education, regulatory initiatives such as food safety controls, and special measures for concentrated vulnerable populations such as children and prisoners. Ranging from microbiological investigation to school nursing and what passes for health inspection at borders, prevention shares the frustrating characteristic of much public health: it can seem to encompass the world.

The conceptual challenges of communicable disease control

Making sense of this complex world is difficult, for policymakers even more than for the scholars who can cheerfully annex or ignore adjacent policy fields to suit their definitions. Even by the standards of health politics and policy, communicable disease control is complex; and by the standards of health politics or any other field, it is underserved by the social sciences literature. Assumptions about communicable disease control have a way of vanishing when subjected to comparative inquiry: it is not always clear what concepts or words mean in different systems, ways of addressing problems are very different, the borders of the policy field are not agreed, and in some countries vital functions do not seem to be carried out at all.

Part of the reason is that communicable disease control involves a great deal of fragmentation and intersectoral coordination. It is a field filled with different actors who have different definitions, interests, and priorities. The coordination, or conflict management, or knowledge management, required to prevent and manage disease is impressive. As argued by Greer and Mätzke (2012) it demands:

- Interprofessional relations. For most of the last century, there has been a significant divergence, and sometimes hostile relationship, between professionals of public health and the medical profession (Fox 2003, 2012). The different outlooks and interests are easy to catalogue or caricature: doctors seek autonomy from the state and public health professionals seek to use it; doctors focus on determinate analyses of single patients, and public health focuses on probabilistic analyses of populations; doctors organize themselves professionally while public health, even where it involves doctors, tends to be a bureaucracy; and doctors of course tend to prize curative work and individual-level prevention, while public health scholars have a tradition of disparaging the contribution of health care to health. Doctors, with their control of vaccines, diagnoses, antibiotics, and prestige, are crucial to the operation of public health systems for which they might have little sympathy. Other professions such as nursing and social work have their own points of disagreement, and even less formed professions such as ambulance crews and "emergency management" have outlooks that can clash with public health approaches (Botoseneanu *et al.* 2011).
- Interorganizational relations. Part of the reason it is so hard to define public health—as attested by the endless boundary-defining conversations that mark the field—is that much of its work is done by others. The border with the health care system is permeable and contested in any system. So are borders with animal health (Grant 2012; Knab 2011) and security (Fidler and Gostin 2008; de Ruijter 2012). Beyond that, many of the most important contributors to public health, once established in the name of communicable disease control or social hygiene, have turned into other fields of work. This includes water and sewage treatment and restaurant inspection, but also much of the work done by other professions such as social work or educationalists. In times of crisis, yet more organizations appear, such as ambulance crews, police and armed forces, as well as specialist coordinators and crisis managers from the top of government. This creates enormous scope for misunderstanding, inconvenience, and coordination failure. And when disputes arise, it is never a good idea to assume that the public health officials will prevail.
- Intergovernmental relations. In addition to dispersing communicable disease control across multiple professions and organizations, it is also dispersed across governments. Environmental health, vaccination, clinics for the most marginal populations, and social work are all likely to be local functions, while public health finance, resources and power are often distributed across

central and regional governments (Adolph *et al.* 2012). As a rule, any significant policy in a state with multiple tiers of government requires intergovernmental interaction and collaboration, and that is the case for communicable disease control.

- International relations. Finally, it is with good reason that public health has been one of the oldest areas of international organization (Liverani and Coker 2012; Zacher and Keefe 2008). The World Health Organization is the center of the world of global health governance, though its weaknesses are many and much documented. It is also surrounded by a *nébuleuse* of partnerships, organizations, charities and governmental activity that scarcely adds up to governance, and the ensemble is prone to turf wars that divert energy. The case of the European Union poses two obvious questions: what role does the EU play vis-à-vis the WHO (since they are obvious competitors in the field of communicable disease control and health systems advice), and what impact does their contentiousness have on the member states' own interactions with the WHO? The answers are not clear (Van Schaik 2011; Guigner 2006, and this volume).

These dynamic, often dramatic, assemblies of actors and states, with vague borders and insuperably complex intellectual and practical communication problems, ricochet between crisis and collective action. There is a permanent collective action problem in public health (Barnett and Sorenson 2011). At each level of coordination, there is incentive for somebody to skimp on key activities, whether it is member states that refuse to core-fund the WHO or individual doctors who do not bother to report cases of this or that disease. The result is stability, and sometimes degeneration, punctuated by crises that inspire reforms of some sort. Crises hit asymmetrically, and the politics and policy debates of different political systems react differently, with the result that any given system's history tends to be one of punctuated equilibrium, but systems show little tendency to converge.

European communicable disease control: A picture of diversity

Different countries handle the conflicts and coordination problems of communicable disease control very differently. This presents the distinctive characteristic of its management in the European Union: its diversity. The best studies of the organization of communicable disease control in Europe over two centuries have found that historical trajectories dominate: countries failed to live up to reputations for authoritarianism, technical expertise, decency or libertarianism, but did reliably repeat with HIV whatever approach they had adopted with cholera a century earlier (Baldwin 2005a,b) In general, the best-studied topic, HIV/AIDS, also demonstrates the differences between national trajectories (Steffen 2000; Berridge 1996; Fox and Fee 1988; Kirp and Bayer 1992).

Given this tradition, we should not be surprised that a large-scale study of public health capacity (Brant *et al.* forthcoming) found not just wide variation, but a complete lack of the patterns social scientists usually expect to see in Europe. Likewise, a study of surveillance found essentially no agreement across countries on the diseases that are tracked and reported or obvious patterns (Reintjes 2012). Even the broadest patterns—in allocation of legal authority, for example—are restricted to variation between Northern, Southern, and Eastern Europe (aka the beer, wine and vodka countries that Cisneros Örnberg mentions in Chapter 12— which seem to be doing better as correlates of organization than of alcohol) (Elliott *et al*. 2012). Such variation seems to make a mockery of proposals for good practice. And indeed, benchmarking against WHO or other public health guidelines tends to find most EU systems sadly wanting (MacLehose *et al*. 2001; Reintjes *et al*. 2007; Mounier-Jack and Coker 2006). These comparative studies show that is untenable to assume that concepts have stable meanings across borders, that functions are all recognized and organized, or even that anybody is formally responsible for carrying out an activity that others might regard as important. They also show that any kind of EU harmonizing, Europeanizing effect will have to overcome a great deal of persistent and largely unexplained diversity.

European Union competencies

European Union public health competencies, narrowly defined, are weak, but its overall "warrants" to act on public health grounds are strong.[2] In the consolidated Treaty incorporating Lisbon, Article 6 gives it a competency for the "protection and improvement of human health." The whole of Title 14 is dedicated to public health—an enormous increase in the importance of a policy field that only entered the EU treaties in 1992.[3] Much of the Title is about patient mobility or involves repeating that member states want to retain control of health care services. But Article 5 is about communicable disease control (and public health promotion), stating:

> The European Parliament and the Council, acting in accordance with the ordinary legislative procedure and after consulting the Economic and Social Committee and the Committee of the Regions, may also adopt *incentive measures* designed to protect and improve human health and in particular to combat the major cross-border health scourges, measures concerning monitoring, early warning of and combating serious cross-border threats to health, and measures which have as their *direct objective* the protection of public health regarding tobacco and the abuse of alcohol, *excluding any harmonisation of the laws and regulations of the Member States*.

Note the prose, especially the (author's added) italics stressing that the EU shall not have executive powers or the ability to force harmonization. This is a limited article.

On the other hand, the basic logic of spillover holds, and means that there is more to EU communicable disease control impact and activity than Article 5 of Title 14. Food safety and animal health, for example, are areas where the

EU's important role fed directly into regulation: once there was a cross-border market in food and animals, it was no surprise that the vCJD ("mad cow") crisis gave scope to create an EU competency in those areas (Grant 2012) as well as in blood and blood products (Farrell 2005). The creation of an EU role and competency in communicable disease control is part of a recent story, discussed in the next section.

European integration in communicable disease control

European Union initiatives emerged as a sequence characteristic of European integration. The secular trend was toward a greater EU role. The punctuations were crises that put communicable disease control on the EU agenda and creating opportunities for entrepreneurs and politicians to make a mark. The actors were the familiar ones of punctuated equilibrium arguments in public policy studies: policy advocates such as the Commission and expert networks, with ideas, and politicians, who had a sudden need for actions when a crisis erupted. The story of European integration intertwines the construction of these networks and the periodic adoption of their suggestions in response to crises. In each case the real policy action happened below the level of the developing EU treaties.

The first step was research: EU-funded investigations of shared problems starting in the 1980s. EU research budgets often lead the expansion of EU competencies. Research funding produces European networks that can lobby for both substantive goals and also for more European funding and action. If people are brought together to study a problem on a Europe-wide level, it stands to reason that they will suggest some Europe-wide actions that the EU might support, and indeed they often do. Even if EU-level change is not induced, the work produced can sensitize governments to European comparisons and European dimensions. So, for example, the earliest program in the EU on cancer research promoted a Europeanization of cancer leadership, lobby for the program's preservation, and real policy changes in some countries (see the chapters by Briatte and Elliott in this book) (Trubek 2007; Trubek *et al.* 2008a). In HIV/AIDS policy, the effect was less reported but very real: the need to provide comparable data for European projects, for example, forced the French to count HIV-positive homeless people— and discover a group that had been invisible to policymakers (Steffen 2012). The low cost, and low profile, of disease programs was an advantage. Low costs allowed actors within states, be they Francois Mitterrand and Bettino Craxi (with cancer research) or ministry officials trying to give their minister a useful agenda on a visit to Brussels, to act and possibly gain credit without incurring much cost. While the EU is not, on the whole, a flexible and responsive political system, it offered officials and ministers opportunities that did not always exist at the right time domestically.

The first and most important research programs were established, though invisible to almost all but experts in the relevant policy areas, by 1992 when the Maastricht Treaty added formal public health powers. These powers were in small part a reflection of the desire to follow up the internal market and the hard-money approach to monetary integration with something of a "social" Europe. They were in large part a response to the vCJD ("mad cow") disease in the UK, which damaged faith in Europe's food supplies, led to temporary import bans that violated the spirit of the internal market, and made it abundantly clear that markets had outrun their regulators. This led negotiators to create a somewhat strange set of competencies over blood and blood products tied to a broader but weak public health power.

That power helped legitimate the ongoing development of functional cooperation, which was starting to take its next step. The second step, in the 1990s, was longer-lasting networks to promote the collection and dissemination of comparable data. The everyday logic is simple: if something is worth doing, then there is no case for doing it as short-term research projects or ad hoc network funding. These networks (Dedicated Surveillance Networks) were created by a 1998 Decision (2119/98/EU) and focused on tracking 17 diseases, investing in epidemiology and surveillance capacity as well as disseminating information and some amount of expertise on handling outbreaks (Lenglet and Hernandez Pezzi 2006). Regional networks also began to emerge: first EPINORTH, which shares information across the Baltic area and as far southeast as Ukraine, and then EPISOUTH for the Mediterranean (there is now talk of an EPIEAST for Russia, a major reservoir of diseases and diplomatic troubles). EPIET, the European Programme for Epidemiology Intervention Training, started in 1995 and focuses on training field epidemiologists.

The third step was an agency: the ECDC, European Centre for Disease Control and Prevention (Greer 2012a).[4] Once again, the everyday logic is clear. If something is still worth doing, then why do it through time-limited networks mixing universities and government organizations, with senior staff working part-time and often focusing on the next bid, and secretariats spread out all over Europe? It starts to make sense to consolidate long-running programs into an agency. In addition to the administrative simplicity of consolidating networks into a single organization with a permanent staff, there are specific advantages in a field prone to emergencies such as communicable disease control. The advantages are those that always come with a decision to make rather than buy; expert staff working for an EU agency can do more, and be more readily available, than outsiders contracted for certain deliverables. This is helpful because emerging infectious diseases, like any crisis, have a way of demanding flexibility and capacity that can be redirected.

EU agencies are an established and increasingly numerous type of organization, with a body of law to shape them (see Rittberger and Wonka 2012). Since their invention, they have become a standard part of European intervention in many fields. Their growth mimics the growth of the agency form in most states, something of a legacy of New Public Management and a form that can depoliticize and strengthen certain activities by setting up a new staff somewhat freer from the constraints of government departments (Pollitt *et al.* 2001; Talbot 2004). In the EU, they also have an advantage familiar to students of US politics: because they are not part of the Commission and have specific accountability and boards, member states trust them more than the Commission. This means that member states will support an agency when they would be reluctant to entrust a power to the Commission—and the Commission and Parliament will propose an agency when they know there is support for the action but not for an expansion of Commission powers (Pollack 2003).

EU agencies' power is limited (Hervey 2012); EU law and Court jurisprudence is quite clear that they cannot have what amount to lawmaking powers. In most cases, what they do is set the standards that EU law makes binding, such as standards for airplane parts or the handling of blood products. In some more powerful cases such as pharmaceuticals (Hauray 2006; Sabel and Zeitlin 2007), EU agencies form the hub of regulatory networks that mix their work with that of member state-level agencies.

The ECDC is not one of the more powerful kinds of EU agency; it is an "observatory" that collects and disseminates information and good practice (Yataganas 2001). There are two functional reasons for this organization type that played out in its creation. First, there is the extent of diversity within the continent; and second, there was nothing like the critical mass of competition regulators or pharmaceutical market access agencies that could be generalized and networked (though they might emerge as a consequence of the initiatives in this chapter, and book). Communicable disease control agencies in the EU are still relatively rare, concentrated around the North Sea, spreading slowly if at all and quite variable in their powers and resources (Elliott *et al.* 2012). The process of creating competition regulators, for example, took decades and big changes in the economics and politics of the EU and key member states (Thatcher 2007; Kelemen 2011); if there is any similar trend in communicable disease control it is weaker and enjoys backing from less powerful interests. In other words, it is harder to Europeanize, or even formulate actions, for such a diverse set of organizations. Member states whose officials want to show off might have interests that coincide with member states whose officials want help, but member states who want to solve domestic problems through EU action (as is often the case with France in public health) meet reticence from member states more concerned about sovereignty (as with the UK and Germany much of the time).

The creation of the ECDC did not involve disputes about the basic idea of an EU agency; that was largely agreed by member states in the wake of academic debates that had suggested its possibility and desirability, and in the aftermath of the SARS crisis some action seemed necessary. The debate was therefore focused on the scope of its duties and its autonomy. There was a broad member state consensus on the idea of a role in risk assessment for an EU agency. France, which embraced public health as a consequence of its sequence of public health disasters including a heat wave in Paris that reflected badly on French society as well as the French state, was the most influential state pushing for a role in risk management. The rest of Europe focused on a more practical issue, namely the scope of the agency: would it deal with emergencies, or ongoing surveillance and capacity, or the identification of future threats? In shorthand, would it be a Center for Disease Control, or for Disease Control *and Prevention*? The result was a Center with a name and some warrants to act widely ("Prevention"), but with a focus on infectious diseases. We can interpret this outcome as the most that advocates of an EU role in health could extract from the political juncture. The inclusion of the word prevention meant that the new agency would have a broad field of action, with permission to engage in a wide variety of public health issues. Its original justification, communicable disease control, was narrower than its warrants, for general public health.

The European Parliament, which typically tries to expand the powers of EU agencies to affect citizens, chose a very savvy rapporteur (John Bowis) who channeled pressure for a bigger ECDC role into language he expected would pass the Council. The resulting Regulation (851/2004) passed on the first reading (a sign of consensus and coordination between the three EU institutions).

The scope of ECDC autonomy was the second topic for the EU policymakers to address. Crafting the board of any agency is an important way to steer it. The ECDC board represents all member states, in a configuration that seems to be regarded as too large to control it. As a result, the executive staff of the ECDC has gained autonomy. The limited scope of ECDC and its small budget meant that member states and the European Parliament were comfortable with a board that represented them all but would be relatively difficult to use to steer the agency.

ECDC's budget is indeed small. Its staff hovers around 150–200. It is not comparable to the vast US Centers for Disease Control and Prevention (CDC), or even the bigger communicable disease units in the member states. The size differential can be attributed to the fact that the role of other disease control agencies includes risk management, much prevention, and a broader range of risk assessment; ECDC's job, at least at present, is to network. Its premise is the same as a lot of other EU policy, namely that influence comes from expanding networks into new parts of Europe, empowering networks by entrusting them with the job of setting European standards, and deepening them with resources and increased prestige and expertise.

The ECDC had the good, or bad, fortune to start its work in the midst of the 2005 H5N1 (avian) influenza crisis and almost immediately proceeded to the 2009 H1N1 (swine) influenza crisis. In addition to slowly folding in the various programs—EPIET, Dedicated Surveillance Networks, overall reporting, the publication Eurosurveillance—hiring staff and coping with Swedish labor regulators at its Stockholm base, it also had to become a credible voice in difficult situations where it was often overshadowed by member state agencies and caught in tensions between and within member states about the distribution of vaccines and antiviral medicines, over which it had no power. Other programs cover the imaginable range, such as annual conferences on epidemiology and vaccines.

Its success is still in the balance. Success as a government agency comes from political diversity and institutional uniqueness (Carpenter 2001). Political diversity means having a wide range of supporters and not being regarded as a tool of a particular interest. ECDC was born with diversity—not much legislation passes on the first reading, which means many diverse actors supported it. In the ECDC's case establishing lasting diversity would mean appealing to experts, member states, the major public health actors in the member states, the Commission, the European Parliament and others. An evaluation early in its career suggested that its future was still in the balance (Oortwijn *et al.* 2008). Anecdotally, it seems that it has not reconciled an imperative to make itself a hub of thriving networks with a politically driven tendency to turn inward. The surveillance networks that it has assimilated, and joint work such as the Euroflu project with the WHO European region, however, are signs of its implantation at the center of major networks that can strengthen its credibility. The risk is that if ECDC becomes too introverted, defensive, or political, it will end up being a drag on these networks rather than a driver.

Institutional uniqueness means that the agency does something nobody else does. In the ECDC's case that means becoming the hub of key networks and establishing a reputation for expertise that neither member states nor the WHO can match. The division of labor between member states and the ECDC is in principle clear: the ECDC can act as a clearinghouse for information, and a mechanism to transfer expertise from the more- to the less-sophisticated systems. The price of failure is that it gets taken less seriously and becomes less able to resist budget cuts or get its views heard in debates.

The obvious rival for institutional uniqueness is the WHO (Guigner 2006, 2009). "The" WHO, in Geneva, is the central worldwide hub for communicable disease control, but is also a severely flawed organization. Its highly autonomous 53-country European region, WHO EURO in Copenhagen, is on paper something less of a rival to ECDC because it is less focused on communicable disease control, though there have been multiple—implausible—suggestions that ECDC subsume it. The political solution has been for a former ECDC director, Szusanna Jakab, to become the Regional Director of the WHO European Region. This move paved the way to a good division of labor that allows both organizations to enhance their reputational uniqueness in the short term. The longer-term relationship will depend on the extent to which the WHO, the ECDC, somebody else or nobody else provides unique and broadly credible information and networks. There is some movement towards a stable division of labor (especially in influenza, the best example of a good relationship and one that no credible agency could ignore in 2009–10). The worst-case scenario would be that the WHO, the WHO European region, and the ECDC never attain a clear division of labor and succumb to the infantilism that afflicts global health governance (Muraskin 1998 presents a superb example).

It is worth noting the salient differences between the ECDC and the WHO. First, the WHO is a long-established international organization and the ECDC is an executive agency accountable only to the EU and its member states. This means it avoids the drag that some regimes exercise within the WHO at the global or the European level and the pressure to "mission creep" that affects the WHO. The consensus in the EU is that the ECDC exists to conduct risk assessment and perhaps communication, and develop epidemiological and public health expertise.

Political tensions derive from arguments about its performance, and extension into risk management and non-communicable diseases. The debates surrounding the ECDC are exemplary of the kinds of discussion that surround any executive agency in any well-functioning political system, which gives ECDC a much clearer remit than the WHO has ever had, in a cleaner and more densely institutionalized environment. Second, because it is an EU agency rather than an international organization, the ECDC is more autonomous than the WHO; ECDC has a stable legal framework and a governance structure that frees its leadership to develop the organization as they see fit without spending so much time managing relations with member states. It also has a stable financing mechanism, something the WHO as a whole lacks. Finally, the ECDC is newer, which means the reasons for its creation are both recent and malleable. This means that the ECDC, if it plays its cards well, can continue to gain reputational uniqueness and political multiplicity by using its autonomy and resources to work out what it does and do it well.

Effects: Europeanization in communicable disease control

There are both methodological and policy problems with assessing the impact of EU policy, or the degree of Europeanization of communicable disease control. The policy problem is that it is still too soon for there to be a significant (measurable) impact on communicable disease control in the member states. The ECDC is still a young organization, whether judged in terms of experience and the number of tests to the system or young in terms of years. The ECDC has only been operating since 2005, after all (and was set up amidst an influenza crisis). It would be a bit early to expect any of its work to influence Europe's epidemiological profile.

What is visible, even at this early stage, is the extent of the Europeanization of communicable disease control policy; that is, the extent to which policy and practice in the member states has changed as a result of the European Union intervention. This is an area with methodological difficulties. In general, Europeanization means some level of harmonization—if not convergence on "one best way," at least convergence on some organizational forms, behaviors, and standards that EU legislation and perhaps associated networks propagate. In an area where the null hypothesis is historically persistent and largely patternless variation, it is unlikely that there will be the wholesale transformation that would be necessary to produce a "European model" of communicable disease control, or even convergence on a putative best practice.

To what extent, then can we identify Europeanization—the effect of the EU on organization, behavior, and standards in communicable disease control? Given that there can be no harmonizing legislation under the Treaties, the effects of the EU will come through the deployment of "softer" tools: networks, data, grants, and the activity of the ECDC above and beyond them. These mechanisms are substantially the same ones covered in other chapters of this book; they are at work with disease networks in the Chapter 4 by Briatte, with comparative health data in the Chapter 3 by Elliott, and with the consensus-building exercises discussed, for example, by Kurzer in Chapter 11.

The more concrete list of activities that ECDC and EU officials will share, and publish in annual reports, works on a technical level: better-trained field epidemiologists thanks to EPIET, better surveillance and networks for surveillance in the Baltic and Mediterranean thanks to EPI-North and EPI-South, some harmonization of surveillance thanks to the DSNs, and whatever gains come from bringing officials and experts together in various EU-centric networks or some convergence of messaging during the H1N1 influenza crisis of 2009. *Eurosurveillance* deserves special notice for its transmission of field epidemiology and new findings on topics of interest to officials across Europe. TESSy ("The European Surveillance System") is a developing surveillance system that exchanges available, albeit imperfect information from the different member states. These epidemiology and surveillance activities are actually the appropriate kinds of outcomes to expect and evaluate. The bigger question, of course, is whether the newly empowered, trained, extended and Europeanized networks shape their member states' behavior and improve public health.

Against these technical successes, there are two obvious failures to remember. One is the nationalism and state autonomy recently furnished by Germany that unnecessarily heightened the politicization of communicable disease control. Germany wrongly blamed an *E. coli* outbreak on Spanish rather than its own foodstuffs in 2011, provoking Spanish outrage, lost sales, and a renewed appreciation of German power among Europeans who scarcely needed such reminders. The other is the multi-stage fiasco of 2009 H1N1 influenza: first, Europe's governments reinforced inequalities when richer governments (even within countries, as in Germany) placed vaccine and medicines orders while others could not; then came localized policy failures if the primary care system resisted public health instructions; then governments looked foolish when the epidemic did not impress the public and much vaccine and antiviral medicine went unused; and finally public health policymakers were accused by a Council of Europe report of being alarmist and under the influence of drug companies (Flynn 2010). The ECDC, working frantically on the same diseases, has been a bystander to most of these episodes. That is by design (and it is hard to see how the ECDC's authority would gain from being implicated in them!). In both episodes, real political power lodged in states mattered more than bureaucratic networks or technical understanding; the European influence was in data and the construction of networks that could, if not harmonize, at least communicate decisions.[5]

Conclusion: Structure, process and outcome

The European Union might be going through a difficult period in its history, and the integrative elan of the Commission is not what it was in the 1980s and 1990s, but the politics of communicable disease control in Europe are being driven by longstanding asymmetries and the very local politics of the little-known organizations involved: ECDC, WHO, and the various member state communicable disease organizations. The "low politics" of networks coincide with the occasional crisis to move communicable disease forward; when politicians in a crisis need a solution, there is more and more of a "European" communicable disease control, and public health community, with advocates who can offer a suggestion.

Health policy analysts often use Avedis Donabedian's conceptual framework of structure, process, and outcome (Wyszewianski 2009). Structure is the allocation of resources and legal authority; process is what is taking place; and outcome is something desirable and ideally measurable. Structurally, the EU's activity is small: networks, research, training, and data collection, consolidated into the ECDC where they can sustain a permanent staff capable of being deployed when new challenges arise. The Treaty base might be rather grand compared to its pre-Maastricht non-existence, but it is still limited. The ECDC's staff remains about 2 percent of the staff of the US CDC.[6]

The process is where the activity, and the Europeanization, is taking place now. Networks, grants and data are at their most visible in the ECDC. The ECDC is the EU's biggest bet on communicable disease control, and by far the most visible; EPIET or disease surveillance might be important and might be slowly rewiring public health in member states, but the ECDC has the profile and centralizes the EU programs. This is the clearest effect, what Guigner calls "cognitive Europeanization" (Guigner 2007). We can watch the ECDC, now incorporating much of what the EU does on an ongoing basis, changing the frames of reference and horizons of European epidemiologists, microbiologists, and officials.

As for outcomes, it is easy to be cynical because it is always easy to be cynical about low politics, because the politically nervous new agency does not always do itself favors in public, and because of the newness of key policies and the mismatch between the EU efforts and the weight of the health care, local government, and public health establishments of the member states, or between the technocracy of the EU and the vicious, expensive, politics of vaccination and antiviral drugs. The evidence of effectiveness can seem like a list of anecdotes.

That is a downbeat note to end on, but it captures the tension in communicable disease control and so much else about European Union politics. "Low politics" European integration such as the work of the ECDC has its effects on the level of the technical experts it involves. There is a very large gap between low politics and high politics; it would take a lot of Europeanization and European integration to lead Germany to pool vaccines with Romania or take Spanish agricultural interests as seriously as its own domestic food scare. Consider what it takes to change the animal quarantine policies of the insular UK. The tension is inescapable, and just as visible when we compare the networks of fiscal and monetary policymakers with the coordination failures of their heads of state in the financial crisis, or the damage done to NATO by the Iraq and Libyan wars, or even the tension between technical networks and ministerial power within states (Geuijen *et al.* 2008; Peters *et al.* 2000). It leads us to the paradox of the European Union today: so integrated by the standards of low politics, so much less integrated at the level of the state and prone to fracture under stress.[7] That is not just a problem of communicable disease control.

Notes

1 I would like to thank Sébastien Guigner for comments and Margitta Maetzke for very helpful conversations about the topic; this chapter is nevertheless my own responsibility.
2 "Warrants," political justifications to act, is a term from Orren and Skowronek (2004).
3 These powers are in addition to two older kinds of discussion of health in the Treaties: the oldest usage, still current in trade law everywhere, in which public health is grounds to make an exception to free trade, and a post-1992 usage in which the Commission and EU legislators are repeatedly urged to have regards to public health when making policy. For the former, see Chapter 8 by Holly Jarman.
4 There is an entirely parochial tendency in public health debates to refer to these agencies as "institutes." Both political science and EU law make it clear: they are agencies. There is no gain to inventing a new category specific to public health publications.
5 For H1N1 as a case study of the development of the EU's health security architecture, see the excellent de Ruijter (2012).
6 Something ECDC officials do not always note when proclaiming their organization's humility relative to the American approach. If CDC had 300 staff and were dependent on state governments for almost everything it did, it might behave differently as well.
7 And therefore so rich in data for both constructivist analyses of European integration and realist analyses of European disintegration.

11 Non-communicable diseases

The EU declares war on "fat"

Paulette Kurzer

For many years, European officials, medical scientists, and nutritionists thought that obesity was a problem on the other side of the Atlantic. By 2005, however, it appeared that a higher percentage of men were obese or overweight in Cyprus, the Czech Republic, Finland, Germany, Greece, Malta and Slovakia than the estimated 67 percent of men in the United States (IOTF 2005). While this discovery may have prompted the European Union (EU) to improve nutrition, enhance consumer information, and strengthen food quality, European institutions have in fact a long tradition of regulating nutrition and food products.

EU officials made their first attempt to regulate nutrition in the 1970s when the principal focus was to ensure the free movement of agricultural items. In the late 1970s, the European Commission adopted legislation to govern food labels (Food Labelling Directive (79/112/EEC)), which was expanded in 1990 with the enactment of the Nutrition Labelling Directive (90/496/EEC).

After 2000, the EU adopted new regulations to guarantee food safety in the wake of the mad cow disease and other food scares (*Salmonella* in eggs and pork, dioxin-contaminated foods, *Campylobacter* in fresh poultry, *E. coli* 0157:H7 in beef, and foot and mouth disease). The outbreak of *Bovine spongiform encephalopathy* (mad cow disease) is commonly regarded as the "trigger" for the wave of new pan-European food safety and nutrition legislation and for establishing new regulatory institutions across Europe, including the European Food Safety Authority (EFSA) (Bernauer and Caduff 2006; Marsden *et al.* 2010; Skogstad 2006). Nevertheless, the *Food Safety Regulation* (EC/178/2002) does not directly address the nutritional composition of food items. Attention to the relationship between nutrition, diet, and health landed on the agenda of the Directorate-General for Health and Consumer Protection (DG Sanco) through a different route in spite of the fact that EU institutions have been engaged in regulating food production, distribution, and marketing since the 1970s.

From the late 1990s, a steady stream of reports and publications called attention to the phenomenon of the rising weight of men, women, and children due to bad eating habits and poor lifestyle choices. Gradually, the Commission responded by proposing different legislative measures in order to improve the nutritional content of packaged food to ward off an obesity crisis, which threatens Europe's public health, its health systems, and even its economic prosperity. Because obesity is associated with higher risks of chronic illnesses, it also adds significantly to health care costs.

A quick glance at European-wide health statistics, published by the OECD, confirms that Europeans have become heavier (like Americans!). The 2010 OECD report shows that obesity, as measured by the Body Mass Index (BMI) of 30 or above, has more than doubled over the past 20 years in most countries and describes approximately 15.5 percent of the adult population in the EU. The member states with the highest proportion of overweight adults are UK, Ireland, Malta, Luxembourg, Lithuania, Hungary and Greece. Moreover, on average 24 percent of the children aged between 6–9 years are overweight or obese across Europe. The highest proportion of overweight children, age 11–15, are found in Malta, Greece, Portugal, Italy, and Spain where more than 17 percent of children have a weight that exceeds the normal BMI range (Lobstein *et al.* 2004; OECD 2010).

These trends date back to the 1980s. Thus the question is why, and how did the Commission and in particular DG Sanco become engaged in the question of obesity and healthy nutrition? Obesity is related to public health nutrition, which in turn is the application of nutrition (and physical activity) to the promotion of good health of a community (Hughes 2003). Obesity is primarily associated with diet and nutrition and refers to a person's relative body fat calculated from his or her height and weight. According to conventional medical wisdom, being overweight heightens the risk of type 2 diabetes, coronary heart disease and stroke, sleep apnea, osteoarthritis, gallbladder disease, and liver diseases, and other chronic conditions. Therefore, it would appear reasonable for the European Commission to enter into this field and push through bundles of legislation to improve healthy food choices, physical activity, and more balanced nutritional content of processed food.

However, it should be noted that multiple factors play a role in the worldwide trend toward obesity. On the surface, the issue seems straightforward: people gain weight when they consume more calories than they burn off. Yet, the causes of weight gain are multifactorial. One of the principal causes behind the rise of obesity is the overabundance of cheap processed foods, which tend to be rich in fat, sugars, and salt and which are heavily marketed by the food industry and allied companies. The technological innovations in the mass production and distribution of food lowered the overall price and the time spent preparing food. In turn, the oversupply of calorie-dense foods creates incentives to over-consume, especially since our daily environment is saturated with commercials, advertisements, and other marketing devices to convince people to consume more than they need.

On top of these structural factors, there are micro-behavioral ones. People are genetically predisposed to enjoy fatty textures and sugary flavors. Food companies exploit this innate craving of such foods to move more products off the retail shelves or restaurant menus (Brownell and Horgen 2004; Nestle 2002; Popkin *et al.* 2012). Fighting obesity is therefore a complex challenge that ultimately may require a radical overhaul of Europe's food production, distribution, and marketing system. There is not one solution. Rather, the "cure" lies in informational education, behavior modification, improved food choices, reformulation of proc-essed food, and expanded opportunities for physical activity. In sum, addressing obesity demands altering an environment that encourages people to over-consume low-cost yet energy-dense foods.

How did obesity get on the policy agenda on the EU? The emergence of obesity and diet/nutrition on the agenda of DG Sanco is largely due to the successful activities of pan-European and international NGOs (Greer 2009b; Lelieveldt and Princen 2011, pp. 215–18). The WHO-Europe office has promoted an anti-obesity action plan since the late 1990s and was instrumental in convincing the EU council (representing the political leaders of the member states) to endorse a new public health program for Europe, in which the war against fat occupied a prominent place. Because of the technical nature of biomedical consequences of nutrition and diet, political leaders and EU officials count on the staff at the WHO-Europe office to supply scientific analysis and policy recommendations (Princen 2007). Policy recommendations, supported by statistical analyses, appear in various reports and are submitted to the WHO's counterparts in the ministries of health in the European member states and officials in DG Sanco.

The WHO research reports are studded with data and analysis of health trends that come from the international biomedical community. Particularly important in supplying information is the International Obesity Task Force (IOTF), a global network of experts on obesity and related morbidity/mortality and the advocacy arm of the International Association for the Study of Obesity (Lang and Rayner 2005). The IOTF has served as a major impetus behind the "medicalization" (Sopal 1995) of obesity, by defining it as a medical problem that requires interven-tion and treatment. Coming from the WHO, the scientific, "medicalized" dis-course on obesity provided EU institutions with a credible rationale for engagement with obesity. Obesity itself is not a medical disease or a condition and requires an interpretive narrative that establishes an association between being overweight or fat and diverse health risks. The WHO and the international public health com-munity are perfectly situated to supply that narrative (Garde 2010; Kurzer and Cooper 2011). At the same time, the EU has a limited mandate to reshape life-styles and living environments. It must cooperate with national and local public authorities, NGOs, and the private sector. Even in the Commission, DG Sanco may encounter resistance for its anti-obesity campaign when its objectives contra-dict the policy mission of the more powerful DG Agriculture, which supports the current food production regime.

In December 2002, the EU Council of health and social ministers first adopted a position on obesity and it specifically referred to the request of the community of international public health experts to take action against obesity. A year later, the EU Council repeated its earlier declaration and called upon the Commission to elevate obesity as a major health threat to the future of EU (Council of the European Union 2003, 2004). In response, DG Sanco in 2004–2005 convened a series of meetings with member states, the WHO-Europe office and a small group of key NGOs and economic operators to explore the different aspects of the growing problem of overweightness and obesity in Europe. This "Obesity

Roundtable" established a general consensus on the main drivers of overweight and obesity; that is, the combination of increasing calorie intake and a more sedentary lifestyle. It also identified the need to take into account national, regional and local dietary differences. The approach which subsequently emerged from these early consultations heavily emphasized a need for a multi-stakeholder approach and for action levels, and the importance of including the private sector (Garde 2010).

The EU Council officially signed off on an anti-obesity action plan in June 2005 by issuing a statement, noting "with concern the rise in obesity prevalence rates . . . [the Council] recognises the potential which the promotion of healthy diets and physical activity has for reducing the risk for a number of diseases and conditions, such as obesity, hypertension, heart disease" (Council of the European Union 2005, p. 3). Soon thereafter, the Commission published its Green Paper (concept draft) *Promoting healthy diets and physical activity: A European dimension for the prevention of overweight, obesity and chronic diseases* (Commission of the European Union 2005). The Green Paper laid out the Commission's most comprehensive framing of the causes and consequences of obesity. In the same year, the Commission had also arranged to create the EU Platform for Action on Diet, Physical Activity, and Health. The aim was to contain or reverse the current trends by developing best practices and encouraging voluntary action on consumer information, labeling, advertising, marketing, food composition, education, and promotion of physical activity.

Two years later, with approval from the Council, the Green Paper turned into a White Paper, which contained a specific list of policy steps. The *White Paper on a Strategy for Europe on Nutrition, Overweight and Obesity related health issues* appeared on May 30, 2007 (Commission of the European Union 2007). It focused on policy responses to the issue of obesity based on the informational foundation laid by the Green Paper and ongoing consultation with stakeholders during the Green Paper process. The White Paper received widespread attention and provoked debate in the food industry, capitals of the member states, and other EU institutions.

The European Parliament initiated its own debate on the obesity report in September 2008, and passed a resolution, which called obesity and diet-related diseases "growing epidemics" and "major contributors to . . . mortality and morbidity in Europe" (European Parliament 2008, p. 2). Furthermore, the European Parliament called on member states to "recognise obesity as a chronic disease" (European Parliament 2008, p. 3). The resolution was accepted with an overwhelming majority of 536 yes votes to 37 no votes and encapsulated the growing sense of urgency to take immediate action against obesity.

In the meantime, the WHO-Europe issued the European Charter on Counteracting Obesity (2006) and developed the WHO European Action Plan for Food and Nutrition Policy 2007–2012 (World Health Organization 2008). WHO-Europe also continued to collect statistics on weight trends and published studies on diet-related diseases, all of which found their way into the official reports of the Commission and the resolution of the European Parliament.

In summary, there were a slew of activities after 2004, which culminated in both informal exchanges of information and concrete measures. Numerous reports and declarations were issued, backed up by the evidence gathered by the WHO, which in turn relied on a network of international public health scientists for documenting the health impact of obesity. Many of these scientists have their home base in the US or UK and are members of the International Association for the Study of Obesity (IASO), which produces studies and collects the biomedical evidence used in the WHO health reports. The IOTF is the advocacy arm of the IASO that aims "to articulate the policy directions needed for obesity prevention and inspire their translation into policy, research and practice." Accordingly, the IASO supplied "definitive evidence for the European Commission's Directorate-General for Health and Consumers" and convened meetings, which resulted in the *Charter on Obesity* in November 2006 that sets out for the first time a coherent approach to obesity management and prevention (Garde 2010; IASO 2009).

What has been accomplished?

In the last few years, the DG Sanco has created several "platforms" in which consumer NGOs, public authorities, and the private sector collaborate on public health issues. In 2005, the Platform on Diet, Physical Activity, and Health was formed to address the conundrum of unhealthy diets, lack of exercise and rising rates of obesity. The underlying logic of this public health platform is to bring together a wide array of stakeholders, urge them to make voluntary "commitments," monitor these commitments, and indirectly generate rules that will tackle obesity and diet (Jarman 2011a). In effect, the Commission hopes that the Platform will generate legislation-like outcomes without actually going through the legislative process while establishing norms and networks (Greer and Vanhercke 2009). The accumulation of commitments in the Platform enables the Commission to instigate action, despite the EU's limited powers in health and universal resistance to expanding them. For DG Sanco, in possession of limited tools, the Platform provides a vehicle for bringing together public and private interests to steer economic operators into the direction of recognizing that they play an important role in solving the obesity crisis.

To keep the Platform at a manageable size, members must be umbrella organizations operating at a European level. The other main criteria for membership is that each member must annually propose and commit to specific activities designed to halt and reverse the obesity trend. These commitments must be recorded, and outcomes monitored and measured in such a way that they can be reported to the Platform. In 2011, the Platform counted 33 stakeholders, and they varied from the International Sport and Culture Association (ISCA), the Standing Committee of European Doctors (CPME), and the World Federation of Advertisers (WFA) to Agricultural Organizations and Cooperatives (COPA-COGECA), the Association of Commercial Television (ACT), the European Confederation Sport and Health (CESS), and the Confederation of the Food and Drink Industries of the EU.[1] In short, the participants range from small NGOs, such as the Standing Committee of European Doctors, to very large private-sector industry lobby groups, such as the Confederation of Food and Drink (now FoodDrink Europe).

Members have to select from a list of categories when submitting a commitment to the Platform. In 2010, stakeholders submitted 136 commitments falling into five different categories of activities: Marketing and Advertising; Reformulation; Labeling; Lifestyles; and Others. These activities comprise a wide range of initiatives: reformulating food products, limiting advertising and marketing to children, designing workplace-based programs aimed at improving employees' health and diet, promoting physical activity, and disseminating awareness of the importance of good nutrition.[2]

All the commitments are voluntary. Most commitments come from industry and an example is "Not to market to children under 12 years in the internet sphere," proposed by FoodDrink Europe. Individual companies also submit commitments through the umbrella federation, FoodDrink Europe. *Danone* promised to assess the nutritional quality of *Danone* dairy, water, and baby nutrition products by the end of 2010. *Mars Inc.*, the candy manufacturer, pledged to develop training activities in the EU to expose its employees to its marketing code. *Carrefour*, the French supermarket chain, agreed to introduce new products with high nutritional value aimed at children. It also expanded its use of organic products and other high-quality ingredients.

NGOs also submit commitments, although this often involves pledging to undertake activities they would have undertaken anyway (Jarman 2011a). For example, the IOTF seeks to establish international standards for marketing food to children, which is the kind of activity it would have undertaken anyway.

Reviewing the list of commitments, the real question is of course whether all these activities amount to anything in particular, whether they address the crux of the obesity crisis, namely the imbalance between food consumption and energy expenditure?

On the one hand, the emergence of less coercive forms of regulation such as soliciting commitments through the EU Platform is a response to the complexity of the obesity issues, as well as the need to recognize the distinctive context of each member state. Considering the multi-dimensionality of the challenges of modern life, officials cope with a degree of uncertainty over how to frame regulatory goals. Therefore, the Commission prefers to work with less precise, non-binding arrangements since they involve lower transaction costs while co-opting powerful stakeholders. This method also facilitates coordination and cooperation when the option of hard regulation (binding laws) is not available due to the legal mandate of the treaties and the power of national jurisdiction. In this sense, the EU Platform on Diet is a deliberate choice in favor of modest progress in order to avoid a legislative stalemate.

However, the effectiveness of the EU Platform, reliant on soft policy instruments, can only succeed if member states, auditing firms, and the EU itself closely supervise the implementation of the stated commitments made by the participating actors (Hervey 2008; Kröger 2008). The European Commission does not possess enforcement capacity to guarantee that private actors keep their promises and comply with the spirit and letter of the stated commitment. It is assumed that industry will comply with its pledges because it may otherwise face the credible threat of direct intervention (Héritier and Lehmkuhl 2011).

However, the Commission has a hard time threatening to step in with real legislation because its legal remit is circumscribed. Moreover, from the beginning, in order to solicit the cooperation of the food business sector, DG Sanco agreed to monitor the execution of the commitment regardless of its actual impact on health. Commitments are not judged on whether they are effective in arresting the growth of the obesity epidemic. Therefore private stakeholders can promise to undertake many measures, none of which may fundamentally tackle the underlying structural determinants of obesity. Food companies can demonstrate their good faith by accepting corporate responsibility yet simultaneously escape any real curbs on their activities and profit margins (Greer 2009b; Garde 2010, pp. 32–34). For this reason, public health advocates and consumer groups are strongly opposed to self-regulation (Garde 2008).

Several countries have taken action, finding the commitments of the private sector insufficient. Denmark has imposed a "fat tax" on fatty foods in an effort to convince Danes to eat healthier. Hungary imposed a tax on all foods with unhealthy levels of sugar, salt and carbohydrates, as well as goods with high levels of caffeine. Denmark, Switzerland and Austria have banned trans-fats, while Finland and Romania are considering fat taxes (Topping 2011). While several EU member states have decided to take stronger action and push through the reformulation of processed foods or tax fatty foods, the Commission has used its authority to regulate the single market to submit two separate proposals to create uniform, consistent nutrition labels to supply consumers with the appropriate information to make healthy choices.

The politics of fighting obesity: Nutritional information labels

There is one area in which EU institutions wield considerable influence, namely the single market. The Commission has used its single market mandate to draft two different food-labeling laws, both of which have a strong public health objectives and sustain fair competition in the European food sector. In each case, the food and drink sectors marshaled unparalleled resources to strip the proposed rules from their most powerful public health features, with the assistance of the European Parliament, which earlier in 2008 had expressed outrage about the rising incidence of obesity.

The first initiative, *Nutrition and Health Claims Regulation* ((EC) 1924/2006) dealt with health and nutrition claims and predated the discussion on obesity. In 2001, the Commission issued a discussion paper in which it proposed restrictions on health and nutrition claims made by food manufacturers (Commission of the European Union 2001). What prompted this initiative was a court case in which the EJC ruled that a total prohibition on all health-related claims from food labels was disproportionate relative to its stated objective of protecting consumers.

In some countries, such as Austria, national law forbade all forms of health claims. The Court decided that such a blanket prohibition impeded the free movement of packaged foods (Smith 2012).

In 2003, the Commission proposed a new regulation that would establish uniform rules by defining the use of health claims on food packaging. The regulation on nutrition and health claims was meant to prevent unfounded claims on food packages such as "rich in vitamin C" or "low in fat" or health claims such as "good for your heart." Food companies would have to support these claims with scientific evidence, which in turn would be tested and analyzed by separate scientific committees organized by the European Food Safety Authority (EFSA). The second part of this new proposed regulation would prohibit food products from making health claims if a product was low in fat but still high in sugar or salt. Such claims mislead consumers into thinking that the product is healthy in spite of its high sugar, salt or fat content. According to Commission officials, the so-called nutrient profiles would avert floods of false health claims that contributed to bad dietary habits (Garde 2010, pp. 150–55).

Commission proposals are first submitted to the relevant European Parliament committee. In this case, the proposal went to two committees: Environment and Public Health (ENVI) and Internal Market (IMCO) in 2004. The ENVI committee was split about the effectiveness of nutrient profiles while the internal market committee was opposed to nutrient profiles. In the end, the European Parliament rejected the section on nutrient profiles in 2005 with the justification that it constituted excessive regulation, violated consumer choice, and undermined fair competition in the food industry. To be sure, fierce industry lobbying influenced British and German members of the European People's party and strengthened the determination of a large number of members of Parliament to dilute the health claim regulation by eliminating nutrient profiles (Europolitics 2005; Euractiv 2004; Smith 2012).

Once the Commission proposal, modified by the European Parliament, arrived at the EU Council of national health ministers, the politicians decided to restore the nutrient profiles. In the process of reconciling the EP and EU council drafts, nutrient profiles re-emerged, although the adopted draft weakened the original intent of the health claims proposal. Industry received greater flexibility and could market a product as "healthy" so long as it reduced the offending nutrient (salt, sugar, or fat) by 30 percent or more compared to similar products. Thus, there was no longer a requirement that a product should be low in salt, sugar, and fat to deserve the label "healthy."[3] It just had to be less unhealthy than similar products on the market (e.g., low-fat yogurt, with large amounts of sugar).

Industry still had the last word. Once the regulation went into force, the Commission was supposed to have in place provisions to test and evaluate nutrients and to compile a list of health function claims based on scientific evidence. By early 2009, the European food industry had submitted about 10,000 requests for approval of health claims to EFSA (EFSA 2011; Mariotti *et al.* 2010). Subsequently, the scientists at EFSA ran into a huge backlog and struggled to find an acceptable definition of what is too much fat, sugar, or salt. The delays and confusion were exploited by the coalition opposed to health claims and led to repeated calls of revising the adopted regulation by deleting nutrient profiles all together. In June 2010, during the first vote on another food labeling issue, some members of the European Parliament inserted an article in the new regulation to remove nutrient profiles from the Nutrition & Health Claims Regulation. The vote on this amendment was a tie, and thus defeated, with 309 in favor and 309 against (Asp and Bryngelsson 2008; Clarke 2010a,b).[4]

This was not the end of the nutrition and health claims regulation story. In September 2011, a consortium of European health product trade groups petitioned the European Commission to pause and rethink its process on the approval of health claims because they claimed that the EFSA method was "breaching the proportionality of the claims regulation." About 80 percent of claims submitted had been rejected (Clarke 2011). Thus, the concept of "honest" health claims has run into an array of obstacles, many of which arose from opposition by the European Parliament, which in turn was subject to intense lobbying by the food industry (Garde 2010, pp. 155–66).

Once the nutrition health claims regulation was out of the way, the Commission decided to go ahead with revising existing food labeling regulations. The proposed law, *Regulation on the Provision of Food Information to Consumers* (2008/0028) (COD) would improve the health and diet of European consumers by supplying them with accessible information about nutrition.

The proposal introduced new consumer information labels on all packaged foods. The Commission's draft mandated that labels must indicate a wide range of nutrients on the front of the package (calories (energy), total fat, saturated fat, salt, carbohydrates), in a minimum font size of 3mm, on a contrasting background for easy readability. The Commission also urged the European Parliament and Council to adopt mandatory "country of origin" labels, and it also left room for member states with extensive nutritional label requirements to continue to require those labels. As a concession to the alcoholic drinks sector, the labeling requirements only extended to processed food and non-alcoholic beverages, with the one major exception of alcopops (sweetened alcoholic drinks marketed to young people).

As with previous measures, the draft proposal of the Commission generated enormous lobbying activity by the food industry and its allies, calling into question their sincerity in seeking to mitigate the obesity crisis. When the draft went to the ENVI committee, the chair stripped the Commission proposal of all its "health impact" components: alcopops were exempted, nutritional information could be placed anywhere on the package, the size of the font of the text was reduced, national variations in labeling rules (by member states with stricter rules) were prohibited, and the number of products subject to "country of origin" labels was limited to meat.

The report was submitted to the EP for its first reading in June 2010. The EP approved the report of the ENVI committee with the exception that it called for mandatory nutritional information (energy, fat, saturated fat, sugar) on the front of the pack expressed per 100g/ml. But it approved the initial amendment to ban national labeling rules and exempt alcopops from labeling rules (EurAktiv 2010a,b; European Parliament 2010).

The largest bone of contention concerned "traffic-light" or color-coded labels (Lang 2006). Such labels use red, yellow or green dots on the front of the food package to show whether the product is high, medium or low in harmful nutrients such as fat or sugar. All NGOs in the medical (Heart, Diabetes, Cancer), public health (EPHA, Eurohealthnet), and consumer advocacy (BEUC) fields strongly supported this scheme, pointing to research findings that color-coding was the easiest label format for consumers to understand, especially when shopping in a hurry (Čuk 2009; Borgmeier and Westenhoefer 2009). From the beginning, the Commission yielded to objections raised by industry and left color-coded labels out of the draft. NGOs, in turn, tried to re-introduce color-coded labels by appealing to members of Parliament to approve such labels alongside Guidelines Daily Amount (GDA) information. Neither the ENVI committee nor the European Parliament supported the concept of color-coded labels in spite of their proven effectiveness (Chafin 2010a).

Beyond the color-coded labels, the food and beverage industry aimed to minimize in general the labels' impact. Therefore, industry representatives made the counter-proposal that companies be required to display only calories on the front of the packaging and list additional information on the back. They also questioned the proposed requirement for minimum font size and pushed for listing quantities of energy/calories and nutrients in discretionary portion sizes, which would give them some room to play with portion sizes. In addition, industry representatives opposed country-of-origin labeling (Kurzer and Cooper, forthcoming).

Again, the European Parliament, which is supposed to be concerned about Europe's health, undid many of the original provisions by accepting many of the counter-arguments offered by industry. Accordingly, in June 2010, members of Parliament voted against color-coding with an astonishing majority of 559 in favor, 54 against, and 32 abstentions (Hickman 2010). The EP's amended draft did not mandate front-of-the-pack listing of ingredients and applied country-of-origin rules to meat only. It also forbade member states from adding their own (stricter) labeling rules. Thus again the EP sided with industry, against the public health community when the labeling regulation was discussed.

The EU Council of health and consumer protection ministers again stepped in and restored some of the elements deleted by the European Parliament, which required a second reading or vote in the European Parliament in July 2011. The final regulation falls short of what the Commission had in mind, but at the same time, introduces uniform nutrition labeling in the EU. In force since December 2011, under the new rules, energy value and amounts of fat, saturates, carbohydrates, protein, sugars and salt must be indicated "in the same field of vision" though not necessarily at the front of the pack. Values must be expressed per 100g or per 100ml, and may also be expressed per portion. A minimum font size of 1.2 mm is required to ensure that the labels are legible. Compulsory country-of-origin labeling only applies to fresh meat like pork, sheep, goat and poultry.[5] Alcopops are excluded for now. However, the Commission will investigate a uniform labeling system for trans fats (associated with high cholesterol and heart disease) and contemplate restrictions on its use. It will also draft proposals to cover alcohol under the nutritional labeling rules (EurActiv 2011).

In the end, the food industry won important battles (Rasmussen 2011). With regard to consumer information legislation, the compromise led to the agreement to make the texts on the labels smaller than originally envisioned, to permit the placement of the labels anywhere on the package instead of on the front of the pack. Both the EP and EU council rejected the color-coded labels and rejected country-of-origin labels for milk and dairy products, for meat when as an ingredient in processed foods, and for single-ingredient products such as coffee.

Each labeling requirement was watered down by members of the European Parliament who appear easily swayed by food interests and have a tendency to prioritize corporate interests over Europe's health. There is an easy explanation for the European Parliament's behavior. The food business is the EU's largest manufacturing sector in terms of turnover and employment, with an annual turnover of €954 billion (12.9 percent of total manufacturing) and employing 4.2 million people (13.5 percent of total manufacturing). It purchases and processes 70 percent of EU agricultural production. As a sector it is both concentrated and fragmented. The top 1 percent (3,000 companies) accounts for slightly more than 50 percent of turnover, but the other 99 percent consist of small- and medium-sized enterprises (CIAA 2010). The food industry's strategy has been to target the EP committees and especially to approach the chair of the committee in charge of preparing the report that will be submitted to a plenary vote in the EP (Kurzer and Cooper forthcoming). Alongside the chair of the committee report, industry also lobbies and approaches regular EP members. Corporate Europe Observatory estimated that the food and drink industry invested more than €1 billion in a lobbying campaign to block the EU-wide traffic light labeling scheme. An anonymous MEP claimed that industry lobbyists managed to "drown out the message from public health campaigners on a scale of 100 to 1," as MEPs were bombarded with thousands of e-mails, letters, phone calls, reports, and conferences (Hickman 2010).

What will the future bring to the fight against diet-related diseases?

Serious efforts to combat obesity have to be society-wide, extensive, and deep. New concepts and categories in health promotion and health development need to be developed, and significant changes in food supply chains, product marketing, daily routines, and cultural environment must be introduced. Certainly, DG Sanco cannot solve the obesity challenge without continuous engagement of other public agencies, private actors, and member states. In the end, the EU may provide templates of best practices, impose benchmarks to steer national and local authorities on what may work, and create networks of professionals and practitioners, but its engagement and impact are constrained by the requirement that its actions are based on EU treaties.

In the 1990s, the EU created EFSA, which is meant to assess risk and to provide independent information, and scientific advice. It is supposed to support EU legislation and policies in all fields, which have a direct or indirect impact on food safety and quality. EFSA relies on independent committees who furnish the agency with specialized scientific and technocratic knowledge and expertise. Nevertheless, it would appear that the committees and EFSA itself are not constructed to vet and approve thousands of different health claims submitted by the private food sector, which resents the introduction of nutrient profiles in the first place. Because EFSA employs strict scientific criteria to evaluate nutrient profiles, many claims which were tested, ended up being rejected. All of this tends to harden the resistance of the food industry against EU legislation to combat obesity.

Because of its limited capacity, DG Sanco must rely on voluntary commitments through the EU DG SANCO platform on Diet, Physical Activity and Health. Food companies join the Platform, possibly, because it ostensibly demonstrates a commitment to addressing obesity. While participating in the Platform, however, food companies pursue measures that do not bite into their bottom line. Their behavior during the deliberations on two separate food labeling regulations suggest that ultimately economic operators are reluctant, to say the least, to acknowledge their responsibility for diet-related health consequences and introduce drastic changes in the way in which foodstuffs are marketed, sold, and processed. This also hurt the EFSA, which does not have the manpower and resources to quickly process and assess hundreds of different health claims of thousands of different food products, and thus draws the ire of the food industry.

In areas where the EU seems to have an advantage—single market regulations—it has been thwarted repeatedly by the combination of lobbying influence of the private sector, the susceptibility by European Parliamentarians to its pressures, and the limited size and authority of EFSA. We would expect the European Parliament to be on the side of consumers and the public health community. It has not been with the public health community, except rhetorically and symbolically, when it issues broad declarations of deep concern. During the policy process, members of the European Parliament have been hostile to legislation that seeks to introduce modest efforts to educate and inform consumers about the nutritional content of packaged foods. National politicians from the health ministries have been more receptive to pan-European rules although they have not aggressively pushed for bolder measures.

The future looks mixed, therefore, especially in light of the economic and financial crisis that probably will drain away attention and energy and make the EU institutions more reluctant to consider legislation opposed by an industry sector that employs directly and indirectly millions of Europeans.

Notes

1 Taken from: http://ec.europa.eu/health/nutrition_physical_activity/docs/platform_members.pdf (accessed September 11, 2012). Some other members are Eurocommerce, European Community of Consumer Cooperatives (Eurocoop), EuroHealthNet, European Association for the Study of Obesity (EASO), European Association of

Communications Agencies (EACA), European Cyclists Federation (ECF), European Consumer Organisation (BEUC), Freshfel Europe, International Baby Food Action Network (IBFAN), and International Diabetes Federation (IDF).

2 The list is found at http://ec.europa.eu/health/nutrition_physical_activity/docs/eu_platform_2011frep_en.pdf (accessed September 11, 2012).

3 The second exemption was that products can tout their health claims if they contain low content in one nutrient even though they are high in other unhealthy nutrients. Thus, breakfast cereals low in fat can advertise that even if their sugar content is high so long as it does not contain other unhealthy nutrients (high salt).

4 Later, it appeared that some MEPs were confused and voted incorrectly. Five MEPs admitted they had in fact voted incorrectly against the amendment, while two other MEPS had said that they had incorrectly voted in favor of it. If the MEPs had voted correctly, the amendment would have passed with 312 votes in favor and 306 votes against, putting pressure on the Council and Commission to review the nutrient profile chapter of the Health Claims regulation. Richard Clarke, "Fate of nutrient profiles in doubt after MEPs reveal voting blunders." *Functional Ingredients* (Aug. 10, 2010). http://newhope360.com/fate-nutrient-profiles-doubt-after-meps-reveal-voting-blunders (accessed September 11, 2012).

5 The new rules also require manufacturers to indicate the origin of vegetable oils used in food. Currently, many ingredient lists for products merely state "vegetable oil," without specifying whether it comes from rapeseed, corn, sunflower or palm. Concerned with palm oil plantations that endanger rainforests and wildlife, EU law-makers insisted that the source of vegetable oil should be indicated on the packaging.

12 Alcohol policy in the European Union

Jenny Cisneros Örnberg

Introduction

Europe has the highest drinking levels, the highest alcohol per capita consumption and the highest rates of alcohol-related harm in the world. Overall, it is estimated that 55 million people in the EU drink alcohol to harmful levels, and of these, 23 million are addicted. More than one-fourth of road traffic accidental deaths are caused by drunk driving, and over a quarter of deaths among young men are linked to alcohol. From a health perspective, alcohol is responsible for more than 60 different types of diseases and conditions including injuries, mental and behavioral disorders, and cancers. Harmful and hazardous alcohol consumption is attributed to an estimated 7.4 percent of all illness and early death in the EU (Babor *et al*. 2010; European Commission).[1]

How, when, and why we drink depend on cultural views and attitudes, historical and individual circumstances, and on how we, as society, have chosen to deal with alcohol and alcohol-related problems (Cisneros Örnberg 2009b). Since the EU has, above all, an economic mission, alcohol has been primarily addressed and defined in market terms within agricultural, tax and trade policy. Alcohol beverages constitute a set of commodities that are produced, distributed and consumed on a large scale in Europe. Alcohol is therefore one of the Union's leading export commodities, and many of the member states have a considerable positive trade balance from their export of wine and spirits. The production and sales of alcoholic beverages play a significant role in the European economy and have done so for a long time (Lubkin 1996). Public health, on the other hand, has been a field for cooperation in the EU only since 1993. Room (1999) argues that alcohol policy as an English term is of recent date and basically an import from the Nordic languages, referring to public policies pertaining to the relation between alcohol, health, and social welfare. A central purpose of such policies is serving the interest of public health and social well-being (Babor *et al*. 2010).

Historically, alcohol has been an unusual or non-existent policy area among many of the member states and the EU, partly due to the diversity of approaches and the cultural differences attached to alcohol policy across Europe (Lubkin 1996). Nevertheless, there has, since the mid-1990s, been a notable increase in policy discussions within the EU relating alcohol as a commodity to its public health implications. In this way, alcohol demonstrates both the fundamentals of the European Union and its internal market, and the growing use of so-called soft law on the European level, resulting in an increased work among the member states with alcohol as a health question.

The following chapter will give an overview of the development of alcohol policy on EU level, and analyze its concomitant opportunities and challenges. How can we understand this development? What have been the driving forces? What does the future look like? On a theoretical level, the chapter will also elucidate the frames, strategies and limits for public health work at the EU level.

Organization of alcohol policy in the EU

With the adoption of the Single European Act in 1986, the European Community started addressing areas that previously had been handled at national or regional levels. During the 1990s, the EU evolved from being an organization focused on economic policy to being a political union expressing interests in social rights on a supranational level (Blomqvist 2003). Policymaking on public health questions increased in importance and extent after the Amsterdam Treaty in 1999, which incorporated a new public health article (Article 152) requiring the Union to promote, as well as protect, the health of EU citizens. The Article calls for European Community action to complement national policies, and to improve public health and prevent disease by encouraging and supporting cooperation and collaboration between member states. The article also lists causes of danger to human health, and articulates the general objective of improving health (Cisneros Örnberg 2009b; European Union 2006).

Given the importance attached to subsidiarity in health matters, the idea of so-called added value—would EU intervention add value to the initiatives contemplated by member states if they had acted alone—has been presented as a criterion for EU actions and policies (Randall 2001).[2] This means that there are few possibilities for relying on legal instruments to foster harmonization between the member states. Instead, the European Commission governs through communications, codes of conduct and guidelines. This approach enables member states to collaborate in areas where the EU-system precludes a common policy or legal framework, and in areas of significant international diversity. Concerted EU actions are therefore possible without interfering with individual member states' legal autonomy and authority. This means that the 27 member states can operate individually and differently while still working towards a common goal of less alcohol-related harm. At the same time, common interests and interdependencies mean that each state has a stake in the behavior of the others. However, there are opportunities for EU-wide policies that could support a public health approach to alcohol; for example, binding legislation could increase minimum excise tax rates or create common rules on marketing and advertising. However, as I will show, policymaking in this arena has faced difficulties in reaching consensus.

The European Commission

The European Commission Services are divided into Directorates General (DG). Until the late 1990s, public health policy was addressed within DG V, which also dealt with employment, industrial relations and social affairs. After reorganization in 1999, the DG for Health and Consumer Protection (SANCO) was formed, an organizational change that reflected, according to Randall (2001), the rising status of health within the Commission. DG SANCO is today divided into seven different directorates (A–G), with directorate C handling public health questions. Directorate C is in turn divided into four subunits, wherein the C4 unit handles health determinants, including so-called "lifestyle determinants" like tobacco, alcohol, drugs, and obesity. In June 2011 the number of DG SANCO staff was 880, of which three desk officers, supported by assistants, have been working full time on alcohol issues. While SANCO C4 is responsible within the Commission Services for alcohol policy development, all major decisions are coordinated with other relevant DGs and in close cooperation with other DG SANCO units.[3]

The European Parliament

The European Parliament is the only directly elected body of the European Union. The citizens of member states elect the 736 members of the European Parliament once every five years. To prepare for the Parliament's plenary sessions, the members are divided into 20 specialized standing committees, where large parts of the overall political discussions occur. The Committee on the Environment, Public Health and Food Safety (ENVI) is responsible for alcohol-related questions. With 64 members, ENVI is one of the largest committees and deals with issues that affect the daily lives of EU citizens. In the field of health, ENVI addresses questions relating to the internal market and issues that have cross-border effects, for example the safety of pharmaceutical and cosmetic products, the fight against counterfeit medicinal products or the defense of patients' rights. In the area of food safety, the Committee mostly deals with advertising and labeling, as well as food hygiene. Most questions that the European Parliament decides are addressed together with the Council of the European Union. This means that the Parliament has the option to block decisions if the two institutions do not agree.

The members of parliament can raise oral or written questions to the Commission or the Council. At the end of 2011, members had used this authority in 34 cases on issues concerning alcohol, such as minimum pricing, warning labels, marketing and advertising, alcohol and pregnant women, rise in cancer cases, EU data collection, discrepancies in import tariffs, underage drinking, alcohol and driving, and the cost of alcohol to the EU.

The Council of the European Union

The Council of the European Union, informally known as the EU Council (hereafter referred to as the Council), is where national ministers from each EU country meet to adopt laws and coordinate policies. The Council represents the govern-ments of the individual member countries and has its meetings in ten different constellations. The Council discusses alcohol as a public health issue primarily in meetings on Employment, Social policy, Health and Consumer Affairs. The presidency of the Council is shared by the member states on a rotating six-month basis. As president, one has the power to shape the agenda and push forward national concerns linked to traditional national priorities. Although predetermined agendas restrict the presidency (Liefferink and Skou Andersen 2002) to some extent, research shows that exploiting the position to defend major interests or to promote national pet projects has become expected behavior (Tallberg 2003). However, before questions reach the ministerial level they have been discussed thoroughly in workgroups and committees comprised of civil servants that negoti-ate on behalf of the member states, and in Coreper (*Comité des représentants permanents*/Committee of Permanent Representatives) negotiations. Coreper I handles Employment, Social policy, Health and Consumer Affairs policy issues.

The Court of Justice of the EU

The Court of Justice of the EU (CJEU) has become an increasingly influential political actor, contributing to what many analysts argue is a "market adjustment" of welfare policy within the Union (Blomqvist 2003). European law is to a great extent directly applicable in the member countries and is supposed to be used in a direct manner by national courts and authorities. European law has, furthermore, a general precedence over national law in case of a conflict between legal systems.

The CJEU has played an important role in strengthening the supranational features of the EU as an organization. However, there is significant disagreement about the extent of the implications of this development. The use of proportionality judgments means that public health is ascribed a small role compared to economic aspects in alcohol-related cases. Given the influence that agriculture and alcohol-producing interests have within the EU, it is doubtful that alcohol will ever be addressed with the same heavy hand as was, for example, tobacco.

Nevertheless, "case law seems to leave quite some discretionary space for the national executive in the interpretations of how to make national law and policy compatible with incremental judicial interpretations of EU law" (Sindbjerg Martinsen and Vrangbæk 2006, p. 6). Furthermore, Baumberg and Anderson (2008) argue that even though there is a partial juridification of alcohol policy, the court is at times prepared to prioritize health over trade concerns. Baumberg and Anderson further assert that pessimistic interpretations of the role EU law can play in alcohol policy should be tempered. Previous research also shows that the impact of EU public policy is contingent on whether a country is already involved in a process of reform or not. The rules that are decided within the EU can therefore only strengthen and accelerate already ongoing processes and give national politicians support in reform proposals (Mörth 2003, 2004; Radaelli 2003).

The CJEU has, when it comes to alcohol, mainly pronounced verdicts in cases concerning taxation (C-86/78; C-168/78; C-170/78; C-171/78; C-68/79; C-216/81;

C-243/84; C-166/98; C-434/97; C-5/05, C-167/05), advertising (C-152/78; C-1/90; C-176/90; C-405/98; C-318/00; C-262/02; C-492/02) and monopolies (C-91/78; C-189/95; C-170/04) (for a discussion of the different cases, see, for example, Baumberg and Anderson 2008).

The development and content of EU alcohol policy

Two circumstances seem to have been important in triggering EU activities to address alcohol. First, there was an increased concern among non-governmental organizations (NGOs) and European politicians about the introduction of alcopops (highly sweetened premixed drinks) (Sutton and Nylander 1999) and second, there was a growing concern about the spread of Northern binge drinking patterns among young people in wine-producing countries (ibid.; European Commission 2000). In 1996 the Commission established a Working Group on Alcohol and Health, consisting of experts from the EU's member countries as a forum for sharing experiences on alcohol-related problems and alcohol policy (Tigerstedt *et al.* 2006).

In December 2000, the Commission delivered a proposed Council Recommendation on youth alcohol consumption (Council 2001a) that encouraged member states to take a multi-sectoral approach to educating young people about alcohol and increasing their involvement in health-related policies and actions. The Commission's proposal was presented during the French presidency, but it was Sweden, with strong support from France, that initiated and completed the work in the following six months. In June 2001, the Health Ministers of the EU adopted the Council Recommendation (2001/458/EC).

On June 5, 2001, the Health ministers invited the Commission to put forward proposals for a comprehensive community strategy aimed at reducing alcohol-related harm (Council 2001b). The same year the Commission recommended measures aimed at abating drunk driving, including an EU-wide Blood Alcohol Concentration (BAC) maximum limit. Also, the Road Safety Action Program 2003–2008 gave special attention to drunk driving, with tighter controls of BAC levels. In 2002 the European Parliament and the Council adopted a program of community action in the field of public health for 2003–2008 (1786/2002/EG), including several areas focusing on drunk driving prevention and awareness in an effort to combat alcohol-related harm (Cisneros Örnberg 2009b).

The work on developing a comprehensive Alcohol Strategy was delayed due to lack of personnel and the more immediate priority to address tobacco consumption (Cisneros Örnberg 2009a). To spur activity on alcohol policy, the Swedish government seconded a national alcohol policy expert to DG SANCO in 2004. Seconded officials from member governments are considered "detached national experts" and are often used to provide additional expertise on salient policy issues (Egeberg 2010). Five years after the invitation from the Council, the Commission's Communication on an Alcohol Strategy was approved on October 24, 2006 (European Commission 2006b).

The EU alcohol strategy focuses on five areas: protecting young people, children and the unborn child; reducing injuries and deaths from alcohol-related road traffic accidents; preventing alcohol-related harm among adults and reducing the negative impact on the workplace; informing, educating and raising awareness on the impact of harmful and hazardous alcohol consumption and on appropriate consumption patterns; and developing, supporting and maintaining a common evidence base. The adopted strategy has been described both as a landmark in alcohol policy development, and as watered down due to alcohol-industry involvement in the process. This outcome is very similar to what is seen in the realm of food labeling and nutrition, as discussed in Chapter 11 on obesity. Both the alcohol industry, with their so-called social aspects groups, and NGOs are considered legitimate stakeholders in EU policymaking. Through networking and lobbying these groups try to affect alcohol policy development. Health Commissioner Kyprianou and the NGOs severely criticized the alcohol industries' involvement and lobbying for amendments that resulted in revisions of the Alcohol Strategy (Cisneros Örnberg 2009b).

The Commission established a structure for implementing the EU Alcohol Strategy in 2007 consisting of three pillars: first, the Committee on National Alcohol Policy and Action (CNAPA), which includes delegates appointed by member states' governments; second, the Committee on Data Collection, Indicators and Definitions, which has representatives from member states, the Commission, WHO, ESPAD and EMCDDA; and third, the European Alcohol and Health Forum (EAHF), a common platform to convene all interested stakeholders at the EU level. Of the three pillars, the EAHF has received the most attention, consisting of more than 60 stakeholders including public health NGOs, alcohol manufacturers and producers, and health professionals. The EAHF has established two task forces, the Task Force on Youth-Specific Aspects of Alcohol and the Task Force on Marketing Communication. An EAHF-appointed Science Group provides scientific guidance to EAHF members.

DG SANCO presented the first progress report on the implementation of the EU Alcohol Strategy in 2009. The report concluded that the recent activity was a promising start, but that more needed to be done (European Communities 2009). The next progress report is due in 2012, the same year that the present strategy ends. In December 2009, at the end of the Swedish presidency, the Employment, Social policy, Health and Consumer Affairs Council meeting adopted *Conclusions on Alcohol and Health*, inviting the Commission to define priorities for the next phase of the Commission's work on alcohol and health after the end of the current strategy. The resolution contains rare formulations that include both marketing and pricing policy (Council 2009). The Council also invites member states and the Commission to "keep public-health-based alcohol policy high on the agenda towards 2012 in order to build sustainable and long-term commitments to reduce alcohol-related harm at EU level" (Council 2009, p. 5).

Clearly there is a general understanding on the EU level for the need of policy measures to prevent alcohol-related harm, but specific solutions lack agreement. The main areas for consensus among member states focus on the protection of young people, drunk driving prevention, pregnancy, hazardous and harmful drinkers, and the need for research and education. Still contentious questions are those involving price and availability such as taxation, restrictions on sales/serving to adults, and advertising. These controversial issues are also those that, according to research, are the most efficient in terms of reducing alcohol consumption and related problems (Babor *et al.* 2010).

Despite research suggesting that alcohol pricing policies are an effective measure to reduce alcohol-related harm, economic measures are rarely used to achieve public health aims. Taxation of alcohol is used primarily for fiscal rather than public health gains in most EU nations (Rabinovich *et al.* 2009). The present minimum excise tax rates on alcoholic beverages came into effect in 1993, and there has been no consensus between the member states to upgrade them since. The last attempt was in 2006 during the Finnish presidency, but the proposal to raise the minimum tax level by 4.5 percent on spirits and beer failed to attain universal support (European Commission 2008a).

The minimum tax rate on wine is zero and was not included in the suggested changes. Member states are free to set excise duty rates at levels above the minimum. This has resulted in great diversity within the Community in the levels of taxation. The Commission has concluded that wide tax differentials between member states constitute both an opportunity for cross-border shopping and an incentive for fraud and smuggling. The issue of wine taxation is particularly controversial and politically sensitive since the current minimum of zero is seen by wine-producing member states as a necessary supplementary measure to the EU's agriculture policies on wine. Other member states that want to see an increase in minimum wine tax rates demand it in the context of any discussions of raising minimum excise taxes (Press release 2004).

Even though the CJEU has concluded that advertising acts as an encouragement to consumption (see for example C-262/02), common rules or even guidelines have been hard to achieve on an EU level when it comes to the marketing and advertising of alcoholic beverages. To date, the discussion on alcohol advertising has mostly focused on industry self-regulation. With the exception of cross-border television advertising, alcohol advertising is regulated differently depending on the country, forum, and the sort of beverage. One aim for the Commission is to reach agreement with stakeholders on codes of commercial communication that can be implemented at national and EU levels. The "Audiovisual Media Services Directive" (Directive 2007/65/EC) states that "audiovisual commercial communications for alcoholic beverages shall not be aimed specifically at minors and shall not encourage immoderate consumption of such beverages." The Council Recommendation 2001/458/EC encouraged member states to cooperate with producers and retailers of alcoholic beverages and relevant NGOs to establish agreements on alcohol promotion, marketing and retailing. The documents demonstrate the EU level-approach is that young people in particular should be protected from exposure to alcohol advertising.

There are currently no considerations at the EU level on a regulatory approach to health warnings on alcoholic beverages. DG SANCO stated in its February 2006 report on labeling that health warnings could be an effective means to inform consumers about risks associated with inappropriate consumption of alcohol

(Health and Consumer Protection Directorate-General 2006). However, in May 2007 the European Parliament failed to introduce standardized EU-wide health warnings on alcoholic drinks, despite recommendations from its own Health Committee and despite its standardization in tobacco products. Some members of Parliament denounced the lack of action as caving to strong lobbying efforts from alcohol producers. Member states can introduce labeling measures, but are then required to notify the Commission and provide justification. The Commission then verifies, on a case-by-case basis, that draft national measures are necessary to achieve stated objectives, such as the protection of public health, while not creating disproportionate barriers to the free movement of goods (Directive 2000/13/EC). Information and warning messages can cover general health warnings, specific health warnings (e.g., liver cirrhosis), information about volume and units of measurement, drinking guidelines, legal age limits for purchasing alcoholic beverages, messages about drinking in moderation, drinking and driving, and the dangers of operating machinery and causing harm to others (family members or other third parties).

France is the first and only EU member state to require warning labels on all alcoholic beverages. As of October 2007, a mandatory warning points out the risk for the fetus of drinking during pregnancy. Under the 2004 Protection of Minors Act, the German Government introduced mandatory labeling for spirit-based alcopops, and prohibited the sale of alcopops for young people under the age of 18 (CRIOC 2011).

On January 30, 2008, the Commission adopted a proposal revising food labeling rules. The proposal combined two previously separate regulations—one for general labeling rules (2000/13/EC) and another addressing nutrition labeling (90/496/EEC). However, as mentioned by Kurzer in Chapter 11, alcoholic drinks containing more than 1.2 percent by volume of alcohol were excluded from the proposal. A Commission official referred to both the "complexity of production methods" and "political choice" as justification for allowing the exclusion of wine, beer and spirits from the directive (EurActiv 2008). The European Parliament adopted the new EU regulation (1169/2011) in July 2011. The Commission is, however, instructed to examine by the end of 2014 whether alcoholic beverages should be labeled with ingredients, caloric, and nutritional value information, and whether the Commission should propose amendments to the rules already adopted (EurActiv 2011).

Converging trends

Previous research has shown a homogenization in drinking patterns, consumption levels, and beverage preferences among the EU15 countries (Leifman 2002; Simpura *et al.* 2002). According to Tigerstedt and Törrönen (2007) the standard concepts and images of different European drinking cultures have therefore become diluted and inappropriate. The validity of the typology between "beer-drinking countries," "wine-drinking countries," and "spirits-drinking countries," and the distinction between wet and dry drinking cultures has weakened during recent decades. Although the total consumption of alcohol generally has decreased in the Mediterranean countries, there has been an increase in binge drinking, especially among youth. This has increased the incentive to work from a social and health perspective, both nationally and on the EU level. Southern European countries' policies have recently moved somewhat closer to Nordic more restrictive positions, particularly on such dimensions as drunk driving, alcohol education, and youth binge drinking (Österberg and Karlsson 2002; Babor *et al.* 2010). Most member states also now have a written alcohol policy in place and there is a trend toward setting an age limit of 18 for selling and serving alcohol (European Communities 2009).

While states are moving towards an increased understanding for stricter alcohol policies, the control of alcohol production, distribution, and sales has decreased in the EU member states. This liberalization of alcohol supply measures has led to an increase in alcohol consumption within the Nordic countries. A RAND report on the affordability (i.e., the net effect of price and income) of alcohol beverages in the European Union finds that they have become more affordable in most EU countries since the mid 1990s—in some countries by over 50 percent (Rabinovich *et al.* 2009). The Report also concludes, as have many previous studies, that there is a positive relationship between alcohol affordability and alcohol consumption in Europe. The real value of excise duty rates for most alcohol beverages has gone down since 1996 among a vast majority of the member states. There has also been a decline in the EU minimum excise duty rates in real terms for alcohol beverages since 1992 as they have not been adjusted for inflation.

The development of European alcohol policy in the future

At the end of 2012, the Commission will report on the implementation of measures to tackle harmful and hazardous alcohol consumption and on the impact of the present EU Alcohol Strategy. It is clear that harmful and hazardous alcohol consumption will continue to be considered an important determinant of health in the context of the wider EU health strategy. Demonstrated added value of the present EU Alcohol Strategy and the experience of member states with EU policy implementation will shape discussions on the continuing work specifically focused on alcohol. Commission representatives have stressed the importance of member states' involvement in the evaluation process, and have invited them to make clear which elements in the current EU Alcohol Strategy are particularly useful, and where there are gaps.

An important feature of the evaluation will be the active involvement of members of the CNAPA in a questionnaire survey and complementary interviews. The evaluation of the Alcohol Strategy will begin during the spring of 2012 and result in a report at the end of the year. This will be followed by Council Conclusions based on the report during the Cyprian presidency in 2012 or the Irish presidency in 2013. Based on the previous engagement of the these two countries in alcohol policy, and the potential for the country that holds the presidency to shape the agenda, the potential for development of alcohol policy is larger if the question is put on the agenda of the Irish presidency.

During the CNAPA meeting in November 2011 the Commission put forward a suggestion that the new alcohol strategy should include only children and adolescents. This was met with strong opposition from all member states representatives, except Greece. Rather, there seemed to be a strong consensus among the member states on the importance of a second alcohol strategy that would include further development and expansion of presently included areas. Third-party harm, cross-border issues, and health in other EU policies (taxation, labeling, and marketing) were discussed as future foci (Flash report 2011). Identifying common indicators in response to calls for regular reporting has also been presented as an important step towards comparability across member states despite immediate challenges to harmonization or standardization of member states' alcohol data gathering approaches (Committee on National Alcohol Policy and Action 2011).

The development and continuation of an alcohol strategy is to be considered a significant step in EU alcohol policy development. Alcohol policy is no longer an exclusively Nordic area of interest, but is also on the agenda for countries such as France, Germany and Ireland. All member states, with a few exceptions, are nonetheless reluctant to give up health as an area of national competence. This means that no one at the EU level is talking about the possibilities for a future framework convention for alcohol, as was achieved for tobacco, or about common legislation. However, the understanding among politicians and civil servants about the benefits of such a development has increased over the years. Nevertheless, there is an expressed concern from Eurocare (The European Alcohol Policy Alliance)[4] about what will happen within the alcohol political field in the coming five years with a new European Parliament, new Commission and expected changes internally within DG SANCO (Ugland 2011).

Alcohol policy within a theoretical frame

As the possibilities for national alcohol policy divergence has shrunk, more public health decisions have moved from a national to an international level. The reluctance among member states to give away important competences to the EU is to a certain extent matched by a conviction that cooperation offers long-term gains (Héritier 1999). A more open market forces member states to collaborate on issues, such as alcohol, they would rather have kept on a national level. This increased cooperation has led to a process of reframing of alcohol on the EU level, from a market and agriculture frame to an increased focus on alcohol as a social and health question (Cisneros Örnberg 2009b).

The introduction of "new modes of governance" (NMG) in the EU context can be seen as a reaction to the imminent risk of deadlock in community decision making (Eberlein and Kerwer 2004). Relying on "soft law," which is not legally binding and has no legal sanctioning mechanisms against non-compliance, leaves the effective policy choice to each individual member state (Kohler-Koch and

Rittberger 2006). By emphasizing "benchmarking," "peer review" and "best practice," NMG engender the assumption that participating actors can learn from assessment and comparison (Eberlein and Kerwer 2004, p. 125).

Critics argue that a big part of the EU's social policy goals often remain only as goals and that implementation seldom is effective. However, Landelius (2001) counters that the formulation of common goals can constitute a first step to a more unified view on a controversial question, and can thereby lay the ground for more concrete political initiatives in the future. Soft law policymaking has led to the establishment of new committees that play a central role in monitoring the policy coordination process. Meetings of civil servants and high-level politicians also have a socializing effect concerning what is seen as appropriate behavior (Jacobsson 2004).

Previous research highlights four strategies to be especially important in developing EU-level alcohol policy decisions. First, keep the question high in priority; second, get support from important actors; third, frame the issue in the form of irrefutable claims, and finally, acknowledge that change takes time, both when it comes to policymaking and to how a problem is perceived (Cisneros Örnberg 2009a). Within a soft-law context, decisions will end up either as determinative of the status quo or the lowest common denominator; for example, a relatively vague policy that leaves room for different national activities.

In the field of alcohol two approaches have been particularly resonant: the protection of children and young people, and the need for research (generally monitoring). When children and young people are perceived to be at risk, the phenomenon is easily constructed as an important problem for which specific measures are defined and implemented (Cisneros Örnberg 2009a). Regarding research, the Commission often starts decision-making processes with distributive measures such as funding research, which meet little political opposition (Héritier 1999). Since the late 1990s, the EU has financed research programs collecting comparable data for the surveillance of alcohol consumption and related social, economic and health indicators (Cisneros Örnberg 2008). This activity has increasingly been done in cooperation with the WHO.

According to Ugland (2011) the European Commission successfully exploited a window of opportunity for alcohol policy development after several EU institutions, member states and NGOs raised concerns about underage binge drinking. The Nordic countries played a crucial role in the early stages of policy development and attention to the issue seemed to increase the years Sweden, and to some degree Finland, held the presidency of the Council (Cisneros Örnberg 2009b; Ugland 2011). Change would not have been possible, however, without the support and influence of important actors such as France. France, as one of the primary wine producers/exporters, has been referred to as an "exception," a "paradox" and a "strange bedfellow" when it comes to alcohol policy both with regard to national legislation, support of other member states right to restrictive rules based on public health considerations, and it its role in the development of a common EU-level alcohol policy (Ugland 2003; Rigaud and Craplet 2004). The change in how alcohol is framed highlights the fact that member states are not only affected by EU decisions but are also part of the creation of new EU norms and regulations.

The change in framing of alcohol highlights that member states are not only affected by EU decisions but also part of the creation of new norms and regulations on the EU level. There is therefore a need to further analyze the interplay and interconnectedness between the member states and the EU and focus on Europeanization as the interaction between European and domestic policy processes. Although the Europeanization concept has been widely used across different disciplines and the views on what the concept contains are not always clear, it could be argued that the dominant perspective in the Europeanization literature still remains "top-down," a view that lacks the focus that, for example, Börzel (2002) or Green Cowles *et al.* (2001) bring into the Europeanization debate, describing Europeanization as a bottom-up or a two-way process.

Previous research supports the notion that future development of EU-level alcohol is contingent on active agenda and priority setting, as well as anchorage and commitment within member states to uphold and expand the field. The development of EU-level alcohol is thereby conditioned on the support from not only politicians but also the general public within each member state.

Conclusions

Alcohol as a social and health question in the EU has risen in prominence since 1999 as exemplified by the establishment of DG SANCO, several court verdicts prioritizing health over trade concerns, the *Council Recommendation of 5 June 2001 on the drinking of alcohol by young people*, the adoption of an EU Alcohol Strategy, and an increased appreciation for, if not enactment of, restrictive measures based on hard law. Policy development can partly be ascribed to the increased competence and interest in health questions in the wake of the Amsterdam Treaty, and the considerable trend toward harmonization in alcohol consumption and drinking patterns across Europe. What is seen is an increased concern for combating alcohol-related harm in many member states, and at the EU level, alcohol is considered to be one of the key health determinants that need to be tackled. However, since most member states have been reluctant to transfer formal welfare policy decision making to the EU, most EU-level alcohol policy is based on the so-called new modes of governance. Relying on soft law at the EU level leaves the effective policy choice to each individual member state.

The development of alcohol policy at the EU level has nonetheless become increasingly important as the possibilities for member states to pursue a differentiated alcohol policy have decreased. This is especially apparent for the Nordic countries that have a tradition of restrictive alcohol policy. Not surprisingly, the Nordic countries exhibit the greatest support and commitment for developing common alcohol political measures. Previous research supports the notion that strategies that are based on priority but also strong anchorage among other member states seem to be of particular importance for the development of areas based on soft-law decision making. These strategies can be identified through initiatives such as secondments and through agenda setting during the presidencies. The influence of the Nordic countries at the EU level shows the importance of analyzing Europeanization processes as a constant interchange of ideas, strategies and policy frames.

Although the total consumption of alcoholic beverages generally has decreased in the Mediterranean countries, there has been an increase in binge drinking, especially among youth. This has further increased the incentive to address alcohol consumption as a social and health issue, both nationally and on the EU level. Southern European countries have moved somewhat closer to the more stringent Nordic position, particularly on problems such as drunk driving, and youth binge drinking. At the EU level, there is a push toward increased monitoring and statistical collection of indicators as a mechanism to introduce a common view of new policy areas. Even though the data so far have methodological and scientific difficulties, the work results in an important benchmarking and agenda setting.

Finally, the increased number of forums and committees has created an organizational structure on EU level resulting in an overall increase in the attention to alcohol policy questions among member states. However, these committees could easily disappear if alcohol is no longer addressed as a single issue but is incorporated in a wider EU health strategy. A long-term commitment to alcohol policy is therefore contingent on the adoption of a new Alcohol Strategy. There is an expressed interest in continued work in this area and increased cooperation among member states and working groups. The implementation report and following council conclusion during late 2012 or early 2013 will ultimately determine how this area will be handled in the future.

Notes

1 See: http://ec.europa.eu/health-eu/my_lifestyle/alcohol/index_en.htm (accessed September 10, 2012).
2 Subsidiarity is intended to determine whether, in an area where there is joint competence, the Union can take action or should leave the matter to the member states. The subsidiarity principle is based on the idea that decisions must be taken as closely as possible to the citizen: the Union should not undertake action (except on matters for which it alone is responsible) unless EU action is more effective than action taken at national, regional or local level.
3 See: http://ec.europa.eu/dgs/health_consumer/chart.pdf (accessed September 10, 2012).
4 EUROCARE is an alliance of approximately 50 public health organizations from 22 European countries dedicated to the prevention and reduction of alcohol-related harm.

13 Tobacco control

The end of Europe's love affair with smoking?

Donley T. Studlar[1]

Traditionally Europe has been closely associated with smoking—culturally (French intellectuals), as a source of fiscal revenue through taxation of manufactured cigarettes (especially important in large-scale tobacco manufacturing countries such as the United Kingdom, Germany, and the Netherlands), and agriculturally through economic benefits (a mainstay of farmers in Mediterranean countries such as Italy and Greece). Yet, over the past half-century, individual countries in Europe have joined, and in some cases led, the attack against smoking. The EU began to combat smoking in the mid-1980s and has progressively moved toward greater tobacco control for its members and associated countries accepting the Single European Act (SEA) in the following instruments: taxation, removal of agricultural subsidies, product regulation, advertising restrictions, protection from secondhand smoke, anti-smuggling enforcement, capacity-building aid to anti-tobacco organizations, and education, especially through health warnings on packages and mass media campaigns.

Through powers granted in the SEA (1987), the Maastricht Treaty (1993) and the Amsterdam Treaty (1999), tobacco policy in the EU has moved from being principally economically promotional toward being restrictive on public health grounds. Almost all major institutions of the EU have been involved in this process. There is evidence that the more prominent role of the EU in tobacco control has functioned in ways congruent with diffusion and Europeanization through multi-level governance. There has been top-down, lateral, and bottom-up diffusion of tobacco control policies among jurisdictions in Europe, including the EU. The EU also has become a principal world actor in tobacco control, taking an active role as an organization in the processes leading to the Framework Convention on Tobacco Control (FCTC). Ideas, institutions, socioeconomic conditions, and interest groups have contributed to this considerable change in tobacco policy in the EU. Thus far, however, policies have changed more than smoking behavior. Tobacco control promises to continue to be prominent among EU public health policies in the future as further challenges arise in dealing with this large-scale disease risk factor that is socially contagious rather than biologically induced.

What is the issue?

In a similar fashion to its member states and other Western industrialized democracies, the EU has moved gradually from tobacco promotion policies based on the economic value of the product to more public health-based tobacco control policies (Cairney *et al.* 2012). All of the contradictions have not been fully reconciled between these two policy directions, which one might expect in an organization so clearly devoted to economic development as the EU. Nevertheless, it is remarkable that the EU has taken advantage of its regulatory powers over the past 25 years to reorient its policy away from an exclusive emphasis on economics. Especially when one considers the fact that several EU member states have been inclined to favor individual freedom of choice over the precautionary principle on the tobacco issue (Strünck 2005), the EU has played an important role in convergence and diffusion of tobacco control policies toward a protective health norm.

The Tobacco Epidemic Model (Lopez *et al.* 1994) distinguishes four stages of development of the tobacco problem, based on Western experience over the past century. After Stage One featuring an increase in male smoking, Stage Two involves a major increase of smoking in both males and females as per capita income rises; this eventually results in an increase in the incidence of tobacco-related disease. Stage Three begins the amelioration of the epidemic through social knowledge of the health hazards of tobacco and government policy. The EU began in the latter part of Stage Three for most of its member countries and has pushed some of them toward Stage Four, the decline of smoking, through measures delineated below (Cairney *et al.* 2012; Tiessen *et al.* 2010).

Tobacco policy as an issue has existed for a long time in Europe, at least since its importation from the New World in the sixteenth century. From the start, it both spread rapidly and was the subject of controversy. King James I's "Counterblast to Tobacco" (1604) is a well-known condemnation, but the habit spread from the upper classes to those below, and governments came to depend on tax revenue from tobacco, especially in wartime when smoking increased. Smoking rates accelerated with the introduction of mass manufacturing of cigarettes (literally, small cigars) in the late nineteenth century (Cox 2000). The modern phases of tobacco control are outlined in Table 13.1 (Studlar 2002). Gradually cigarettes, which were extremely portable and convenient to use, displaced other inhaled and chewable forms. European anti-tobacco groups resisted this change based on concerns about the moral and physical effects of smoking in the early twentieth century (Welshman 1996; Hilton 2000). The use of cigarettes among troops in World War I dissipated cultural mores against smoking, and it spread more widely through the use of advertising, including appeals to women. These developments were little questioned until the 1950s, except in Germany (Proctor 1999).

The German concerns about the health effects of smoking were lost in post-war anti-Nazism (Cooper and Kurzer 2003) until the publication of seminal articles on the topic in the United Kingdom in 1950, as well as similar articles in the US at

Table 13.1 Eras of tobacco control in Europe

Period	Theme
Paradigm: Tobacco Promotion (Political Economy)	
Phase 1: 1885–1914	Consolidation of the Cigarette Industry and Early Controversies over Morality and Public Health
Phase 2: 1914–1950	Tobacco Growing and Manufacturing Promoted by Governments
Phase 3: 1950–1964	The Gathering Storm of Health Concerns
Paradigm: Tobacco Restriction (Public Health)	
Phase 4: 1964–1985	Regulatory Hesitancy
Phase 5: 1985–2011	Tobacco as Social and Global Menace
Phase 6: Current	The Future: Neo-prohibitionism vs. Harm Reduction

Source: Adapted from Studlar (2002); Cairney *et al.* (2012).

the same time (Doll 1998). This began the long controversy about whether cigarettes were sufficiently hazardous to people's health that the government should discourage their use, irrespective of the economic effects. Even in the face of major reports reporting the cumulative dangers of smoking, such as that from the British Royal College of Physicians (1962) and the US Surgeon General (1964), governments were hesitant to engage in policy that would have broad social and economic effects, especially given that approximately half the population smoked (larger numbers of men than women). Thus early efforts were limited to educational efforts, including health warnings on cigarette packages, and limitations on broadcast advertising. The only exceptions to this trend were the Nordic countries of Sweden, Finland, and Iceland, who adopted early innovative policies on cessation, broad advertising bans, and rotating picture warnings (Roemer 1982). Only with the rise of scientific evidence about the effects of secondhand smoke in the 1980s did governments end their policy hesitancy and engage in a broader range of measures to reduce smoking, including stronger warning labels, greater advertising restrictions, cessation, limits on indoor smoking, and even higher taxes to reduce smoking (Studlar 2004).

Today the EU countries constitute the fifth-largest producers of tobacco leaf and the second-largest manufacturers of cigarettes (25 percent) in the world. The tobacco industry varies by country, usually a mixture of domestic producers and branches of transnational corporations. All EU members have a tobacco industry presence, either through a domestic or transnational company (European Commission 2004c). EU tobacco agriculture amounts to 4 percent of world production. Although 13 EU countries grow tobacco, Italy and Bulgaria produce most of it, followed by Poland, Greece, and Spain (Advisory Group on Tobacco 2011b). Since the quality is generally low, European leaf has been losing market share to foreign growers. Estimated employment in tobacco agriculture across the EU is 300–400,000 although figures are difficult to obtain from some countries. Because of its strong tobacco-manufacturing sector, the EU is the world's largest tobacco leaf importer (European Commission 2004c; Advisory Group on Tobacco 2011b).

The dominant manufacturers in the EU are part of a transnational oligopoly— Philip Morris International (PMI), British American Tobacco (BAT), Imperial Tobacco, and Japan Tobacco International (JTI). Although Poland manufactures more cigarettes than any other member state, the three world centers of tobacco manufacturing and export within the EU are the United Kingdom, Germany, and the Netherlands (European Commission 2004c, p. 71; Shafey *et al*. 2009; Eurostat 2009). Today, tobacco manufacturing remains highly profitable but has become a more capital-intensive, less employment-based sector. With a €48 billion gross turnover in 2006, EU manufacturing employed 64,000 while 150,000 were employed in 64,000 tobacco retail outlets in Europe. In 2007 tobacco tax revenues amounted to some €67 billion, but almost four times that amount, €230 billion, was estimated as being lost to smuggling, contraband, and counterfeiting (Tiessen *et al*. 2010; Eurostat 2009).

Smoking prevalence rates vary considerably across Europe, but have generally been converging downward. In the 1960s about half of the European population smoked. In the mid-1980s smoking prevalence remained at approximately 40 percent across Europe, including Communist countries. Generally, smoking is higher in Central and Eastern European countries than in Western ones. In all geographic regions and across times, smoking rates have been highest among men.

The most recent data indicate that smoking rates have been reduced to around 30 percent overall, still higher for men than for women and for those in the older EU than in the accession countries (Frisbee 2010). Rates range from 42 percent in Greece and 39 percent in Bulgaria to 21 percent in Finland and 16 percent in Sweden in 2009 (Tiessen *et al*. 2010). Countries that were stronger on tobacco control restrictions generally had lower prevalence rates and greater reductions in smoking over time (Wilensky 2002, p. 566; Studlar 2004; European Commission 2004c; Frisbee 2010). Nevertheless, European rates are still relatively high compared to other parts of the industrialized world such as Canada, Australia, the US, and New Zealand, where smoking rates are around 20 percent. Only a few European countries, mainly Nordic ones, had comparably low rates to these non-European leaders. Socioeconomic differences in smoking prevalence have become more pronounced as rates decrease (Tiessen *et al*. 2010).

The morbidity and mortality costs of tobacco use are substantial, including both direct health care costs, indirect losses in productivity, welfare provision, and smoking-related accidents, and intangible costs in pain and suffering. Costs have been estimated to be €363 billion in 2000, some 3.9 percent of EU GDP (Tiessen *et al*. 2010). It has been estimated that as much as 15 percent of deaths within the EU-25 in 2000 (650,000) were attributable directly to smoking (Peto *et al*. 2006), and another 79,000 due to environmental tobacco smoke (Scoggins *et al*. 2009).

Since the 1980s, European countries' responses to the tobacco epidemic have converged on policies of greater control, but there has been considerable variation across countries and over time. The accession of new members from Central and Eastern Europe in 2004 and 2007 brought into the EU even heavier-smoking populations from the former Communist bloc, where there had been almost no efforts to combat smoking (Frisbee 2010). The health and financial consequences of diseases caused by tobacco were the subject of increasing documentation. Smoking became identified as by far the largest contributor to premature death. Nevertheless, countries spent less on tobacco control measures than on more publicly visible and salient drug problems, such as illicit drugs and drunk driving. With anti-smoking campaigns and policies taking off, smoking became more concentrated in the lower socioeconomic classes of society, and the gender gap in smoking became narrower within the more industrialized democracies, even reversing the usual male dominance in Sweden. Nevertheless, these changes have been slow and in most European countries civil society movements against tobacco use were relatively weak. Until recently, most governments were reluctant to support de-normalization crusades against tobacco use similar to those undertaken in English-speaking countries (Marmor and Lieberman 2004; Wilensky 2002).

Tobacco companies have retained their corporate headquarters in various European countries, but have become increasingly transnational in their operations. Not only did they come to rely more on cheaper tobacco leaf purchased from developing countries rather than European sources, but they also sought more customers abroad as smoking declined in the industrialized democracies.

Taxes were a popular policy tool for two reasons. First, there were public health benefits due to slightly reduced numbers of smokers sensitive to the price increase. Second, any lost revenue due to fewer tobacco purchasers was more than offset by the fact that most smokers in fact remained addicted and simply purchased cigarettes at the higher price (Lewit and Coate 1982). International evidence, widely diffused by a few tobacco control political entrepreneurs such as Stan Glantz and governmental and non-governmental organizations such as the International Union Against Cancer (UICC), the World Health Organization (WHO), the World Conference on Tobacco Or Health (WCTOH), and the World Bank (WB) indicated that while price increases were the most effective policy instrument for reducing tobacco use, other instruments contributed as well (Jha and Chaloupka 2000).

By the first decade of the twenty-first century, European countries were ranked by public health specialists for their policies on media campaigns, advertising, cessation, health warnings, and public place bans as well as taxation (Joossens and Raw 2008). There remained considerable variation in policies, ranging from the United Kingdom and Ireland at the top to several Mediterranean, German-influenced countries, and Luxembourg on the bottom (see also Studlar *et al.* 2011). Public opinion has moved broadly in tandem with restrictive state measures. Over the past 25 years, opinion toward tobacco has remained highly negative in some countries and has become more uniformly unfavorable across EU members (Studlar 2009; Cairney *et al.* 2012).

EU policy

The uneven progress of tobacco control policy across European countries has led the EU to act as a facilitator and coordinator. The SEA (1987) provided for regulatory measures, such as the harmonization of health and safety standards for products, to create a single market among the then-12 member states. In order to prevent lowest common denominator policies, a "high level of health protection" was included as part of the SEA, insuring an EU role in public health. Over the past two decades there has been shared responsibility between the EU and member states for tobacco control policies. While member states retain most authority, the EU has the capacity to coordinate, complement, and support public health efforts.

In the EU system, the institutional responsibility for tobacco control policy is complex. In the executive cabinet branch of the EU, the Commission, is the main EU body for proposing tobacco control measures (Princen 2009), but other institutions also are involved. Even within the Commission, there are several directorate-generals with roles in tobacco policy. The Directorate General for Health and Consumers (DG Sanco) is the main ministry responsible, with some participation by several others, including the ministries of (1) Agriculture and Rural Development, (2) Competition, (3) Trade, (4) Regional Policy, (5) Justice, (6) Employment, (7) Social Affairs and Inclusion, and (8) Taxation and Customs Union, Audit and Anti-Fraud (though the EU does not benefit directly from tax harmonization) (Guigner 2006). A Regulatory Committee of the Commission, established under the 2001 Tobacco Products Directive (TPD), is composed of representatives of member states as well as DG Sanco civil servants. This committee meets twice per year to consider all dimensions of tobacco control, especially those concerning implementation issues and future possible proposals (Faid and Gleicher 2011).

The Council of Ministers and the EP must approve all directives. Within the Council of Ministers, the meetings of Health Ministers are frequent, and the rotating Presidency of the Council is important for moving issues to resolution (Faid and Gleicher 2011). The European Council, the meeting of member state chief executives, can also play a role by setting long-term agendas. The European Court of Justice (ECJ) becomes involved in tobacco policy if there is litigation over the legality of legislation or persistent implementation failures by states after warnings by the EU Commission. The process becomes even more complicated in the case of the EU's FCTC participation since that involves both member states and the EU developing positions for international negotiations (Faid and Gleicher 2011).

Table 13.2 presents a chronology of the major developments in EU tobacco policy. Until 1985, EU tobacco policy was almost completely concerned with promotion rather than control. Tobacco growing was included in the Common Agricultural Policy (CAP) in 1970. Although constituting only about 2 percent of CAP spending, tobacco became proportionately the most heavily EU-subsidized crop, with much greater financial support than tobacco reduction efforts (Elinder *et al.* 2003; European Commission 2004c; Guigner 2006). Starting in 1972, the EU attempted a tax harmonization regime for cigarettes in order to combat smuggling and standardize prices, but relatively little progress was made on this until the late 1980s when the entrance of three poor agrarian Mediterranean tobacco-growing countries—Spain, Greece, and Portugal—made tax harmonization more

Table 13.2 Chronology of tobacco policy in the EU

1970	Tobacco growing subsidized in Common Agricultural Policy countries (CAP)
1972	First attempts at harmonization of cigarette taxes
1985	First European anti-tobacco campaign announced
1987	*Single European Act*
1989	First EU health warnings; Television ad ban; Limits on product labeling; First EU non-binding resolution on tobacco control, second-hand smoke
1990	First limits on toxic ingredients
1992	Tax harmonization for cigarettes becomes renegotiated every few years; smokeless tobacco banned (later exceptions for Sweden and Norway)
1993	Maastricht Treaty expands EU role in health, also emphasizes markets and subsidiarity; EU-level tobacco industry became more organized
1994	First EU financing of NGO capacity-building projects
1995	First advisory body on tobacco control, BASP, ends, eventually replaced by ENSP (1997)
1996	First general EU statement on tobacco control policy (others 1999, 2002)
1997	First EU general ad ban approved (TAD1)
1999	Amsterdam Treaty, Article 129, "A high level of human health level protection shall be assured in the definition and implementation of all Community policies and activities." EU recommended policies for member states
2000	ECJ strikes down TAD1; Lisbon Process
2001	Larger health warnings: Bans on "light and mild" descriptors
2002	EU sues tobacco companies for smuggling in the US: Council recommendation on improving tobacco control.
2003	Revised EU print, telecast, and internet ad and sponsorship ban (TAD2): Graphic warning labels approved
2004	EU signs FCTC; ten new accession countries join EU
2005	Agricultural price support for tobacco reduced, to end by 2010; 10 Accession countries given delays for *acquis* on tobacco tax; Ratification of FCTC
2006	Commission refers Germany to the ECJ for lack of advertising ban transposition; Finnish Presidency emphasizes health in all policies, including tobacco.
2007	Green Paper on second-hand smoke restrictions; Two new accession members EU mandates fire-safe cigarettes
2009	Council Recommendation on Smoke-Free Environments
2010	Revised tax harmonization for tobacco products
2011	Fire-safe (reduced ignition propensity, RIP) cigarettes approved as safety standard; Consultation on revision of Tobacco Products Directive

Source: Adapted from Asare *et al.* (2009)

imperative. In 1985, at a European Council meeting, two major chief executives, François Mitterrand of France and Bettino Craxi of Italy, pushed through a resolution establishing the Europe Against Cancer program. Smoking became the principal target of this policy. The program became a major touchstone of the new EU competence in public health, enshrined in the SEA, and the Maastricht and Amsterdam Treaties.

EU policies took the form of directives, regulations, and recommendations. In the mid-1980s most of the authority for policy adoption lay with the Council of Ministers, with a qualified majority necessary to adopt policies. With responsibility for public health expanding, the Commission added a separate Directorate-General for Health and Consumer Affairs in 1999 to prepare legislation and monitor enforcement (Guigner 2004). Early (1980s and 1990s) policies included minimum cigarette tax harmonization for EU members, a standardized warning label, a television advertising ban, published limits on toxic ingredients, a ban on some smokeless forms of tobacco, (e.g., snus), and recommendations for states to restrict smoking indoors. Today, the minimum tax has reached nearly 60 percent of the product price (with transition schedules for some accession members) (Cnossen and Smart 2006), a black-and-white "tombstone" label on almost half of a pack of cigarettes, front and back), and, perhaps most famously, a general advertising ban, initiated by the EP in 1991 and finally passed in 1997. This decade-long battle over control efforts temporarily ended with the ECJ overturning the first directive in 2000, based upon Germany and tobacco companies' contention that the EU had exceeded its authority, but a more limited replacement ban, covering only transborder activities, was adopted in 2003 (Khanna 2001). The Tobacco Advertising Directive (TAD) of 2001 covered a broad array of regulations on cigarette content, labeling, oral tobacco, and descriptors. On the latter, the EU was one of the first jurisdictions in the world to ban "light and mild" cigarettes (Cairney *et al.* 2012).

In addition to its own policy interventions, the EU has provided grants to tobacco control non-governmental organizations or "public interest groups." The EU has also financed mass media campaigns for tobacco control, sued tobacco companies for cigarette smuggling, and attempted to combat smuggling, contraband, and counterfeiting through law enforcement in other ways as well.

Anti-tobacco groups found the "new realm" of EU institutions, especially the Commission and the Parliament, a more favorable venue for getting their views adopted into legislation than did tobacco manufacturers (Princen 2009). In contrast, the Council of Ministers is composed of member states, more subject to domestic political pressures from locally based tobacco interests. The four countries most opposed to the first TAD (United Kingdom, Germany, Netherlands, and Denmark) each have strong domestic tobacco industries. More generally, however, there has been a strong consensus for EU action in the Council, with the UK, Netherlands, and Denmark becoming more supportive over time while Austria joined Germany in resisting tobacco control measures (Duina and Kurzer 2004).

The tobacco industry and its allies have worked to influence the EU from within through sympathetic states (principally Germany) and front groups (European Commission 2004c; Neuman *et al.* 2002). For example, they have sought to alter the EU's excise tax policy on tobacco (Bingham 1988), opposed the Tobacco Advertising and Tobacco Products directives, tried individually (and collaboratively through the Tobacco Manufacturing associations) to weaken EU influence during the FCTC negotiations (Mamudu and Studlar 2009), and tried to block further EU tobacco control measures under the rubric of "better, less burdensome regulation." Tobacco companies also used the European Tobacco Growers' Association (UNITAB), which is an affiliate of International Tobacco Growers' Association (ITGA), to lobby the EU on tobacco control and the FCTC. Tobacco companies have also received grants from the EU regional development program to equip cigarette factories and fund training projects, which contradicts the EU commitment to reduce its citizens' economic dependence on tobacco (Barr 2010).

Princen (2009) argues that the establishment of the EU as a new venue for tobacco control policy has been to the advantage of anti-tobacco civil society groups, especially for those in member states where tobacco companies were more influential. Furthermore, those countries where corporatist interest groups, including the tobacco industry, are highly entrenched found a new, more pluralist structure in the EU and have had to adapt their strategies accordingly.

Since 1997, anti-tobacco groups in EU Member States have coalesced under a common umbrella organization, the European Network on Smoking Prevention (ENSP), set up under EU initiative and financing and based in Brussels. ENSP replaced the disbanded European Bureau of Action on Smoking Prevention (BASP), which had been the first EU-level non-state advisory body on tobacco control, and had had its EU funding withdrawn. ENSP is made up of 28 member state-level coalitions, with hundreds of member organizations and international networks active in tobacco control in Europe. ENSP's mission is to develop a strategy for coordinated action among tobacco control organizations to promote comprehensive tobacco-control policies (Gilmore and McKee 2004). More recently, ENSP's influence may have been eclipsed by the more independent Smokefree Partnership, an alliance of the European Heart Network, the European Respiratory Society, Cancer Research UK, and until 2010 the French National Cancer Institute (Smokefree Partnership 2009). Other networks such as Association of European Cancer Leagues have also become actively involved in EU tobacco control policymaking processes and programs.

The incorporation of new members, especially those from Central and Eastern European countries now freed from Soviet-style Communism, presented further opportunities for EU tobacco control. Accession conditions included developing public health infrastructure and adopting tobacco control policies congruent with EU directives, although in some cases there were derogations, especially for tax harmonization (Cnossen and Smart 2006). By 2004 the first wave of ten new entrants was accepted into the EU, followed by two more in 2007 (Szilágyi 2006; Zatoński 2003; Lipand 2007; Gilmore and McKee 2004). Under Communism there had been almost no tobacco control, yet the adoption of EU-mandated measures led to substantial improvement in the health figures for these countries over the next decade (Frisbee 2010). A further example of the wide reach of the EU "regulatory state" is that non-EU members who have treaties with the EU allowing them to access the Single Market (mainly Norway, Iceland, and Switzerland) are required to adopt EU directives on tobacco control in the interests of leveling competition (Majone 1997).

When the FCTC was negotiated in 2003, the EU and WHO, the only international organizations involved in the process, worked with states and some nongovernmental tobacco control organizations. The EU provided the largest amount of funding for conference. There was division of labor between the EU and its individual member states, with the EU speaking for its members, with consultations, when issues within EU competence were discussed. When issues were within the remit of individual members, they were free to address those in their own ways. The EU was considered a leader in the negotiations (Guigner 2009), supported the final FCTC document, and became one of the signatories in 2004; it has also participated in the ongoing WHO "Conferences of the Parties" for implementation of the treaty (Mamudu and Studlar 2009; Faid and Gleicher 2011). Nevertheless, NGOs have criticized the EU for falling short of its FCTC obligations as evidenced by its weak labeling policies, lack of stringent secondhand smoke law enforcement, and opaque decision-making ("Out of Step" 2011).

Subsequent to the TPD and the 2003 TAD, the EU has maintained its tobacco regime, but with few dramatic developments. With the policy role of the EU challenged through renewed nationalism and euro-skepticism in individual countries, DG Sanco has been most interested in small-scale initiatives. In this spirit, the EU has developed model pictorial health warnings for possible adoption by individual countries, urged members to adopt stronger clean indoor air policies, adopted fire-safe (reduced ignition propensity, self-extinguishing) cigarettes as a mandatory standard, and updated its taxation policies. Furthermore, it has phased out direct agricultural subsidies for tobacco growing.

In general, there has been a process of Europeanization of tobacco control policies since the mid-1980s. The EU generally sets a minimum regulatory standard for tobacco control. Leader countries are free to pursue more stringent measures while others only comply with the minimum, sometimes after warnings from Commission and even litigation (Joossens and Raw 2008; Studlar *et al.* 2011; European Commission 2004c; Scoggins *et al.* 2009). EU influence is especially evident in the case of the 12 recent accession members (Gilmore *et al.* 2004; McKee *et al.* 2004). Eight of the accession countries had no tobacco control instruments in place before they shed Communism; by the time of their accession, all of these countries had a full array of anti-tobacco measures. Recent EU applications for membership and later accession was associated with swift and significant policy downloading and convergence in tobacco control (Frisbee 2010). EU influence also extends to countries, such as Germany, that often resist tobacco control measures but in most cases eventually have to comply.

Existing studies indicate that the EU has had a considerable influence on the domestic tobacco control policies of its members, both through top-down and horizontal policy diffusion by the member states learning from each other in EU councils, not only the Council of Ministers but also the participation of domestic civil servants in expert committees and consultations within the EU Commission (Studlar 2009; Studlar *et al.* 2011). For instance, Finland has been the prime mover in fire-safe cigarettes implementation. Thus in tobacco control, while the EU may not have reached all of its ambitions since its role is largely limited, by the 2000 ECJ decision, to economically-related matters, it has been, as Bulmer and Padgett (2005) envisioned, "a giant transfer platform" within a structure of MLG. More recently, it has extended this role to the FCTC as well (Mamudu and Studlar 2009; Guigner 2009; Faid and Gleicher 2011).

Issue trajectory

While it is difficult to make precise assessments of the impact of EU policies, especially because of their interaction with social trends and member states policy companies, one can discuss trends and possible policy impacts. Smoking in member countries has been declining, especially over the past decade. Increasingly, EU countries are adopting more stringent regulatory measures on various policy instruments, ranging from indoor smoking to pictorial health warnings on packages. Despite minimum EU tax harmonization, there remain considerable price differences across the EU, which leads to smuggling and tax avoidance (Tiessen *et al.* 2010). Although the EU ended direct subsidies for tobacco growing in 2010, leaf producers are still able to qualify for indirect subsidies rather be compelled to grow other crops (European Parliament 2009).

The EU has become a major actor in European and global tobacco control. The EU has emerged as a leader in pictorial health warnings as well as in ingredient disclosure and product regulation. Its high minimum levels of taxation are a notable achievement. Through requiring serious movement toward tobacco control in accession countries, it has influenced a broader area of Europe. There is also the prospect that EU tobacco control policies, especially minimum taxation, may have to be accepted by neighboring countries in the negotiation of new Association Agreements ("Out of Step" 2011). The EU also has had a strong role in the financing and policy development and implementation in the FCTC (Guigner 2009).

What is left to do? With the worldwide diffusion of tobacco control movements and policy, the issues facing the EU are similar to those elsewhere on the globe (Cairney *et al.* 2012). The major dilemma is whether countries are going to continue to follow neo-prohibitionist policies designed to drive the number of smokers down, eventually to zero, or whether they will pursue policies for harm reduction and minimization. The latter option will involve cooperation, rather than confrontation, with the tobacco industry. Neo-prohibitionist policies would include plain packaging (initiated by Australia), stronger restrictions on indoor and perhaps outdoor smoking, further measures to raise taxes, establishing more uniform cigarette prices, combating smuggling, and more generally, closer compliance with the provisions of the FCTC. Altogether, this would amount to further denormalization of behavior (smoking), product (cigarette), and even producers (the industry) through interventions of prevention, protection, and cessation.

Harm-reduction/minimization policies would aim to limit smoking to a die-hard group of addicted smokers through "safer cigarettes," limited sales outlets, and alternative nicotine delivery products, such as e-cigarettes (ENDS) and snus. Harm regulation issues have created new alliances in tobacco control. Major tobacco companies have lobbied the EU to lift the snus ban, based on the favorable results for lower risks of some types of cancer for users. This move has been endorsed by some anti-smoking groups and the UK Royal College of Physicians but remains controversial. There is also the possibility of new "cigarette-like" products that might have an impact upon tobacco control. Upon an "urgent need" from the member states, in 2008 DG Sanco issued an "orientation note" on ENDS and possible EU legislation to help guide members' policy on this issue, as some had treated them as medicinal devices because of nicotine content while others had not (European Commission 2008d; Scoggins *et al*. 2009). This suggests a division in anti-tobacco ranks on the issue of harm reduction may be developing in Europe.

As of 2011, the EU had engaged in a broad public consultation and internal review of the goals and instruments of the TPD, with recommendations for revisions expected in 2012. The topics for consideration are the range of nicotine delivery products covered, labeling requirements (including possibly plain packaging), reporting and market control mechanisms, cigarette ingredients, and sales arrangements (including vending machines, regulations of promotions and displays at retail outlets, package size, minimum age, and internet sales) (Tiessen *et al*. 2010). Public consultation has occurred with unprecedented participation, much of it orchestrated from Italy by pro-tobacco interests (European Commission 2011d), and has included an impact assessment evaluating five modeled changes in policy, ranging from "no change" to the most restrictive legal changes (Tiessen *et al*. 2010).

Conclusions

Over the past 25 years, the EU has engaged in a remarkable policy transformation from economically centered tobacco promotion to a more public health tobacco control orientation. The fact that tobacco growing constituted such a small share of the economy of most member countries helped this process, as did the fact that tobacco fit into the EU Single Market regulatory realm, with no entrenched industry and grower interests represented in Brussels mainly through the CAP (Princen 2009).

The EU thus is part of the MLG network for tobacco control, extending from the WHO and FCTC on the global level to individual countries and even sub-state jurisdictions (Mamudu and Studlar 2009; Asare *et al*. 2009). The EU shares responsibility with member states for policies on taxation, health warnings, advertising and tobacco product regulation. Sub-state jurisdictions often have a large role in health education, smoking cessation, and indoor non-smoking legislation. Non-governmental organizations are an important part of this network, both as lobbyists and partners/subsidiaries of the EU. This structure allows for potential shifts of policy agendas across different venues.

The EU acts increasingly as a hub for policy diffusion, both coercive and voluntary. It sets policy frameworks, passes regulations that member states are often obliged to adopt, encourages the wider process of voluntary transfer when member states and interest groups share ideas, and engages directly with the WHO and its regional office in Europe (Guigner 2006, 2009). The effect of the EU as a source of policy diffusion has varied. Its role is relatively limited with "leader" states that have demonstrated a willingness to go beyond the consensus-based EU agenda. In contrast, its role is significant for "laggard" states that are obliged to implement EU regulations beyond their current requirements, as well as accession states mandated to engage in tobacco control as a condition of EU membership (Cairney *et al.* 2012). Overall, there has been significant policy convergence in the use of regulatory, financial, educational, and capacity-building instruments across Europe, which the EU has facilitated (Studlar *et al.* 2011).

Note

1   Thanks to Alessandro Cagossi (West Virginia University) for expert research assistance.

14 Conclusion

Paulette Kurzer

This volume on the European Union and public health has sought to examine the way in which the EU shapes European and global public health policies and outcomes and assess its impact on the national health systems of the EU member states. The findings presented in this book point out that Community provisions—the single market—were the principal dynamic in furthering the expansion of a European public health domain. Careful scrutiny of the developments of the last two decades reveals that European public health programs and policies recorded substantial progress.

EU health policy is a question of establishing a common ground with other areas of EU policymaking, in particular the EU's internal market regime. In this volume, mobility of patients and health care services, uniform nutritional labels, pan-European tobacco control, increased Community-wide standards for treatment protocols, and European health data sources and collection confirm the steady expansion of a public health domain. In addition, new European regulatory and supervisory agencies and the greater authority of the Commission to engage international health organizations also emerged in response to pressures to secure and preserve a single market.

At the same time, many authors stress the numerous limits and constraints on deepening existing programs and widening the EU's authority in public health. On the one hand, in many different areas—infectious diseases, non-communicable diseases, international presence, regulatory agencies—European institutions behave like a single actor and have left a policy or institutional trail. On the other, in every case study ranging from alcohol, global infectious diseases, to new public health agencies the EU could have achieved more if it had not faced political, financial, and legal barriers and constraints.

In this chapter, I will first summarize the divergent paths that resulted in the rise and consolidation of a European public health domain. In the next section, I will delineate some of the greatest barriers and obstacles to further growth. I conclude with some speculative thoughts on what we should expect in the near future.

The high politics of low politics

The authors of the chapters collectively point out that there are several pathways through which public health has become embedded in the European landscape.

The chapters in this volume highlight at least three separate trajectories although they often exist side by side and are mutually reinforcing. The first and most obvious route is through a legal mandate derived from the Lisbon Treaty and intergovernmental agreements. The next pathway is through the eruption of a "crisis" that severely shakes the confidence of consumers and generates political conflicts and contestation, which then opens space to propose new measures or programs that national politicians would not have found acceptable during normal times. The final trajectory is through an informal process of expert networking and collaborative research projects often linked to formal or informal committees and financed by the European Commission or DG Sanco.

Of the three pathways, there is little doubt that the surest trajectory is through legal integration and the extension of EU jurisdiction to regulate public health.

Legal integration and EU jurisdiction

Logically, the most direct pathway flows through a direct legal mandate, granted through an intergovernmental treaty and endorsed by the member governments. Occasionally, national politicians succeeded in reaching a consensus to transfer new competencies to EU institutions (European Commission) and authorize EU officials to draft and implement new programs that often address shortfalls in the single market. The free movement of goods or services may require a level of harmonization or uniformity, in order to guarantee the safety, information, and product standards are consistent for both consumers as well as producers. At the same time, divergent health and safety standards are often excuses for non-trade barriers and justify subtle discrimination against services or products from other member states. Nevertheless, as Scott Greer in Chapter 1 points out, the official treaty base is extremely thin and serves more like a declaratory statement than an established set of legislative powers. Wolfram Lamping in Chapter 2 discusses the formal treaties that endow the EU with limited competence to secure "good health for all" and "access to medical care," while the EU Charter of Fundamental Rights, incorporated in the Lisbon Treaty (2009), affirms the right of EU residents to have access to preventive health care. Yet the official treaties do not tell us how or why the public health field has expanded during the last two decades.

As many of the chapters suggest the actual momentum animating the development of different public health measures and programs is the obligation carried by the EU institutions to preserve and promote the single market. The legal foundation of the EU constitutes a weak source of policy instruments and powers; however, the EU is in charge of monitoring the proper functioning of the internal market, with the implication that it supervises the free movement of goods, persons, services and capital. It is through this legal dynamic that the EU has become an actor in the field of public health. Accordingly, over time, we see that the European Commission has managed to claim authority to pass legislation on nutritional labeling, on the sale and marketing of tobacco products, and on securing new surveillance and regulatory tools. The free movement of goods requires consistent and transparent labeling rules, nutritional information, and pan-European marketing and advertising rules with regard to alcoholic beverages and tobacco products. Paulette Kurzer, Jenny Cisneros Örnberg, and Donley Studlar (Chapters 11, 12, and 13) show how DG Sanco was able to marry "the integrity of the single market" to public health objectives. Tobacco control has moved the furthest because the public health angle was the strongest while smokers had become a minority in many European societies (Studlar *et al.* 2011; Kurzer 2011). Changes in norms and behavior influenced member governments to approve tobacco control regulations and influential NGOs and the WHO have kept pressure up on the EU and member states to abide by the anti-tobacco rules and to continue to pursue tobacco control policies.

Nutritional labeling arose to address the growing obesity crisis and required pan-European agreements on how to list ingredients on packaged food and how to regulate health claims made by food industry (Smith 2012). After much wrangling, the EU adopted uniform nutritional information labels that list calories, fat, sugar, and salt. To date, it has been hardest to reach a consensus on how to combat alcohol-related harm because numerous national governments question the authority of the EU to draft alcohol control policies while many governments have their own national approach to regulating drinking and alcohol consumption.

A legal mandate also granted the institutions of the EU the exclusive jurisdiction to represent the EU member governments in the World Trade Organization and World Health Organization. Several chapters in this volume provide intriguing examples of how the Commission manages to represent the member states in different international trade and public health fora. The WTO has numerous additional agreements governing pharmaceuticals and their intellectual property rights and also covers the trade of health services. European officials participate in these venues, representing the agenda of the EU after having aggregated and formalized the collective interests of the member states.

Holly Jarman looks at the global trade in health services where patients, professionals, and providers move both across EU borders and interact with the rest of the world. Although the treaties restrict the autonomy of the EU to conclude international trade agreements on health services, in fact, the market liberalization in the EU has generated new sources of tension between member governments, EU law and agreements, and trade with third countries. The movement of health services and medical personnel are a fact of contemporary life and will eventually compel national leaders to accept greater EU powers so that the EU can draft a common governance regime.

Both Sébastien Guigner and Elize Massard da Fonsesca examine the EU's role in global health. Officially, the EU has the right to address global health by strengthening international governance, by promoting the concept of universal health, by coupling the many different developments which influence global health—migration, trade, climate change—together and by diffusing knowledge. Massard da Fonsesca discusses the involvement of different EU agencies in the International Agreement on Trade-Related Aspects of Intellectual Property Rights (TRIPS), demonstrating that the EU has been a firm proponent of such agreements to combat fake or counterfeit trade in pharmaceuticals. She argues, moreover, that EU officials struggle to bridge the tension between "doing good"—guaranteeing access to critical medication to developing countries—and "doing right"—suing third parties suspected of possibly violating pharmaceutical patents (see also Dür and De Bièvre 2007). Health priorities are trumped by commercial considerations.

Guigner explores the partnership between the EU and WHO since both institutions are committed to promoting global health. Whereas he agrees with Studlar and Massard da Fonseca that DG Sanco established a good working relationship with the Europe regional office of the WHO, he points out that the EU is held back by its internal organizational structure and decision-making procedures, which tend to undermine its direct influence in international venues. The EU is divided into different directorate generals (departments) and the policy domain of public health is spread out over several different and competing directorate-generals.[1] At the same time, member states continue to exert influence through the EU council of ministers, which often subordinates public health to other priorities. The central tension is that the EU is neither an international public health organization (like the WHO) nor a nation state. It lacks the expertise, resources, and experiences of an international health agency and it lacks the administrative capacity of a state to deliver cohesive policies (McKee *et al.* 2010). Nonetheless, in spite of these hurdles and its limited jurisdiction, the EU has played a critical role in advancing tobacco control through the ratification of the WHO Framework Convention on Tobacco Control (FCTC) and the International Medical Products Task Force (IMPACT).

In addition, the EU has had another legal venue through which it has become increasingly engaged in health. According to the principles of the single market, health care is a service and numerous opinions issued by the Court of Justice of the EU have repeatedly affirmed the free movement of patients, providers, and health services. To be sure, member governments have no intention of Europeanizing health care and health systems, but competition law and the free movement of people and services have yielded outcomes that EU member governments did not anticipate and probably would have wished to avoid. According to the relevant articles listed in the Lisbon Treaty (2009), health belongs to the member states because national and local authorities understand better how to address health care and health system issues. Health systems and their governance belong to the member states and decisions are taken at the lowest level of policymaking and appropriate to its implementation.

However, treaty articles are no guarantee that the status quo will prevail. As both Wolfram Lamping (Chapter 2) and Holly Jarman (Chapter 8) suggest, various decisions by the Court of Justice concerning patient mobility, derived from the application of single market rules, have provided citizens with wider choice in medical care and have put pressure on national health care services to accept patients and providers from other jurisdictions or alternatively lose patients and providers to other jurisdictions (see also, Hervey and McHale 2004; Palm and Glinos 2010; Gekiere *et al.* 2010).

European officials dream of creating a true multinational European space (Ellinas and Suleiman 2012; Shore 2000). By applying the principles of free movement to health services, officials in Brussels would be instrumental in promoting a borderless European health care market. Their desire is to specify the rights of consumers and patients in terms of quality and safety standards, something which does not yet exist but may emerge in the course of further liberalization of medical and health services. EU patient mobility law is an example of informal legal integration because it is forged from a legal body of opinion based on discrete cases brought by individuals. The end result is piecemeal and incremental integration through liberalization and deregulation.

In sum, public health has taken advantage of the European legal framework in spite of its weak treaty mandate. European integration is defined by a process of market building that emphasizes deregulation, liberalization, and privatization. Market-building policies give rise to externalities that spur a new set of programs to correct or soften the impact of deregulation and liberalization. In health, market-creating policies are rare but the EU has embraced a fair number of market-correcting policies. The latter refers to new rules and regulations that protect consumers or patients from the full impact of liberalization (see Chapter 1 by Scott Greer).

Health and safety crises and their ramifications

Wolfram Lamping and Monika Steffen (2005) remind us how crises can be exceptionally productive moments for political entrepreneurs who exploit the uncertainty and political void to press for further expansion of EU competences. A crisis gives the Commission a compelling narrative with a hook to anchor pan-European initiatives and coordination. A crisis also boosts the credibility of medical, health, and national experts who may have been advocating closer European cooperation for years. The history of consumer and health regulatory activity is full of examples in which a scandal resulted in a collapse of consumer confidence and calls for closer European integration. The most famous example is obviously "mad cow disease" followed by an earlier crisis relating to blood products contaminated with the HIV/Aids virus (Ansell and Vogel 2006; Everson and Vos 2009).

Crises are great entrepreneurial opportunities for Commission officials and many rules and programs came about to guarantee that there will not be a repeat of such incidences in the future. This book describes several instances that explain why the EU became involved in health issues in spite of previous political and technical opposition. Therefore, the second trajectory outlined in the chapters of this volume locates the EU's growing involvement in public health in response to the eruption of a health or safety crisis. Stepping into this morass of conflicting signals and solutions are advocacy groups who had been lobbying for a pan-European programs and agencies from the beginning and seize the opportunity to call for consolidation and further integration of national legal systems and policy processes.

Food regulation was strengthened after the discovery of mad cow disease and after revelations about inept responses by national and European officials at the onset of the crisis. Other events which spurred new legislation and consensus came about due to food radiation, trade in organ donors and blood products, all of which generated major controversies and an erosion of consumer confidence (Farrell 2005, 2009; Meins 2003). To defuse political feuding and restore consumer anxiety, member governments signed off on new supervisory and regulatory agencies delivering more transparent and consistent systems of surveillance and intervention. For example, the European Centre for Disease Prevention and Control and European Medicine Agency arose to systematize surveillance, data collection, and craft policy options in case of a future crisis. Scott Greer explains how political leaders finally agreed to provide funding for the creation of the ECDC, which monitors and collects data and information and is supposed to prepare Europe in case of an outbreak of flu epidemic or other infectious diseases such as *Salmonella*, SARS, or *Legionella*.[2] Greer traces the agreement to establish the ECDC to the crisis and lack of confidence in European-wide food safety and animal health. The European market in livestock and agriculture/food meant that zoonoses (food-borne diseases) crossed borders unchecked, quickly spreading disease throughout the EU. Member governments concluded that it made sense to delegate the task of surveillance and diffusion of information and data to a separate (small) agency. Much of the momentum for establishing a separate entity came from the Commission, which together with advocacy groups and scientific expert networks insisted on pan-European cooperation and the institutionalization of that cooperation.

The discussions on the final mandate and jurisdiction of the ECDC took place right after the outbreak of SARS (severe acute respiratory syndrome) and its founding coincided with an outbreak of the 2005 H5N1 (avian) influenza crisis. Soon thereafter, in 2009, Europeans faced yet another epidemic, 2009 H1N1 (swine) influenza. Expectedly, the ECDC was ignored by member state authorities who refused to pool resources and determined the distribution of vaccines and antiviral medicines without consulting the staff of the ECDC. In turn, the ECDC did not have the capacity to overrule the actions of member states. However, the ECDC's main task is risk assessment and it has invested in improving the EU's capacity to observe and address future crises. It has been successful in promoting the collection of health information and health statistics, as Heather Elliott discusses in Chapter 3. In the absence of comparable and quality health figures and statistics, it would be foolish to even consider a European public health strategy. Until new programs came into being, member states operated their own information system, using their own standards and criteria and selecting different health indicators. The Commission displayed considerable leadership in pressing for a single accessible system of data reporting in order to monitor and observe European-wide health and medical trends. One of the important contributions of the ECDC is to survey and aggregate national health trends and statistics.

The EU is full of small, understaffed and underfinanced agencies (Rittberger and Wonka 2011; Groenleer 2009). Often, this is what government leaders will agree to when forced to compromise and expand EU jurisdiction in a new area. Small agencies are in fact cost effective and eventually have an impact on European health policy and health care systems. Since these agencies are literally small, their weight on the EU budget is correspondingly small. This way, European officials and national governments avoid increasing the EU budget and deflect complaints from euro-skeptic voices that tax-payers' money is spent to support the cozy lifestyle of Eurocrats.

Boris Hauray in Chapter 6 comes to a similar conclusion. The European Medicines Agency came about after lengthy political fights to establish a pan-European agency to assess and evaluate new medication released into the European market. Repeatedly, member states opposed transferring competence to the EU level and European officials could not justify the creation of a separate agency. Eventually, the consolidation of the single market required unified stand-ards for medicines. The decision to fund EMA emerged slowly, as national experts with a background in medicine pressed for its establishment. But the agency is financed and administered by the pharmaceutical sector and EMA is therefore off the budget of the Commission. An unexpected outcome of this arrangement is that the pharmaceutical sector funds its assessment and evaluations and EMA may not genuinely represent consumer and health interests.

Expert networks and research funding

A third pathway is through the funding and organization of European-wide networks of experts. Presently, this pathway may be the most common kind of European Union politics. Policy diffusion through ongoing discussions among experts, professionals, civil servants, and officials is a bottom-up process. It encourages debates and inspires new thinking and new willingness to try different arrangements and policy instruments. Informal and formal networks influence the EU agenda and generate reports, recommendations, comparative assessments, benchmarks, and policy options. Subsequently, the participants in the networks carry home new ideas and templates and attempt to convince politicians to experiment with new programs, helping to close the strikingly diverse patchwork of different institutional and policy configurations among the member states. Once differences in thinking and policies have been narrowed, political leaders may be more willing to transfer new responsibilities to the Commission since they are less likely to fight to maintain their national arrangements. This informal system of policymaking is found in many areas of regulation and decision making, which fall outside the official treaty base. It is used in pension policy, employment policy, civil liberties and minorities, and of course health policy. The Commission cultivates a community of experts and organizes workshops or establishes advisory committees to reach out to national officials and scientists who may be receptive to European intervention and who may be able to lobby the political elite back home.

The meetings and workshops, resulting in publications and follow-up meet-ings, socialize experts and officials participating in these networks to adopt a stronger Europe focus. The activities linked to networks encourage a cognitive transformation where decision makers begin to appreciate the European dimen-sion of an issue. Exposure to different lines of inquiry and different practices is a learning process that fosters greater convergence in attitudes and decision making among policy officials. In the process, professionals, experts, and officials acquire new knowledge and learn about new policy options while being subject to pressures to cooperate and collaborate (Zeitlin *et al*. 2005; Heidenreich and Bischoff 2008; Radaelli 2008).

The Commission is an important player in the establishment and funding of networks. For European officials, it is a way to push forward new initiatives. Since it is always looking for new projects that will elevate its visibility, it needs collaborators both in the national governments and European scientific community to bring any initiative to fruition.

The chapters in this book supply many examples of learning by diffusion through the existence of networks and scientific collaboration.

The chapters on smoking, alcohol, and anti-obesity measures feature the type of health projects that are often led by the Commission in consultation with biomedical experts and NGOs. Commission officials identify a health issue— drinking by young people, rising rates of obesity, uneven mortality cancer rates, divergent treatment protocols—and tap the expertise and knowledge of scientists to define and describe the exact parameters of the health issue. Advocacy groups or NGOs are often in league with the Commission and assist with the formulation of the problem and possible range of policy prescriptions. If NGOs, advocates, experts, and Commission officials succeed then the issue will land on the European agenda.

Arriving on the EU agenda is only the very first phase in a convoluted and cumbersome decision-making process (Princen 2009). Once the Commission receives the green light, the next step may be to invite a larger group of stakeholders to deliberate on possible European-wide collaboration. Because the Commission's legal mandate is weak in public health, it invites representatives of the private sector to join the deliberations with the goal of increasing voluntary compliance with new norms and objectives. That is why the Commission creates "platforms" in the field of diet/nutrition and alcohol. They are instruments to solicit a positive reaction from the private sector and a commitment to change their behavior voluntarily without actual legislation.

Policymaking through networking does not always involve the private sector or the adoption of informal rules.

François Briatte illustrates how the collection of simple health statistics and mortality rates became a venue for cross-national dissemination and learning, especially for the member states with diverging and widely digressing mortality rates. Aggregate measures, published by the EU with the assistance of local experts and scientific communities, shamed lagging member states to admit to failing to meet EU expectations. Officials in national health departments were willing to adopt new treatment protocols and evidenced-based policymaking in order to improve mortality rates of certain common cancers.

Loes Knaapen in Chapter 5 provides another example of how the EU may get involved in standards and protocols though with unexpected results. The original plan was to try to promote the formulation of standardized medical care by funding treatment guideline projects. Once that ran into numerous difficulties, Commission officials switched track and ended up fostering a template for how to address divergent treatment guidelines by funding the creation of professional networks.

As Greer mentions in the introduction, the European Commission has a limited budget. Its money gets the "biggest bang for its bucks" by nurturing scientific communities, by providing seed money for the collection of data, and by promoting transnational networks to disseminate information and expertise. It lends support to the growth of a specific European body of knowledge and it exposes decision makers to the European norms and ideas while funding European-wide professional interactions and collaboration.

Because the EU needs allies, both in the European Parliament and EU Council, another smart move is to support consumer, public health, and professional lobby groups or non-governmental organizations. The Commission provides seed money and organizes meetings and exchange of ideas in the hope of generating positive energy to justify action. NGOs and civil society organizations may not carry as much influence as industry groups, but they can publicize an issue, bring a legal case to the Court of Justice, mobilize voters, and bridge the gap between EU institutions and national or subnational organizations and authorities. Many of the chapters provide examples of this type of outside mobilization. NGOs and advocacy coalitions were critical drivers in tobacco control, obesity, alcohol, and TRIPS.

The limits to a European public health

While many of the chapters describe progress and success, the authors are not starry-eyed dreamers. Clearly, there are limits to what the EU has achieved and what it can possibly achieve in the field of public health. The limits are due to the fact that the European project is driven by economic or market integration. It involves the dismantlement of national institutions, structures, and procedures to erect a European economic space. The treaties prioritize economic integration and discourage the design of compensatory (market-correcting) or supplementary (market-creating) policies and institutions. At times, there are windows of opportunity to introduce market-correcting or market-softening policies but proponents face a gamut of political and legal obstacles until a final piece of legislation has been approved by the EU council of ministers, the European parliament, and key stakeholders. Commission officials, public health advocates, and scientific experts must anchor their action plans to a legal framework, but that legal framework does not favor investing in designing new institutions, programs, or agencies.

What is left for the EU to do is to push for programs and policies that enhance the functioning of the market. Certainly, as analyzed in this volume, on the one hand such a scenario brings about ample opportunities for innovative measures and programs because the free movement of goods and services presumes uniform standards and consistent rules. On the other, limits on Europe's public health ambitions come from the widely held belief (enshrined in the treaties) that measures proposed by the European Commission must be "proportionate." What is "proportionate" is open to interpretation and opponents of harmonization or of the Europeanization of national regulatory tasks can always claim that the EU exceeds its boundaries and should delegate its proposed mission to national authorities or agencies. As many of the chapters point out, the private sector is usually the first to argue that Brussels exceeds its authority and should refrain from meddling in the marketplace. Furthermore, private sector actors have the resources and connections to lobby both national authorities and sympathetic EU officials in rival Directorate Generals (e.g., Industry and Enterprise, Trade, or Internal Market) in order to thwart European coordination in the public health field.

Nutritional labeling, anti-smoking rules, and alcohol policy encountered serious obstacles as the private sector mobilized their allies in national governments and in other DG's in the hope of blocking pan-European measures. Tobacco interests exerted more weight in some countries than others. National officials from these countries together with tobacco companies continued to maneuver behind the scene after the EU had adopted tobacco control measures to foil the next phase of tobacco control measures centering on second-hand smoke, cigarette vending machines, cigarette displays at retail outlets, and tobacco sales over the internet (see Studlar in Chapter 13). The deliberations on combating alcohol-related harm, mainly underage drinking and drunken driving, have not been able to move beyond the admission that alcohol causes harm. Beyond that, there is much disagreement on specific solutions, precise objectives, and policy instruments, reflecting different public health traditions and definitions of harm. In no small way, however, the commercial and political weight of the European alcoholic beverage industry interfered with the formulation of European anti-drinking measures (see Cisneros Örnberg in Chapter 12).

Another example is the establishment of the European Medicines Agency (EMA), whose roots can be traced to the famous thalidomide tragedy when it was discovered that medication against morning sickness of pregnant women caused severe birth defects. In 1965, the EU adopted the very first rule requiring pre-marketing approval of the new pharmaceutical products taking into consideration their quality, safety, and efficacy. However, it took years, if not decades, before the member states agreed to create a specific agency to perform risk assessment in 1995. That agreement, moreover, granted the pharmaceutical sector the right of running that agency. While the European Medicines Agency regulates medical devices and pharmaceuticals, national governments have delegated this task to the pharmaceutical sector, which dominates its procedures and decision making. Originally created to protect the competitiveness of the European pharmaceutical industry as well as the health of European citizens, in the end, the agency is a partner of industry, not an independent regulator, as Hauray persuasively demonstrates in Chapter 6.

It is difficult to avoid the conclusion that public health is subservient to commercial interests and subject to a strict cost-benefit analysis. The European Commission assembles a board of director-generals to assess every proposal for its impact on employment, environment, enterprise, health, the regions, and so forth. But DG SANCO has no representative on that board even though the impact assessment is supposed to take into consideration health. This is indicative of how the EU bureaucracy views health and reflects its lowly status both in the Commission and among EU institutions (Greer, Elliott, Wismar, and Palm, forthcoming).

Elize Massard da Fonseca in Chapter 9 reviews the tension between the EU's commitment to strengthen the enforcement of intellectual property rights and the WHO and DG Sanco's interests in supplying generic drugs to developing countries, with limited capacity to produce their own medicine to combat malaria, HIV/AIDS, and tuberculosis. In this impasse, DG Enterprise and Industry prevailed in spite of considerable pressures from public health and consumer NGOs, who asked for a resolution that would have been more supportive of public health. The European Commission took the side of the pharmaceutical sector because DG Enterprise and Industry carries more clout than DG Health and Consumer Protection.

Private actors also help explain why the free movement of health services, providers, and patients has not (yet) undermined the integrity of national health care systems. Member governments and economic operators in the health sector have no interest in fostering a European health care field although patients use access to the Court of Justice to challenge the status quo and pressure reluctant member countries to open up the national health care system. However, individual legal cases can only make modest progress because the reality is that this initiative lacks political support in the national capitals and in national health care organizations. National governments have made it clear that health systems and services are excluded from Europeanization. Both Lamping and Jarman point out that with no support for patient mobility and patient shopping in the member states, patients encounter stubborn and difficult challenges and cross-border care is modest. Providers are not interested in treating them and insurance companies are not interested in reimbursing for care outside the national system.

In sum, public health is constrained by the same dynamics that furnishes public health proponents and advocates the opportunity to lobby for new programs and rules: the internal market.

In addition, EU public health is constrained by its modest and small budget. In the EU most funding goes to agriculture and regional development. Other EU agencies and institutions have only limited resources to engage in policy projects. In health, the European Commission cannot launch and finance traditional public health programs or policy such as vaccination or new supervisory and regulatory agencies. Manpower, resources, and budget are dwarfed by the resources available to national health systems.

EU officials must rely on member state officials to implement and enforce EU public health programs and decisions. Compliance with EU rules is, to say the least, mixed but the EU can bring member states to court for failure to implement and administer. EU institutions delegate much of the public health education information and mobilization to national agencies since there is no common language and cultural repertoire. However, it can fund research projects, workshops, scientific exchanges, data gathering and analyses, and publishes the sum total of all these efforts.

The way ahead

The EU exerts influence on national health care systems, public health, and global health in different ways while relying on a different array of instruments and policies. Certain rules and programs are driven by the internal market and provisions to establish uniform consistent standards. In some areas, the EU has scored victories—for example, tobacco control, health claims—and in other areas it has been less successful—alcohol policy. The provisions of the internal market generate opportunities for new legislation but also impose constraints and restrictions since the measures must be proportionate to the desired outcome. Many public health initiatives founder because they generate controversy and fail due to a lack of funding, the absence of a clear legal mandate, and political intervention.

Because of its modest budget, the European Commission cannot engage directly in health care or public health and has used its finite resources to establish networks of experts, gathering data centers, coordination, and voluntary participation in public health projects. What will the future bring? To be sure, the eurozone crisis and the corresponding electoral and political fall-out will crimp the latitude of the Commission to undertake bold and ambitious programs. If resources were constrained in the past, they may be even more limited in the future. Europe's political leaders are not in the mood to increase spending on health activities decided in Brussels. Thus, the future will mean more of the same in that funding for public health will be limited and the political will to deepen this area of Europeanization is absent.

However, the chapters in this volume tell us that public health in spite of its lowly status in the political machinery of the EU has in fact spread its wings in many different directions and by fortuitous accident has laid down a sturdy foundation for future policies and programs.

Scott Greer in the introduction mentions "permissive dissensus," which underpinned the gradual emergence of a European public health that is less than what it could be but more than what we would have anticipated. National governments and voters do not see eye to eye on public health, public health objectives and targets, and instruments and tools. Support for any particular program has tended to be concentrated among a small group of member states while the majority pays little attention and holds no strong opinions in favor or against. Officials in Brussels count on Europe's elite group of experts to develop an agenda and they dip into their modest budget to fund research and data collection, which tends to strengthen the networks and diffuse shared norms and knowledge. As most of Europe is focused on other more pressing issues, it ignores the day-to-day activities of the Commission, much of which is focused on such matters as how to prepare the EU for the next epidemic, how to combat harm related to lifestyle-diseases, how to improve the gathering of population statistics or other detailed information. Because member states pay little attention to public health and disagree about the importance and urgency of different programs and rules, Commission officials focus on their day-to-day routine and quietly perform their tasks by working on building up a genuine European public health domain.

Public health is low politics. Few politicians or governments care deeply one way or the other, but there are now structures, procedures, and institutions in place that facilitate the drafting of new measures and rules or programs. To answer the question of what will the future bring, it seems safe to say that it will bring more of the same: small incremental programs, tempered by an occasional setback, and capped by rare triumphs.

Notes

1 Drug addiction falls under drug policy and is mostly directed by the DG on Freedom, Security, and Justice. Food safety is under the authority of a separate agency, European Food and Safety Agency (EFSA). Public health statistics and information are collected by Eurostat. Pollution—air, water, noise, waste—fall under the auspices of the DG Environment.
2 The weird incidence of anthrax sent in letters through the US mail in 2001 was also a wake-up call for EU political leaders.

Bibliography

Abbott, F. (2002) The Doha Declaration on the TRIPS Agreement and Public Health: Lighting a Dark Corner at the WTO, *Journal of International Economic Law* 5(2), pp. 469–505.

Abbott, F. (2004) The Doha Declaration on the TRIPS Agreement and Public Health and the Contradictory Trend in Bilateral and Regional Free Trade Agreements, Occasional Paper 14, Geneva, Quaker United Nations Office.

Abbott, F. (2009) Seizure of Generic Pharmaceuticals in Transit Based on Allegations of Patent Infringement: A Threat to International Trade, Development and Public Welfare, *WIPOJ* 1, pp. 43–50.

Abraham, J. and Lewis, G. (2000) *Regulating Medicines in Europe: Competition, Expertise and Public Health*, London and New York: Routledge.

Adolph, C., Greer, S.L. and Massard da Fonseca, E. (2010) Allocation of Authority in European Health Policy, *Social Science & Medicine* 75(9), pp. 1595–603.

Advisory Group on Tobacco (2011a) Draft minutes of the Advisory Group on Tobacco, held on May 24, 2011, Agriculture and Rural Development, European Commission, available at: http://ec.europa.eu/agriculture/consultations/advisory-groups/tobacco/2011-05-24_en.pdf (accessed February 11, 2012).

Advisory Group on Tobacco (2011b) Draft minutes of the Advisory group on Tobacco, held on November 21, 2011, Agriculture and Rural Development, European Commission, available at: http://ec.europa.eu/agriculture/consultations/advisory-groups/tobacco/2011-11-21_en.pdf (accessed February 11, 2012).

AGREE Collaborative Group (2000) Guideline Development in Europe: An International Comparison, *International Journal of Technology Assessment in Health Care* 16, pp. 1039–49.

AGREE Collaborative Group (2003) Development and Validation of an International Appraisal Instrument for Assessing the Quality of Clinical Practice Guidelines: The AGREE Project, *Qual Saf Health Care* 12, pp. 18–23.

Allen, D. and Smith, M. (1990) Western Europe's Presence in the Contemporary International Arena, *Review of International Studies* 16(1), pp. 19–37.

Allin, S., Mossialos, E. and McKee, M. (2005) *Making Decisions in Public Health: A Review of Eight Countries*, Brussels: European Observatory on Health Systems and Policies.

Ansell, Christopher and Vogel, David (eds) (2006) *What's the Beef? The Contested Governance of European Food Safety*, Cambridge, MA: MIT Press.

Arunanondchai, J. and Fink, C. (2007) Trade in Health Services in the ASEAN Region, World Bank Policy Research Working Paper No. 4147, available at: http://ssrn.com/abstract=965075 (accessed February 11, 2012).

Asare, B., Cairney, P. and Studlar, D.T. (2009) Federalism and Multilevel Governance in Tobacco Policy: The European Union, the United Kingdom, and UK Devolved Institutions, *Journal of Public Policy* 29, pp. 79–102.

Asp, N.-G. and Bryngelsson, S. (2008) Health Claims in Europe: New Legislation and PASSCLAIM for Substantiation, *Journal of Nutrition* 138, pp. 1210–15.

Azevedo, R. (2009) Intervention by Brazil at WTO General Council on Seizure of 500 Kilos of Generic Medicines by Dutch Customs Authorities, *Knowledge Ecology International*, 3 February.

Babor, T., Caetano, R., Casswell, S., Edwards, G., Giesbrecht, N., Graham, K., Grube, J. *et al.* (2010) *Alcohol: No Ordinary Commodity: Research and Public Policy,* 2nd ed., Oxford: Oxford University Press.

Baggott, R. (2011) *Public Health: Policy and Politics*, 2nd ed., Basingstoke: Palgrave Macmillan.

Baldwin, P. (2005a) *Contagion and the State in Europe, 1830–1930*, Cambridge: Cambridge University Press.

Baldwin, P. (2005b) *Disease and Democracy: The Industrialized World Faces AIDS*, Berkeley, CA: University of California Press.

Barnett, T. and Sorenson, C. (2011) Infectious Disease Surveillance in the United States and the United Kingdom: From Public Goods to the Challenges of New Technologies, *Journal of Health Politics, Policy and Law* 36(1), pp. 165–85.

Barr, C. (2010) Cigarette Factories Suck in €1.5m of Funds, *Financial Times*, 2 December.

Barrett, G., Cassell, J.A., Peacock, J.L. and Coleman, M.P. (2006) National Survey of British Public's Views on Use of Identifiable Medical Data by the National Cancer Registry, *British Medical Journal* 332, no. 7549, pp. 1068–72.

Barry, A. (2001) *Political Machines: Governing a Technological Society*, London: The Athlone Press.

Baumberg, B. and Anderson, P. (2008) Health, Alcohol and EU Law: Understanding the Impact of European Single Market Law on Alcohol Policies, *European Journal of Public Health*, 18(4), pp. 392–8.

Baumgartner, F. and Jones, B. (1993) *Agendas and Instability in American Politics*, Chicago, IL: The University of Chicago Press.

Bauschke, R. (2012) Regulatory Agencies, Pharmaceutical Information and the Internet: A European Perspective, *Health Policy* 104(1), pp. 12–18.

Berg, M. (1997) Problems and Promises of the Protocol, *Soc Sci Med* 44, pp. 1081–8.

Bernauer, T. and Caduff, L. (2006) Food Safety and the Structure of the European food Industry, in C. Ansell and D. Vogel (eds) *What's the Beef? The Contested Governance of European Food Safety*, Cambridge, MA: MIT Press, pp. 81–96.

Berridge, V. (1996) *AIDS in the UK: The Making of Policy, 1981–1994*, Oxford: Oxford University Press.

Bingham, P. (1988) Tobacco Strategy Review Team: EEC Single Internal Market: 1992, available at: http://bat.library.ucsf.edu/tid/hmb08a99 (accessed September 11, 2012).

Birt, C. (2008) Response to The European Health Strategy: So What Next? *European Journal of Public Health* 18, no. 6, pp. 556–7.

Blomqvist, P. (2003) EU och välfärdens gränser [The EU and welfares borders], in P. Blomqvist (ed.) *Den gränslösa välfärdsstaten: Svensk socialpolitik i det nya Europa* [The borderless welfare state: Swedish social policy in the new Europe], Stockholm: Agora, pp. 6–33.

Black, N. (1996) Why We Need Observational Studies to Evaluate the Effectiveness of Health Care, *British Medical Journal* 312, pp. 1215–21.

Blank, R. and Burau, V. (2010) *Comparative Health Policy*, 3rd ed., Basingstoke: Palgrave Macmillan.

Bloem, B.R., van Laar, T., Keus, S.H.J., de Beer, H., Poot, E., Buskens, E., Aarden, W. and Munneke, M. on behalf of the Centrale Werkgroep Multidisciplinaire Richtlijn Parkinson 2006–2009 [Central Working Group Multidisciplinary Guideline Parkinson 2006–2009] (2010) *Multidisciplinaire richtlijn ziekte van Parkinson*, Alphen a/d Rijn, the Netherlands: Van Zuiden Communications.

Bloomberg (2009) Brazil Protests Seizure of Dr Reddys Drugs in the Netherlands, *Bloomberg*, 23 January.

Blouin, C., Drager, N. and Smith, R. (eds) (2006) *International Trade in Health Services and the GATS: Current Issues and Debates*, Washington, DC: World Bank.

Borgmeier, I. and Westenhoefer, J. (2009) Impact of Different Food Label Formats on Healthiness Evaluation and Food Choice of Consumers: A Randomised-Controlled Study, *BMC Public Health* 9, pp. 184–96.

Borraz, O. (2007) Governing Standards: The Rise of Standardization Processes in France and in the EU, *Governance* 20(1), pp. 57–84.

Börzel, T. (2002) *States and Regions in the European Union: Institutional Adaptation in Germany and Spain*, Cambridge: Cambridge University Press.

Bossy, T. and Briatte, F. (2011) Les formes contemporaines de la biopolitique, *Revue internationale de politique comparée* 18(4), pp. 7–12.

Botoseneanu, A., Wu, H., Wasserman, J. and Jacobson, P.D. (2011) Achieving Public Health Legal Preparedness: Views on Public Health Law Threaten Emergency Preparedness and Response, *Journal of Public Health* 33(3), pp. 361–8.

Bourdieu, P. (2012) *Sur l'Etat: Cours au College de France (1989–1992)*, Paris: Seuil.

Bowker, G.C. and Star, S.L. (1999) *Sorting Things Out: Classification and Its Consequences*, Cambridge, MA: MIT Press.

Bradley, E.H., Elkins, B.R., Herrin, J. and Elbel, B. (2011) Health and social Services Expenditures: Associations with Health Outcomes, *British Medical Journal Quality & Safety* 20(10), pp. 826–31.

Branch, J. (2011) Mapping the Sovereign State: Technology, Authority, and Systemic Change, *International Organization* 65(1), pp. 1–36.

Brand, H. (2010) From "Public Health in Europe" to "European Public Health," *European Journal of Public Health* 20(2), pp. 127–9.

Brand, H. (2012) Public Health Capacities in Europe (Preliminary results), Maastricht, the Netherlands: Maastricht University.

Brasil (2009) Intervention by Brazil at WTO TRIPS Council in June 2009, Ministry of Foreign Affairs.Brender, J., Christensen, J.P., Scherrer, J.R. and McNair, P. (eds) (1996) *Medical Informative Europe 96: Human Facets in Information Technologies*, Amsterdam: IOS Press.

Bretherton, C. and Vogler, J. (1999) *The European Union as a Global Actor*, London: Routledge.

Briatte, F. (2010) The Europeanization of Health System Performance: The EUROCARE study and Cancer Control in England, paper presented at the Seventeenth International Conference of the Council for European Studies (CES), Montreal, Canada, 15–17 April.

Brodscheid, A. and Coen, D. (2003) Insider and Outsider Lobbying of the European Commission: An Informational Model of Forum Politics, *European Union Politics* 4(2), pp. 165–91.

Brouwers, M. and Charette, M. (2001) Evaluation of Clinical Practice Guidelines in Chiropractic Care: A Comparison of North American Guideline Reports, *Journal of the Canadian Chiropractic Association* 45, pp. 141–53.

Brouwers, M.C., Somerfield, M.R. and Browman, G.P. (2008) A for Effort: Learning from the Application of the GRADE Approach to Cancer Guideline Development, *J Clin Oncol* 26, pp. 1025–6.

Brownell, K. and Horgen, K.B. (2004) *Food Fight: The Inside Story of the Food Industry, America's Obesity Crisis, and What We Can Do About It*, Chicago, IL: Contemporary Books.

Bruno, I. (2008) Y a-t-il un pilote dans l'Union ? Tableaux de bord, indicateurs, cibles chiffrées: les balises de la décision, *Politix* 82, pp. 95–117.

Bruno, I., Jacquot, S. and Mandin, L. (2006) Europeanization Through Its Instrumentation: Benchmarking, Mainstreaming and the Open Method of Co-Ordination . . . Toolbox or Pandora's Box? *Journal of European Public Policy* 13(4), pp. 519–36.

Bulmer, S. and Padgett, S. (2005) Policy Transfer in the European Union: An Institutionalist Perspective, *British Journal of Political Science* 35, pp. 103–26.

Buonanno, L. (2006) The Creation of the European Food Safety Authorities, in C. Ansell and D. Vogel (eds) *What's the Beef? The Contested Governance of European Food Safety*, Cambridge, MA: MIT Press, pp. 259–77.

Burau, V. (2010) *Comparative Health Policy*, 3rd ed., Basingstoke: Palgrave Macmillan.

Burgers, J.S., Bailey, J.V., Klazinga, N.S., Van Der Bij, A.K., Grol, R. and Feder, G. (2002) Inside Guidelines: Comparative Analysis of Recommendations and Evidence in Diabetes Guidelines from 13 Countries, *Diabetes Care* 25, pp. 1933–9.

Burgers, J., Cluzeau, F., Hanna, S., Hunt, C. and Grol, R. (2003) Characteristics of High-Quality Guidelines: Evaluation of 86 Clinical Guidelines Developed in Ten European Countries and Canada, *International Journal of Technology Assessment in Health Care* 19, pp. 148–57.

Busch, L. (2011) *Standards: Recipes for Reality*, Cambridge, MA: MIT Press.

Business Standard (2009a) Dealing with Nasty EU Customs, New Delhi, 10 June.

Business Standard (2009b) India Takes Drug Seizure Issues to the WTO Council, New Delhi, 4 November.

Cairney, P., Studlar, D.T. and Mamudu, H. (2012) *Global Tobacco Control: Power, Policy, Governance, and Transfer*, London: Palgrave Macmillan.

Callon, M. (1986) Some Elements of a Sociology of Translation: Domestication of the Scallops and the Fishermen of St Brieuc Bay, in John Law (ed.) *Power, Action and Belief: A New Sociology of Knowledge*, London: Routledge and Kegan Paul, pp. 196–233.

Cambrosio, A., Keating, P., Schlich, T. and Weisz, G. (2006) Regulatory Objectivity and the Generation and Management of Evidence in Medicine, *Soc Sci Med* 63, pp. 189–99.

Carpenter, D.P. (2001) *The Forging of Bureaucratic Autonomy: Reputations, Networks, and Policy Innovation in Executive Agencies, 1862-1928*, Princeton, NJ: Princeton University Press.

Carpenter, D., Chattopadhyay, J., Moffitt, S. and Nall, C. (2012) The Complications of Controlling Agency Time Discretion: FDA Review Deadlines and Postmarket Drug Safety, *American Journal of Political Science*, 56(1), pp. 98–114.

Caudron, J., Ford, N., Henkens, M., Mace, C., Kiddle-Monroe, R. and Pinel, J. (2008) Substandard Medicines in Resource-Poor Settings: A Problem That Can No Longer Be Ignored, *Tropical Medicine and International Health* 13(8), pp. 1062–72.

Chaffin, J. (2010a) Big Food Groups Win Labeling Fight, *Financial Times*, 16 March.

Chaffin, J. (2010b) Nutrition Labels Give Brussels an Awkward Case of Indigestion, *Financial Times*, 16 March.

Chanda, R. (2011) India-EU Relations in Health Services: Prospects and Challenges, *Globalization and Health* 7(1), doi: 10.1186/1744-8603-7-1.

Charlesworth, K., Galsworthy, M.J., Ernst, K., Irwin, R., Wismar, M. and McKee, M. (2011) Health Research in the European Union: Over-Controlled but Under-Measured? *European Journal of Public Health* 21(4), pp. 404–6.

Checkel, J. (2005) International Institutions and Socialization in Europe: Introduction and Framework, *International Organization* 59, pp. 801–26.

CIAA (2010) *Promoting Balanced Diets and Healthy Lifestyles: Europe's Food and Drink Industry in Action*, 2nd edition, 28 April, available at: http://www.ciaa.be/ documents/ brochures/hls2_brochure.pdf (accessed May 19, 2010).

Cisneros Örnberg, J. (2008) The Europeanization of Swedish Alcohol Policy: The Case of ECAS, *Journal of European Social Policy* 18(4), pp. 395–407.

Cisneros Örnberg, J. (2009a) Escaping Deadlock: Alcohol Policy-Making in the EU, *Journal of European Public Policy* 16(5), pp. 755–73.

Cisneros Örnberg, J. (2009b) *The Europeanization of Swedish Alcohol Policy*, Doctoral Thesis in Political Science at Stockholm University, Stockholm: US AB.

Clarke, R. (2010a) Nutrient Profiles Face Axe from Nutrition and Health Claims Regs, *Functional Ingredients*, 30 April, available at: http://newhope360.com/nutrient-profiles-face-axe-nutrition-health-claims-regs (accessed November 14, 2011).

Clarke, R. (2010b) MEPs Reject Bid to Delete Nutrient Profiles from Health Claims Regulation, *Functional Ingredients*, 21 June, available at: http://newhope360.com/ meps-reject-bid-delete-nutrient-profiles-health-claims-regulation (accessed November 14, 2011).

Clarke, R. (2011) Late Bid to Change European Commission's Mind over Health Claims, *Functional Ingredients*, 13 September, available at: http://newhope360.com/regulation-and-legislation/late-bid-change-european-commission-s-mind-over-health-claims (accessed November 14, 2011).

Cluzeau, F. (1998) Strengthening Effective Practice: Promoting the Rigorous Development of Clinical Guidelines in Europe through the Creation of a Common Appraisal Instrument, EU BIOMED2 Programme application (BMH4-98-3669), available at: http://cordis.europa.eu/data/PROJ_BIOMED/ACTIONeqDndSESSION eq22904200595ndDOCeq18ndTBLeqEN_PROJ.htm (accessed August 3, 2009).

Cnossen, S. and Smart, M. (2006) Taxation of Tobacco, in S. Cnossen (ed.) *Theory and Practice of Excise Taxation: Smoking, Drinking, Gambling, Polluting, and Driving*, Oxford: Oxford University Press.

Coen, D. (ed.) (2007) *EU Lobbying: Empirical and Theoretical Studies*, London: Routledge.

Coen, D. and Richardson, J.J.R. (eds) (2009) *Lobbying in the European Union*, Oxford: Oxford University Press.

Coker, R., Atun, R. and McKee, M. (eds) (2008) *Health Systems and the Challenge of Communicable Diseases: Experiences from Europe and Latin America*, Open University Press and European Observatory on Health Care Systems and Policies.

Coleman, M.P., Alexe, D., Albreht, T. and McKee, M. (eds) (2008) *Responding to the Challenge of Cancer in Europe*, Ljubljana, Slovenia: Institute of Public Health of the Republic of Slovenia.

Collins, Harry M. ([1985] 1992) *Changing Order: Replication and Induction in Scientific Practice*, Chicago, IL: University of Chicago Press.

Commission of the European Union (2001) *Nutrition Claims and Functional Claims*, (DG SANCO/1341/2001), available at: http://ec.europa.eu/food/fs/fl/fl03_en.pdf (accessed June 30, 2011).

Commission of the European Union (2005) *Promoting Healthy Diets and Physical Activity: A European Dimension for the Prevention of Overweight, Obesity and Chronic*

Diseases, COM(2005) 637 final, available at: http://europa.eu/legislation_summaries/public_health/health_determinants_lifestyle/c11542b_en.htm (accessed June 5, 2011).

Commission of the European Union (2007) *White Paper on a Strategy for Europe on Nutrition, Overweight and Obesity Related Health Issues* COM(2007) 279 final, Brussels, 30 May.

Committee on National Alcohol Policy and Action (2011) 8th Meeting, Luxembourg, 1–2 March, Summary Report, available at: http://ec.europa.eu/health/alcohol/docs/ev_20110301_mi_en.pdf (accessed December 13, 2011).

Community Research and Development Information Service (2011) Joint Technology Initiatives, available at: http://cordis.europa.eu/fp7/jtis/about-jti_en.html#criteria (accessed November 2011).

Cooper, A.H. and Kurzer, P. (2003) Rauch ohne Feuer: Why Germany Lags in Tobacco Control, *German Politics and Society* 68, pp. 24–47.

Corporate Europe Observatory (2010) *Patient Groups Need a Strong Dose of Transparency: How a Lax Conflict of Interest Policy Allows Patient Groups to Hide Pharma-Industry Funding*, avaialble at: http://www.corporateeurope.org/ (acccessed September 11, 2012).

Council (2001a) Council Recommendation of 5 June 2001 on the Drinking of Alcohol by Young People, in Particular Children and Adolescents, *Official Journal of the European Communities*, L 161, 16 June.

Council (2001b) Council Conclusion of 5 June 2001 on a Community Strategy to Reduce Alcohol-Related Harm, *Official Journal of the European Communities*, L 161, 16 June, (2001/C 175/01).

Council (2009) Council Conclusions on Alcohol and Health, available at: http://www.consilium.europa.eu/uedocs/cms_data/docs/pressdata/en/lsa/111638.pdf (accessed December 13, 2011).

Council of Europe (2002) *Recommendation Rec(2001)13 on Developing a Methodology for Drawing up Guidelines on Best Medical Practices*, Strasbourg: Council of Europe Publishing, available at: http://www.g-i-n.net/index.cfm?fuseaction=download&fusesubaction=template&libraryID=50 (accessed July 30, 2009).

Council of the European Union (2003) Council Conclusions of 2 December 2002 on obesity (2003/C 11/02), *Official Journal of the European Communities* C 11 Vol. 46, 17 January, available at: http://eur-lex.europa.eu/LexUriServ/LexUriServ.do?uri=OJ:C:2003:011:0003:0003:EN:PDF, (accessed June 10, 2011).

Council of the European Union (2004) Council Conclusions: On Promoting Heart Health, *Official Journal of the European Communities* C 22, January 27, available at: www.ehnheart.org/downloads/699.html (accessed September 10, 2012).

Council of the European Union (2005) *Press Release 2663rd Council Meeting Employment, Social Policy, Health and Consumer Affairs 8980/05* (Presse 117), 2–3 June, available at: http://www.consilium.europa.eu/ueDocs/cms_Data/docs/pressData/en/lsa/85263.pdf (accessed September 11, 2012).

Council of the European Union (2009) Council Conclusions on Safe and Efficient Healthcare Through eHealth, Brussels, 1 December.

Council of the European Union (2010a) Council Conclusions on Investing in Europe's Health Workforce of Tomorrow: Scope for Innovation and Collaboration, 3053rd Employment, Social Policy, Health and Consumer Affairs Council Meeting, Brussels, 7 December.

Council of the European Union (2010b) *Proposal for a Regulation of the European Parliament and of the Council on the Provision of Food Information to Consumers*

2008/0028 (COD), 22 November, available at: http://register.consilium.europa.eu/pdf/ en/10/st16/st16505.en10.pdf (accessed July 17, 2011).

Cox. H. (2000) *The Global Cigarette: Origins and Evolution of British American Tobacco 1880-1945*, Oxford: Oxford University Press.

Cozendey, C. (2009) Interview with Elize Massard da Fonseca, digital recording. Ministry of Foreign Affairs (Palacio do Itamaraty), Brasilia.

CRIOC—Centre de Recherche et d'Information des Organisations de Consommateurs (2011) PROTECT: Health Warnings and Responsibility Messages on Alcoholic Beverages: A Review of Practices in Europe. WP5 Report: Member State Experiences, available at: http://protect-project.eu/wp-content/uploads/2011/03/WP5-Alcohol-labelling-practices-in-Europe-23-03-11.pdf (accessed September 10, 2012).

Cronje, R. and Fullan, A. (2003) Evidence-Based Medicine: Toward a New Definition of Rational Medicine, *Health* 7, pp. 353–69.

Čuk, M. (2009) *Graphic Alternatives to Numerical Representation of Nutrition Facts on Food Labels*, University of Reading/Master's thesis, available at: http://www.dmagazin. si/Nutrition%20labelling.pdf (accessed June 4, 2011).

Culpepper, P.D. (2008) The Politics of Common Knowledge: Ideas and Institutional Change in Wage Bargaining, *International Organization* 62(1), pp. 1–33.

Daemmrich, A. (2004) *Pharmacopolitics: Drug Regulation in The United States and Germany*, Chapel Hill, NC: The University of North Carolina Press.

Daly, J. (2005) *Evidence Based Medicine and the Search for a Science of Clinical Care*, Berkeley: University of California Press.

Daly, Mary (2006) EU Social Policy after Lisbon, *Journal of Common Market Studies* 44(3), pp. 461–81.

Daly, Mary (2007) Whither EU Social Policy? An Account and Assessment of Developments in the Lisbon Social Inclusion Process, *Journal of Social Policy* 37(1), pp. 1–19.

Davis, K., Kingsbury, B. and Merry, S. (2011) Indicators as a Technology of Global Governance, Working Paper 2010/2 Rev., New York: Institute for International Law and Justice.

Dehousse, R. (2008) Delegation of Powers in the European Union: The Need for a Multi-Principals Model, *West European Politics* 31(4), pp. 789–805.

Delanty, G. and Rumford, C. (2005) *Rethinking Europe: Social Theory and the Implications of Europeanization*, London: Routledge, pp. 37–54.

Demortain, D. (2008) Institutional Polymorphism: The Designing of the European Food Safety Authority with Regard to the European Medicines Agency, London School of Economics: Centre for Analysis of Risk and Regulation, Discussion Paper 50.

Demortain, D. (2011) *Scientists and the Regulation of Risk: Standardising Control*, Cheltenham, UK and Northampton, MA: Edward Elgar Publishing.

de Ruijter, Anniek (2012) Moving Beyond Coordination: Health Emergencies as an Impetus for Expanding EU Public Health Policy, paper presented at the University Association for Contemporary European Studies annual conference, Passau, 3–5 September.

Desrosières, A. (2008) *Gouverner par les nombres*, Paris: Presses des Mines ParisTech.

Desrosières, A. (2010) *La politique des grands nombres: Histoire de la raison statistique*, 3rd ed., Paris: La Découverte.

DG Enterprise and Industry (2008a) *Public Consultation in Preparation of a Legal Proposal to Combat Counterfeit Medicines for Human Use: Key Ideas for Better Protection of Patents agaisnt the Risk of Counterfeit Medicines*, Brussels: Europen Commission.

DG Enterprise and Industry (2008b) *Preparation of a Legislative Proposal to Combat Counterfeit Medicines for Human Use: Summary of Responses to the Public Consultation Document*, Brussels: European Commission.

DG Trade (2005) *Strategy for the Enforcement of Intellectual Property Rights in Third Countries*, Brussels: European Commission.

DG Trade (2010) *Independent Evaluation of the Intellectual Property Rights Enforcement Strategy in Third Countries*, Brussels.

Doll, R. (1998) The First Reports on Smoking and Health, in S. Lock, L. Reynolds and E.M. Tansey (eds) *Ashes to Ashes: The History of Smoking and Health*, Amsterdam: Rodopi.

Duina, F. and Kurzer, P. (2004) Smoke in Your Eyes: The Struggle over Tobacco Control in the European Union, *Journal of European Public Policy* 11, pp. 57–77.

Dunlop, D. (1962) The Safety of Drugs, *British Medical Journal* 2(5318), pp. 1487–91.

Dür, Andreas and de Bièvre, Dirk (2007) Inclusion without Influence? NGOs in European Trade Policy, *Journal of Public Policy* 27, pp. 79–101.

Eberlein, B. and Kerwer, D. (2004) New Governance in the European Union: A Theoretical Perspective, *Journal of Common Market Studies* 42(1), pp. 121–42.

Eeckhout, P. (2011) *EU External Relations Law*, 2nd ed., Oxford: Oxford University Press.

EFSA (2011) General Guidance for Stakeholders on the Evaluation of Article 13.1, 13.5 and 14 Health Claims, *EFSA Journal* 9(4) 2135, pp. 1–24.

Egeberg, M. (2010) The European Commission, in M. Cini (ed.) *European Union Politics*, New York: Oxford University Press, pp. 125–40.

Eggers, B. and Hoffmeister, F. (2006), UN-EU Cooperation on Public Health: The Evolving Participation of the European Community in the World Health Organization, in J. Wouters, F. Hoffmeister and T. Ruys (eds) *The United Nations and the European Union: An Ever Stronger Partnership*, The Hague, the Netherlands: TMC Asser Press.

Elgström, O. and Smith, M. (eds) (2006) *New Roles for the European Union in International Politics: Concepts and Analysis*, London: Routledge.

Elinder, L.S., Joossens, L., Raw, M., Anreasson, S. and Lang, T. (2003) *Public Health Aspects of the EU Common Agricultural Policy*, Stockholm: National Institute of Public Health.

Ellinas, Antonis and Ezra Suleiman, A. (2012) *The European Commission and Bureaucratic Autonomy: Europe's Custodians*, New York: Cambridge University Press.

Elliott, H.A., Jones, D.K. and Greer, S.L. (2012) Mapping Infectious Disease Control in the European Union, *Journal of Health Politics, Policy, and Law* 37(6), pp. 933–52.

Elster, J. (1983) *Sour Grapes: Studies in the Subversion of Rationality*, New York: Cambridge University Press.

Epstein, S. (2007) *Inclusion: The Politics of Difference in Medical Research*, Chicago, IL: University of Chicago Press.

Ernst, K., Irwin, R., Galsworthy, M., McKee, M., Charlesworth, K. and Wismar, M. (2010) Difficulties of Tracing Health Research Funded by the European Union, *Journal of Health Services Research and Policy* 15(3), pp. 133–6.

Espeland, W. and Stevens, M. (2008) A Sociology of Quantification, *European Journal of Sociology (Archives Européennes de Sociologie)* 49, pp. 401–36.

EurActiv (2004) Nutrition and Health Claims Made on Foods, available at: http://www.euractiv.com/health/nutrition-and-health-claims-made-foods-linksdossier-188315 (accessed December 6, 2004).

EurActiv (2008) Industry Bashes Commission Proposals on Food Labelling, 3 March, available at: http://www.euractiv.com/print/health/industry-bashes-commission-proposals-food-labelling/article-169973 (accessed July 15, 2011).

EurActiv (2010b) Food Industry Wins Battle on Traffic Light Labels, 22 June, available at: http://www.euractiv.com/en/food-industry-wins-battle-traffic-light-labels-news-495324 (accessed February 10, 2012).

EurActiv (2010a) EU Agreement on Food Labelling Taking Shape, 2 December, available at: http://www.euractiv.com/en/specialweek- foodandresponsiblemarketing/eu-agreement-food-labelling-taking-shape-news-500201 (accessed February 10, 2012).

EurActiv (2011) Parliament to Rubber-Stamp New Food Labelling Rules, 5 July, available at: http://www.euractiv.com/cap/parliament-rubber-stamp-new-food-labelling-rules-news-506067 (accessed March 28, 2012).

EURO-PERISTAT (2008) European Perinatal Health Report, available at: www.europeristat.com (accessed September 11, 2012).

Europa Press Release (2008) Customs: Millions of Illegal Medicines Stopped by MEDI-FAKE Action, Press Release, Brussels: RAPID.

European Centre for Disease Prevention and Control (2010) *Annual Epidemiological Report on Communicable Diseases in Europe*, Stockholm, available at: http://ecdc.europa.eu/en/publications/publications/1011_sur_annual_epidemiological_report_on_communicable_diseases_in_europe.pdf (accessed June 23, 2011).

European Commission (2000) Proposal for a Council Recommendation on the Drinking of Alcohol by Children and Adolescents, COM (2000) 736 Final, 27 November.

European Commission (2002) Communication on Health and Poverty Reduction in Developing Countries, COM (2002)129, Brussels, 22 March.

European Commission (2004a) Access to Medicines: Commission Proposes to Allow Export of Generic Medicines to Poor Countries, IP/04/1332, Brussels, 29 October.

European Commission (2004b) e-Health: Making Health Better for European Citizens: An Action Plan for a European e-Health Area, SEC(2004)539.

European Commission (2004c) Strategy on European Community Health indicators (ECHI): The Short List, Luxembourg: European Commission (SANCO/C/2), available at: http://ec.europa.eu/health/ph_information/documents/ev20040705_rd09_en.pdf (accessed February 29, 2012).

European Commission (2004c) *Tobacco or Health in the European Union: Past, Present and Future*, Luxembourg: Office for Official Publications of the European Commission.

European Commission (2005) Communication: A European Programme for Action to Confront HIV/AIDS, Malaria and Tuberculosis through External Action (2007–2011), COM (2005) 179, Brussels, 27 April.

European Commission (2006a) Communication: A European Programme for Action to tackle the critical shortage of health workers in developing countries (2007–2013), COM (2006) 870, Brussels, 21 December.

European Commission (2006b) Communication from the Commission to the Council, the European Parliament, the European Economic and Social Committee and the Committee of the Regions an EU strategy to Support Member States in Reducing Alcohol Related Harm, available at: http://eur-lex.europa.eu/smartapi/cgi/sga_doc?smartapi!celexplus!prod!DocNumber&lg=en&type_doc=COMfinal&an_doc=2006&nu_doc=625 (accessed December 13, 2011).

European Commission (2007) Accelerating the Development of the eHealth Market in Europe, eHealth Taskforce Report.

European Commission (2008a) Activities of the European Union (EU) in the Tax Field in 2007, available at: http://ec.europa.eu/taxation_customs/resources/documents/taxation/gen_info/info_docs/tax_reports/report_activities_2007_en.pdf (accessed December 13, 2011).

European Commission (2008b) Communication on Telemedicine for the Benefit of Patients, Healthcare Systems, and Society, COM(2008)689 Final.

European Commission (2008c) Green Paper on the European Workforce for Health, COM (2008) 725, Brussels, 10 December.

European Commission (2008d) Orientation Note: Electronic Cigarettes and the EC Legislation, Brussels: Health and Consumer Protection Directorate-General.

European Commission (2008e) Pharmaceutical Sector Inquiry: Preliminary Report, DG Competition Staff Working Paper.

European Commission (2008f) *The State of Health in the European Community: Towards a Healthier Europe*, Luxembourg: Office for Official Publications.

European Commission (2009a) The EU Role in Global Health, Issues paper, Brussels, 14 October.

European Commission (2009b) *Communication GDP and Beyond: Measuring Progress in a Changing World*, Brussels, available at: http://eur-lex.europa.eu/LexUriServ/LexUriServ.do?uri=COM:2009:0433:FIN:EN:PDF (accessed June 24, 2011).

European Commission (2009c) *Communication Solidarity in Health: Reducing Health Inequalities in the EU*, Brussels, available at: http://ec.europa.eu/eahc/documents/news/technical_meetings/ComCom.pdf (accessed June 28, 2011).

European Commission (2010a) A Digital Agenda for Europe, COM(2010) 245, May 19th.

European Commission (2010b) A Strategy for Smart, Sustainable and Inclusive Growth, COM(2010) 2020 Final, March 3rd.

European Commission (2010c) Communication on the EU Role in Global Health, COM (2010) 128, Brussels, 31 March.

European Commission (2010d) *Global health: Responding to the Challenges of Globalization,* Commission staff working document, SEC(2010)380, 31 March.

European Commission (2010e) Health Trends and Challenges in the European Union, presentation by Paola Testori Coggi from Director-General for Health and Consumers, 23 November, Antwerp: Connaissance & Vie, available at: http://ec.europa.eu/dgs/health_consumer/information_sources/docs/speeches/ptc_connaissance_vie_en.pdf (accessed December 13, 2011).

European Commission (2010f) Possible Revision of the Tobacco Products Directive 2001/37/EC, Public Consultation Document, Brussels: DG Sanco.

European Commission (2011a) Commission Implementing Decision, providing the rules for the establishment, the management and the functioning of the network of national responsible authorities on eHealth. 2011/890/EU, December 22nd.

European Commission (2011b) Establishing a Health for Growth Programme, the Third Multi-Annual Programme of EU Action in the Field of Health for the Period 2014-2020, COM(2011) 709 Final, November 9th.

European Commission (2011c) Proposal for a Regulation of the European Parliament and of the Council on Establishing a Health for Growth Programme, the Third Multi-Annual Programme of EU Action in the Field of Health for the Period 2014–2020, Brussels, available at: http://ec.europa.eu/health/programme/docs/prop_prog2014_en.pdf (accessed August 20, 2012).

European Commission (2011d) Report on the Public Consultation on the Possible Revision of the Tobacco Products Directive (2001/37/EC), Brussels: Health and Consumer Protection Directorate-General.

European Commission (2011e) Single Market Act: Twelve Levers to Boost Growth and Strengthen Confidence, Working Together to Create New Growth, SEC(2011)467 Final.

European Commission (2012a) ICT for Better Healthcare in Europe, available at http://
ec.europa.eu/information_society/activities/health/index_en.htm.

European Commission (2012b) Proposal for a Regulation of the European Parliament and
of the Council on the Protection of Individuals with Regard to the Processing of
Personal Data and on the Free Movement of Such Data (General Data Protection
Regulation) COM (2012) 11, Brussels, available at: http://eur-lex.europa.eu/Lex
UriServ/LexUriServ.do?uri=COM:2012:0011:FIN:EN:PDF (accessed August 4, 2012).

European Commission, Directorate General Health & Consumers (2012a) Data Collection,
available at: http://ec.europa.eu/health/data_collection/tools/mechanisms/index_en.
htm (accessed March 15, 2012).

European Commission, Directorate General Health & Consumers (2012b) *Rare Diseases*,
available at: http://ec.europa.eu/health/rare_diseases/policy/index_en.htm (accessed
March 2, 2012).

European Commission, Directorate General Health & Consumers (2012c) *Indicators*,
available at: http://ec.europa.eu/health/indicators/echi/list/index_en.htm (accesed
March 16, 2012).

European Commission, Taxation and Customs Union (2010) Report on EU Customs
Enforcement of Intellectual Property Rights Results at the EU border 2010, Brussels.

European Community (2003), Council regulation (EC) No 953/2003 of 26 May 2003 to
Avoid Trade Diversion into the European Union of Certain Key Medicines, *OJ L* 135,
3 June.

European Community (2006), Regulation (EC) 816/2006 of the European Parliament and
of the Council of 17 May 2006 on Compulsory Licensing of Patents Relating to the
Manufacture of Pharmaceutical Products for Export to Countries with Public Health
Problems, *OJ L* 157, 9 June.

European Communities (2009) First Progress Report on the Implementation of the EU
Alcohol Strategy, September, Directorate-General for Health and Consumers.

European and Developing Countries Clinical Trials Partnership (2007) Independent
External Review Report, IER, 12 July.

European Federation of Pharmaceutical Industries and Associations (2010) White Paper on
the Anti-Counterfeit of Medicines, Position Papers, Brussels.

European Member States. (2012) Treaty on Stability, Coordination and Governance in the
Economic and Monetary Union, 31 January, available at: http://www.european-council.
europa.eu/media/579087/treaty.pdf (accessed March 17, 2012).

European Parliament (2006) European Parliament on Counterfeiting of Medicinal Products,
Session Document RC\629338EN.

European Parliament (2008) European Parliament Resolution of 25 September 2008 on the
White Paper on Nutrition, Overweight and Obesity-Related Health Issues, (2007/
2285(INI)), available at: http://www.europarl.europa.eu/sides/getDoc.do?type=TA&
language (accessed June 10, 2011).

European Parliament (2009) Alternative and Sustainable Production for Tobacco Cultivated
Areas in the European Union, Directorate General for Internal Policies, Policy
Department B: Structural and Cohesion Policies, Agriculture and Rural Development,
Brussels.

European Parliament (2010) *Food Information to Consumers*, 16 June, available at: http://
www.europarl.europa.eu/sides/getDoc.do?type=TA&language=EN&reference=P7-TA-
2010-0222 (accessed June 6, 2011).

European Parliament (2011) Directive 2011/62/EU of the European Parliament and of the
Council, *Official Journal of the European Union*, 2011/62/EU.

European Parliament and Council, Commission of the European Communities (1993) *Commission Communication on the Framework for Action in the Field of Public Health* (Cm. (93) 559).

European Public Health Alliance (2003) *Europe Against Cancer Programme Saves Lives*, available at: http://www.epha.org/a/591 (March 28, 2012).

European Statistical Office EUROSTAT (2009) *Health Statistic: Atlas on Mortality in the European Union*, Luxembourg: Office for Official Publications of the European Communities.

European Union (2006) Consolidated Versions of the Treaty on European Union and the Treaty Establishing the European Community, C 321 E/1, *Official Journal of the European Union*, 29 December, available at: http://eur-lex.europa.eu/LexUri Serv/LexUriServ.do?uri=OJ:C:2006:321E:0001:0331:EN:PDF (accessed December 13, 2011).

Europolitics (2005) Consumer Affairs: Parliament Set to Vote on Key Nutrition Claims Regulation, 23 May, available at: http://www.europolitics.info/consumer-affairs-parliament-set-to-vote-on-key-nutrition-claims-regulation-artr176225-24.html (accessed June 10, 2011).

Eurostat (2009) Tobacco Processing Statistic: NACE Rev. 1.1. E, available at: http://epp.eurostat.ec.europa.eu/statistics_explained/index.php/Tobacco_processing_statistics_-_NACE_Rev._1.1#Further_Eurostat_informationuropean Commission (accessed February 12, 2012).

Everson, Michelle and Vos, Ellen (2009) The Scientification of Politics and the Politicisation of Science, in M. Everson and E. Vos (eds) *Uncertain Risks Regulated*, New York: Routledge-Cavendish.

Evidence Based Medicine Working Group (1992) Evidence-Based Medicine. A New Approach to Teaching the Practice of Medicine, *JAMA* 268, pp. 2420–5.

Fahy, N. (2012) Who Is Shaping the Future of European Health Systems? *British Medical Journal* 344, p. 1712.

Fahy, N., McKee, M., Busse, R. and Grundy, E. (2011) How to meet the challenge of ageing populations, *British Medical Journal* 342, p. 3815.

Faid, M. and Gleicher, D. (2011) *Dancing the Tango: The Experience and Roles of the European Union in Relation to the Framework Convention on Tobacco Control*, Geneva: Graduate Institute, Global Health Programme.

Fairchild, A. L., Bayer, R. and Colgrove, J. (2007) *Searching Eyes: Privacy, the State, and Disease Surveillance in America*, Berkeley, CA: University of California Press.

Falkner, Gerda (1998) *EU Social Policy in the 1990s: Towards a Corporatist Policy Community*, London: Routledge.

Farani-Azevedo, M. (2009) Statement by Ambassador Maria Nazareth Farani Azevado of Brazil to WHO Executive Board on Counterfeit Medical Products IP-Health. January 27, 2009.

Farrell, Anne-Maree (2005) The Emergence of EU Governance in Public Health: The Case of Blood Policy and Regulation, in M. Steffen (ed.) *Health Governance in Europe: Issues, Challenges, and Theories*, London: Routledge, pp. 135–6.

Farrell, Anne-Maree (2009) The Politics of Risk and EU Governance of Human Material, *Maastricht Journal of European and Comparative Law* 16, pp. 41–64.

Faucher-King, F. and Le Galès, P. (2010) *The New Labour Experiment: Change and Reform under Blair and Brown*, Palo Alto, CA: Stanford University Press.

Feigenbaum, H.B., Henig, J.R. and Hamnett, C. (1998) *Shrinking the State: The Political Underpinnings of Privatization*, Cambridge: Cambridge University Press.

Ferrera, M. (2003) European Integration and National Social Citizenship: Changing Boundaries, New Structuring? *Comparative Political Studies* 36(6), pp. 611–52.

Ferrera, M. (2005) *The Boundaries of Welfare: European Integration and the New Spatial Politics of Social Protection*, Oxford: Oxford University Press.

Fervers, B., Remy-Stockinger, M., Mazeau-Woynar, V., Otter, R., Liberati, A., Littlejohns, P., Qureshi, S. *et al.* (2008) CoCanCPG: Coordination of Cancer Clinical Practice in Europe, *Tumori* 94, pp. 154–9.

Fidler, D.P. and Gostin, L.O. (2008) *Biosecurity in the Global Age: Biological Weapons, Public Health, and the Rule of Law*, Stanford, CA: Stanford University Press.

Field, M.J. and Lohr, K.N. (eds) (1990) *Clinical Practice Guidelines: Directions for a New Program, Institute of Medicine*, Washington, DC: National Academy Press.

Flash Report (2011) High-Level Meeting of the Committee on National Alcohol Policy and Action (CNAPA), Brussels, 17 November, available at: http://ec.europa.eu/health/alcohol/docs/cnapa_flashreport_en.pdf (accessed December 13, 2011).

Flynn, P. (2010) The Handling of the H1N1 Pandemic: More Transparency Needed, Report of the Council of Europe, Parliamentary Assembly, Social Health and Family Affairs Committee, 24 June.

Foucault, M. (2004) *Naissance de la biopolitique: Cours au Collège de France, 1978–1979*, Paris: Seuil.

Ford, N., Hoen, E., Adelman, C. and Norris, J. (2002) Generic Medicines Are Not Substandard Medicines, *The Lancet* 9314, p. 1351.

Fox, D.M. (2003) Population and the Law: The Changing Scope of Health Policy, *Journal of Law, Medicine and Ethics* 31, pp. 607–14.

Fox, D.M. (2012) Commentary: The Governance of Disease Control in Europe, *Journal of Health Politics, Policy, and Law* 37(6), pp. 1119–30.

Fox, D.M. and Fee, E. (eds) (1988) *AIDS: The Burdens of History*, Berkeley, CA: University of California Press.

Frau, S., Font Pous, M., Luppino, M. and Conforti, A. (2010) Risk Management Plans: Are They a Tool for Improving Drug Safety? *European Journal of Clinical Pharmacology* 66(8), pp. 785–90.

Frenck, J., Lincoln, C., Zulfiqar, A.B., Cohen, J., Crisp, N., Evans, T., Fineberg, H. *et al.* (2010) Health Professionals for a New Century: Transforming Education to Strengthen Health Systems in an Interdependent World, *The Lancet* 376, pp. 1923–58.

Frisbee, S.J. (2010) *Comprehensive Tobacco Control Policy Regimes and Population Health: Assessing Causal Loops*, Unpublished dissertation, West Virginia University.

Galsworthy, M.J., Hristovski, D., Lusa, L., Ernst, K., Irwin, R., Charlesworth, K., Wismar, M. and McKee, M. (2012) Academic Output of Nine Years of EU Investment into Health Research, *The Lancet* 380 (9846), pp. 971–2.

Garattini, S. and Bertele, V. (2010) Europe's Opportunity to Open Up Drug Regulation, *British Medical Journal* 340.

Garde, Amandine (2008) Advertising and Obesity Prevention: What Role for the European Union? *Journal of Consumer Policy* 31, pp. 25–44.

Garde, Amandine (2010) *EU Law and Obesity Prevention*, Alphen aan den Rijn, the Netherlands: Kluwer Law International.

Garrett, L. (2007) The Challenge of Global Health, *Foreign Affairs* 86(1), pp. 14–38.

Gehring, T. and Krapohl, S. (2007) Supranational Regulatory Agencies between Independence and Control: The EMEA and the Authorization of Pharmaceuticals in the European Single Market, *Journal of European Public Policy* 14(2), pp. 208–26.

Gekiere, Wouter, Baeten, Rita and Palm, Willy (2010) Free Movement of Services in the EU and Health Care, in E. Mossialos, G. Permanand, R. Baeten and T.K. Hervey (eds) *Health Systems Governance in Europe: The Role of European Union Law and Policy*, Cambridge: Cambridge University Press, pp. 461–508.

Geuijen, K., t Hart, P., Princen, S. and Yesilkagit, K. (2008) *New Eurocrats: National Civil Servants in EU Policy-Making*, Amsterdam: Amsterdam University Press.

Geyer, R. and Lightfoot, S. (2010) The Strengths and Limits of New Forms of EU Governance: The Cases of Mainstreaming and Impact Assessment in EU Public Health and Sustainable Development Policy, *European Integration* 32(4), pp. 339–56.

Gilmore, A. and McKee, M. (2004) Tobacco-Control Policy in the European Union, in E.A. Feldman and R. Bayer (eds) *Unfiltered: Conflicts over Tobacco Policy and Public Health*, Cambridge, MA: Harvard University Press.

Gilmore, A.B., Österberg, E., Heloma, A., Zatoński, W., Delcheva, E. and McKee, M. (2004) Free Trade Versus the Protection of Health: The Examples of Alcohol and Tobacco, in M. McKee, L. MacLehose and E. Nolte (eds) *Health Policy and European Union Enlargement*, Maidenhead: Open University Press.

Glinos, I. (2012) Worrying about the Wrong Thing: Patient Mobility versus Mobility of Health Care Professionals, *Journal of Health Services Research and Policy* 17, pp. 264–56.

Glinos, I.A., Baeten, R., Helble, M. and Maarse, H. (2010) A Typology of Cross-Border Patient Mobility, *Health & Place* 16(6), pp. 1145–55.

Global Fund to fight AIDS, tuberculosis and malaria (2011) Pledges and Contributions, available at: http://www.theglobalfund.org/en/about/donors/ (accessed January 10, 2012).

Goldenberg, M.J. (2009) Iconoclast or Creed? Objectivism, Pragmatism, and the Hierarchy of Evidence, *Perspectives in Biology and Medicine* 52, pp. 168–87.

Graham, I.D., Beardall, S., Carter, A.O., Glennie, J., Hébert, P.C., Tetroe, J.M., McAlister, F.A., Visentin, S. and Anderson, G.M. (2001) What Is the Quality of Drug Therapy Clinical Practice Guidelines in Canada? *Canadian Medical Association Journal* 165, pp. 157–63.

Grant, W. (2012) Agricultural Policy, Food Policy and Communicable Diseases Policy, *Journal of Health Politics, Policy, and Law* 37(6), pp. 1029–46.

Green Cowles, M., Caparaso, J. and Risse, T. (eds) (2001) *Transforming Europe: Europeanization and Domestic Change*, Ithaca, NY: Cornell University Press.

Greenwood, J. (1997) *Representing Interests in the European Union*, Basingstoke: Macmillan.

Greenwood, J. (2007) Organized Civil Society and Democratic Legitimacy in the European Union, *British Journal of Political Science* 37(2), pp. 333–57.

Greer, S.L. (2006a) *Responding to Europe: Government, NHS and Stakeholder Responses to the EU Health Policy Challenge*, London: The Nuffield Trust.

Greer, S.L. (2006b) Uninvited Europeanization: Neofunctionalism, Health Services and the EU, *Journal of European Public Policy* 13(1), pp. 134–52.

Greer, S.L. (2008) Choosing Paths in European Union Health Policy: A Political Analysis of a Critical Juncture, *Journal of European Social Policy* 18(3), pp. 219–31.

Greer, S.L. (2009a) The Changing World of European Health Lobbies, in D. Coen and J. Richardson (eds) *Lobbying the European Union: Institutions, Actors, and Issues*, Oxford: Oxford University Press, pp. 189–211.

Greer, S. L. (2009b) *The Politics of European Union Health Policies*, Maidenhead/ Philadelphia: Open University Press.

Greer, Scott L. (2011) The Weakness of Strong Policies and the Strength of Weak Policies: Law, Experimentalist Governance, and Supporting Coalitions in European Union Health Care Policy, *Regulation & Governance*, pp. 187–203.

Greer, S.L. (2012a) The European Centre for Disease Prevention and Control: Hub or Hollow Core? *Journal of Health Politics, Policy, and Law* 37(6), pp. 999–1028.

Greer, S.L. (2012b) Health in All Policies: Entrenching political will, Manuscript, University of Michigan Ann Arbor

Greer, S.L. (2012c) Polity-Making Without Policy-Making: European Union Health Care Services Policy, in J.J. Richardson (ed.) *Constructing a Policy-Making State? Policy Dynamics in the European Union*, pp. 270–91.

Greer, S.L. and Sokol, T. (Forthcoming) Rules for Rights: European Law, Health Care, and Social Citizenship, *European Law Journal*.

Greer, Scott L., Elliott H, Wismar M, and Willy Palm (Forthcoming) *European Union Health Policies*, Brussels: European Observatory on Health Systems and Policies.

Greer, Scott, Hervey, Tamara, Mackenbach, Johan P. and McKee, Martin (Forthcoming 2012) Health Law and Policy in the European Union, *The Lancet*.

Greer, S.L., and Jarman, H. (2012) Managing Risks in EU Health Services Policy: Spot Markets, Legal Certainty and Beauracratic Resistance, *Journal of European Social Policy*, 22(3), pp. 259–72.

Greer, S.L. and Mätzke, M. (2009) Introduction, in S.L. Greer (ed.) *Devolution and Social Citizenship in the United Kingdom*, Bristol: Policy Press, pp. 1–20.

Greer, S.L. and Mätzke, M. (2012) Bacteria without Borders: Communicable Disease Politics in Europe, *Journal of Health Politics, Policy and Law*, doi: 10.1215/03616878-1813763.

Greer, Scott L. and Rauscher, Simone (2011a) Destabilization Rights and Restabilization Politics: Policy and Political Reactions to European Union Healthcare Services Law, *Journal of European Public Policy* 18(2), pp. 220–40.

Greer, Scott L. and Rauscher, Simone (2011b) When Does Market-Making Make Markets? EU Health Services Policy at Work in the United Kingdom and Germany, *Journal of Common Market Studies* 49(4), pp. 797–822.

Greer, S. and Vanhercke, B. (2010) The Hard Politics of Soft Law: The Case of Health, in E. Mossialos, G. Permanand, R. Baeten and T. Hervey (eds) *Health Systems Governance in Europe: The Role of EU Law and Policy*, New York: University Press Cambridge, pp. 186–230.

Groen, L. and Niemann, A. (2010) EU Actorness under Political Pressure at the UNFCCC COP 15 Climate Change Negotiations, Paper prepared for the UACES conference, Bruges, 6–8 September.

Groenleer, M. (2009) *The Autonomy of European Union Agencies: A Comparative Study of Institutional Development*, Delft, the Netherlands: Eburon.

Groenleer, M. (2011) The Actual Practice of Agency Autonomy: Tracing the Developmental Trajectories of the European Medicines Agency and the European Food Safety Authority, *CES Papers: Open Forum* 5, pp. 1–28.

Grol, R., Cluzeau, F.A. and Burgers, J.S. (2003) Clinical Practice Guidelines: Towards Better Quality Guidelines and Increased International Collaboration, *British Journal of Cancer* 89, Sup.1, pp. 4–8.

Grol, R., Eccles, M., Maisonneuve, H. and Woolf, S. (1998) Developing Clinical Practice Guidelines: The European Experience, *Disease Management and Health Outcomes* 4, pp. 255–66.

Grossman, E. (2004) Bringing Politics Back In: Rethinking the Role of Economic Interest Groups in European Integration, *Journal of European Public Policy* 11(4), pp. 637–54.

Guidelines International Network (2002) *Position Paper*, available at: http://www.g-i-n.net/about-g-i-n/history-of-g-i-n (accessed March 22, 2010).

Guigner, S. (2004) Institutionalizing Public Health in the European Commission: The Thrills and Spills of Politicization, in A. Smith (ed.) *Politics and the European Commission: Actors, Interdependence, Legitimacy*, London: Routledge and Kegan Paul.

Guigner, S. (2006) The EU's Role in European Public Health: The Interdependence of Roles within a Saturated Space of International Organizations, in O. Elgström and M. Smith (eds) *The European Union's Roles in International Politics: Concepts and Analysis*, London: Routledge, pp. 225–44.

Guigner, S. (2007) L'européanisation cognitive de la santé: entre imposition et persuasion, in O. Baisnée and R. Pasquier (eds) *L'Europe telle quelle se fait*, Paris: CNRS Editions, pp. 263–82.

Guigner, S. (2008) *L'institutionnalisation d'un espace européen de la santé. Entre intégration et européanisation*, PhD dissertation, Rennes: Université de Rennes 1.

Guigner, S. (2009) The EU and the Health Dimension of Globalization: Playing the World Health Organization Card, in J. Orbie and L. Tortell (eds), *The European Union and the Social Dimension of Globalization: How the EU Influences the World*, Routledge, London, pp. 131–47.

Guigner, S. (2011a) L'influence de l'Union européenne sur les pratiques et politiques de santé publique: européanisation verticale et horizontale, *Sciences Sociales et Santé* 29(1), pp. 81–106.

Guigner, S. (2011b) L'Union européenne, acteur de la biopolitique contemporaine: les mécanismes d'européanisation normative et cognitive de la lutte contre le tabagisme, *Revue internationale de politique comparée* 18(4), pp. 78–90.

Guth, E. (2009) Statement of the European Comission Intervention at the WTO General Council, 3 February, available at: http://www.ip-watch.org/files/WTO_GENERAL_COUNCIL.doc (accessed October 2011).

Guyatt, G.H., Oxman, A.D., Vist, G.E., Kunz, R., Falck-Ytter, Y., Alonso-Coello, P. and Schunemann, H.J. (2008) GRADE: An Emerging Consensus on Rating Quality of Evidence and Strength of Recommendations, *British Medical Journal* 336, pp. 924–6.

Haas, E.B. (1958) *The Uniting of Europe: Political, Social and Economical Forces 1950-1957*, London: Stevens & Sons.

HAI Europe, ISDB and MiEF (2010) *The European Medicines Agency Road Map to 2015: Independence Should Be the Priority*, available at: http://www.isdbweb.org/documents/uploads/press/JointAns_EMAFiveYearPlan2010.pdf (accessed September 10, 2012).

Hall, P. (2005) Preference Formation As a Political Process: The Case of Monetary Union in Europe, in I. Katznelson and B. Weingast (eds) *Preferences and Situations: Points of Intersection between Historical and Rational Choice Institutionalism*, New York: Russell Sage Foundation.

Haltern, Ulrich (2004): Integration Through Law, in A. Wiener and T. Diez (eds) *European Integration Theory*, Oxford: Oxford University Press, pp. 177–96.

Hancher, L. (1990) *Regulating for Competition: Governement, Law, and the Pharmaceutical Industry in the United Kingdom and France*, Oxford: Clarendon Press.

Hancher, L. (2004) The European Community dimension: Coordinating Divergence, in E. Mossialos, M. Mrazek and T. Walley (eds), *Regulating Pharmaceuticals in Europe: Striving for Efficiency, Equity and Quality*, Maidenhead: Open University Press, pp. 55–79.

Hancher, L. (2010) The EU Pharmaceuticals Market: Parameters and Pathways, in E. Mossialos, G. Permanand, R. Baeten and T.K. Hervey (eds) *Health Systems Governance in Europe. The Role of European Union Law and Policy*, Cambridge: Cambridge University Press, pp. 635–82.

Hankin, R. (1996) Integrating Scientific Expertise Into Regulatory Decision-Making, *EUI Working Paper RSC*, 96(7).

Hannes, K., Van Royen, P., Aertgeerts, B., Buntinx, F., Ramaekers, D. and Chevalier, P. (2005) La validation systémique de guides de pratique clinique: l'instrument AGREE, elaboration et diffucion d'une liste internationale de critères, *Rev Med Liege* 60, pp. 949–56.

Hanson, B.T. (1998) What Happened to Fortress Europe? External Trade Policy Liberalization in the European Union, *International Organization* 52(1), pp. 55–85.

Harman, S. (2012) *Global Health Governance*, London: Routledge.

Harrison, S., Moran, M. and Wood, B. (2002) Policy Emergence and Policy Convergence: The Case of Scientific-Bureaucratic Medicine in the United States and United Kingdom, *British Journal of Politics and International Relations* 4(1), pp. 1–24.

Hatzopoulos, Vassilis G. (2002) Killing National Health and Insurance but Healing Patients? The European Market for Health Care Services after the Judgment of the ECJ in Vanbraekel and Peerbooms, *Common Market Law Review* 39(4), pp. 683–729.

Hatzopoulos, Vassilis (2008) Public Procurement and State Aids in Public Health Care Systems, *Euro Observer* 10(3), pp. 3–5.

Hatzopoulos, Vassilis G. and Stergiou, Hélène (2010) Public Procurement Law and Health Care: From Theory to Practice, *European Legal Studies*, Research Papers in Law 2/2010, Brugge.

Hauray, B. (2005a) Concurrence réglementaire contre santé publique? Le contrôle des médicaments dans l'Union européenne, *Critique Internationale* 29 (novembre), pp. 87–106.

Hauray, B. (2005b) Politique et Expertise scientifique: L'évaluation européenne des médicaments, *Sociologie du travail*, 47(1), pp. 57–75.

Hauray, B. (2006) *L'Europe du médicament. Politique – Expertise – Intérêts privés*, Paris: Presses de Sciences Po.

Hauray, B. (2007) Les laboratoires pharmaceutiques et la construction dune régulation européenne des médicaments, *Revue Française des Affaires Sociales* 3(4), pp. 235–56.

Hauray, B. and Urfalino, P. (2009) Mutual Transformation and the Development of European Policy Spaces: The Case of Medicines Licensing, *Journal of European Public Policy* 16(3), pp. 426–44.

Health and Consumer Protection Directorate-General (2006) *Labelling: Competitiveness, Consumer Information and Better Regulation for the EU* (DG SANCO Consultative Document February 2006), available at: http://ec.europa.eu/food/food/labellingnutrition/betterregulation/competitiveness_consumer_info.pdf (accessed September 11, 2012).

Heidenreich, Martin and Bischoff, Guenther (2008) The Open Method of Co-ordination: A Way to the Europeanization of Social and Employment Policies? *Journal of Common Market Studies* 46, pp. 497–532.

Héritier, A. (1999) *Policy-Making and Diversity in Europe: Escaping Deadlock*, Cambridge: Cambridge University Press.

Héritier, A. and Lehmkuhl, D. (2011) Governing in the Shadow of Hierarchy: New Modes of Governance in Regulation, in A. Héritier and M. Rhodes (eds) *New Modes of Governance in Europe: Governing in the Shadow of Hierarchy*, New York: Palgrave Macmillan, pp. 48–74.

Hervey, Tamara K. (2007) EU Law and National Health Policies: Problem or Opportunity? *Health Economics, Policy and Law* 2(1), pp. 1–6.

Hervey, T. (2008) The European Union's Governance of Health Care and the Welfare Modernization Agenda, *Regulation & Governance* 2, pp. 103–120.

Hervey, T. (2010) The Impacts of European Union Law on the Health Care Sector: Institutional Overview, *Eurohealth* 16(4), pp. 5–7.

Hervey, T. (2011) If Only It Were So Simple: Public Health Services and EU Law, in M. Cremona (ed.) *Market Integration and Public Services in the European Union*, Oxford: Oxford University Press, pp. 179–250.

Hervey, T. (2012) The Role of the European Court of Justice in the Europeanization of Communicable Disease Control: Driver or Irrelevance? *Journal of Health Politics, Policy, and Law* 37(6), pp. 975–98.

Hervey, T. and McHale, J. (2004) *Health Law and the European Union*, Cambridge: Cambridge University Press.

Hervey, T.K. and Vanhercke, B. (2010) Health Care and the EU: The Law and Policy Patchwork, in E. Mossialos, G. Permanand, R. Baeten and T.K. Hervey (eds) *Health Systems Governance in Europe: The Role of European Union Law and Policy*, Cambridge: Cambridge University Press, pp. 84–133.

Hickman, M. (2010) Food Companies in Massive Lobby to Block Colour-Coded Warnings, *The Independent*, 15 June, available at: http://www.independent.co.uk/life-style/food-and-drink/news/food-companies-in-massive-lobby-to-block-colourcoded-arnings-2000523.html?service=Print (accessed October 20, 2011).

Hill, S. and Johnson, K. (2004) Emerging Challenges and Opportunities in Drug Registration and Regulation in Developing Countries, Issues paper – Access to Medicines, London: Department for International Development (DFID) Health Systems Resource Centre.

Hilton, M. (2000) *Smoking in British Political Culture 1800–2000*, Manchester: Manchester University Press.

Hirsch, J. and Guaytt, G. (2009) Clinical Experts or Methodologists to Write Clinical Guidelines? *The Lancet* 374, pp. 273–5.

Hoeyer, K. (2010) An Anthropological Analysis of European Union (EU) Health Governance as Biopolitics: The Case of the EU Tissues and Cells Directive, *Social Science and Medicine* 70, pp. 1867–73.

Hooghe, L. and Marks, G. (2009) A Postfunctional Theory of European Integration: From Permissive Consensus to Constraining Dissensus, *British Journal of Political Science* 39(1), pp. 1–23.

Hughes, R. (2003) Definitions for Public Health Nutrition: A Developing Consensus, *Public Health Nutrition* 6, pp. 615–20.

Humpherson, E. (2010) Auditing Regulatory Reforms, in D. Oliver, T. Prosser and R. Rawlings (eds) *The Regulatory State: Constitutional Implications*, Oxford: Oxford University Press, pp. 267–82.

Hurdowar, A., Graham, I.D., Bayley, M., Harrison, M., Wood-Dauphinee, S. and Bhogal S. (2007) Quality of Stroke Rehabilitation Clinical Practice Guidelines, *Journal of Evaluation in Clinical Practice* 13, pp. 657–64.

IASO (2009) Annual Report 2009, available at: http://www.iaso.org/site_media/ uploads/ IASO_Summary_ Report_2009.pdf (accessed November 2, 2011).

Igo, S.E. (2007) *The Averaged American: Surveys, Citizens, and the Making of a Mass Public*, Cambridge, MA: Harvard University Press.

IMPACT (2007) Draft Principles and Elements for National Legislation against Counterfeit Medical Products, Geneva: WHO.

IMPACT (2011) International Medical Products Anti-Counterfeiting Taskforce: The Handbook, Geneva: International Medical Products Anti-Counterfeiting Taskforce.

India (2009) TRIPS Council June 2009, Intervention by India: Agenda Item M – OTHER BUSINESS – Seizure of Generic Drug Consignments at EC Ports.

Institute of Medicine (1997) *America's Vital Interest in Global Health: Protecting Our People, Enhancing Our Economy, and Advancing Our International Interests*, Washington, DC: National Academy Press.

Institute of Medicine (2010) *Infectious Disease Movement in a Borderless World*, Washington, DC: National Academies Press.

IOTF (2005) Obesity in Europe, *International Obesity Task Force*, 3 March, available at: http://www.iaso.org/site_media/uploads/March_2005_IOTF_Briefing_paper_Obesity_in_Europe_3.pdf (accessed November 3, 2011).

IP Watch (2009) Hope for Consensus on WHO and Counterfeits Moves to May Assembly IP Watch, 29 January.

Jacobsson, K. (2004) Between Deliberation and Discipline: Soft Governance in EU Employment Policy, in U. Mörth (ed.) *Soft Law in Governance and Regulation: An Interdisciplinary Analysis*, Cheltenham: Edward Elgar Publishing Limited, pp. 81–101.

Jarman, H. (2011a) Collaboration and Consultation: Functional Representation in EU Stakeholder Dialogues, *Journal of European Integration* 33, pp. 385–99.

Jarman, H. (2011b) Responding to the Shrinking State: Defining Public Services in the EU, Paper Prepared for Adversarial Legalism à l'Européen? Workshop, York University EU Centre of Excellence, Toronto, April.

Jarman, H. and Greer, S.L. (2010) Crossborder Trade in Health Services: Lessons from the European Laboratory, *Health Policy* 94, pp. 158–63.

Jennings, M.K. (1999) Political Responses to Pain and Loss, *American Political Science Review* 93(1), pp. 1–13.

Jha, P. and Chaloupka, F. (eds) (1999) *Curbing the Epidemic: Government and the Economics of Tobacco Control,* Washington, DC: World Bank.

Johansson, L.A. (2008) *Targeting Non-Obvious Errors in Death Certificates*, Uppsala, Sweden: Acta Universitatis Upsaliensis.

Joossens, L. and Raw, M. (2008) Avancées du contrôle du tabac dans 36 pays européens, du 2005 à 2007, *Bulletan épidémiolgique hebdomadaire* 27 May, no. 21–22, pp. 198–200.

Jupille, J. and Caporaso, J.A. (1998) States, Agency and Rules: The European Union in Global Environmental Politics, in C. Rhodes (ed.) *The European Union in the World Community*, Boulder, CO: Lynne Rienner.

Katz, R. and Fischer, J. (2010) The Revised International Health Regulations: A Framework for Global Pandemic Response, *Global Health Governance* 3(2), available at: http://blogs.shu.edu/ghg/files/2011/11/Katz-and-Fischer_The-Revised-International-Health-Regulations_Spring-2010.pdf (accessed January 10, 2012).

Katznelson, I. and Weingast, B. (eds) (2005) *Preferences and Situations: Points of Intersection between Historical and Rational Choice Institutionalism*, New York: Russell Sage Foundation.

Keating, P. and Cambrosio, A. (2009) Who's Minding the Data? Data Monitoring Committees in Clinical Cancer Trials, *Sociology of Health & Illness* 31, pp. 325–42.

Keating, P. and Cambrosio, A. (2012) *Cancer on Trial: Oncology as a New Style of Practice*, Chicago, IL: The University of Chicago Press.

Kelemen, R.D. (2011) *Eurolegalism: The Transformation of Law and Regulation in the European Union*, Cambridge, MA: Harvard University Press.

Kentikelenis, A., Karanikolos, M., Papanicolas, I., Basu, S., McKee, M. and Stuckler, D. (2011) Health Effects of Financial Crisis: Omens of a Greek Tragedy, *The Lancet* 378, pp. 1457–8.

Kermani, F. (2009) The Increasing Rapprochement between the EMEA and the FDA, *RAJ Pharma*, 21 August.

Khanna, D. (2001) The Defeat of the European Tobacco Advertising Directive: A Blow for Health, *Yearbook of European Law* 20(1), pp. 113–138.

Kickbusch, I. (2011) How Foreign Policy Can Influence Health, *British Medical Journal* 342, pp. 1345–46.

Kickbusch, I. and Lister, G. (eds) (2006) *European Perspectives on Global Health: A Policy Glossary*, Brussels: European Foundation Centre.

Kickbusch, I. and Payne, L. (2003) Twenty-First Century Health Promotion: The Public Health Revolution Meets the Wellness Revolution, *Health Promotion International* 18(4), p. 275.

Kilpeläinen, K., Aromaa, A. and the ECHIM Project (eds) (2008) *European Health Indicators: Development and Initial Implementation: Final Report of the ECHIM Project*, Publications of the National Public Health Institute, available at: http://www.echim.org/docs/ECHIM_final_report.pdf (accessed April 2, 2012).

Kilpeläinen, K., Tuomi-Nikula, A., Thelen, J., Gissler, M., Sihvonen, A., Kramers, P. and Aromaa, A. (2012) Health Indicators in Europe: Availability and Data Needs, *European Journal of Public Health* 22(2), pp. 1–6.

Kirp, D.L. and Bayer, R. (eds) (1992) *AIDS in the Industrialized Democracies: Passions, Politics, and Policies*, New Brunswick, NJ: Rutgers University Press.

Kittel, Bernhard (2002) EMU, EU Enlargement, and the European Social Model: Trends, Challenges, and Questions, Working Paper 02/1, Cologne: Max Planck Institute for the Study of Societies.

Klein, R. (2003) Evidence and Policy: Interpreting the Delphic Oracle, *Journal of the Royal Society of Medicine* 96(9), pp. 429–31.

Knab, C. (2011) Infectious Rats and Dangerous Cows: Transnational Perspectives on Animal Diseases in the First Half of the Twentieth Century, *Contemporary European History* 20(3), pp. 281–306.

Knowledge Ecology International (2009) Press Advisory: NGO Letters to WHO and WTO on Dutch Seizures of Generic Medicines In-Transit from India to Brazil, Colombia and Peru, Knowledge Ecology International, 19 February.

Kohler-Koch, B. and Rittberger, B. (2006) The Governance Turn in EU Studies, *Journal of Common Market Studies* 44, pp. 27–49.

Kokott, Juliane. (2009) Opinion of Advocate General Kokott, delivered on March 26, 2009, Case C-13/07 (Case withdrawn), reprinted in C. Herrmann and J.P. Terhechte (eds) *European Yearbook of International Economic Law 2011*, Berlin/Heidelberg: Springer-Verlag.

Koplan, J.P., Bond, C., Merson, M.H., Reddy, K.S., Rodriguez, M.H., Sewankambo, N.K. and Wasserheit J.N. (2009) Towards a Common Definition of Global Health, *The Lancet* 373(9679), pp. 1993–5.

Krapohl, S. (2008) *Risk Regulation in the Single Market: The Governance of Pharmaceuticals and Foodstuffs in the European Union*, Basingstoke: Palgrave Macmillan.

Kröger, S. (2008) Nothing But Consultation: The Place of Organized Civil Society in EU Policy-Making across Policies, *European Governance Papers* (EUROGOV), C-08-03, available at: http://ceses.cuni.cz/CESES-136-version1-7B_NMG _civil_society _ nothing_but_ consultation_kroger.pdf (accessed July 2, 2011).

Kurzer, Paulette (2011) Beyond the Boundaries of Social Policy: How Austria Copes with New Consumer Challenges, in B. Ansell, P. Cohen, R. Cox and J. Gingrich (eds) *Social Policy in the New Europe: Small European States Experiences*, New York: Berghahn.

Kurzer, P. and Cooper, A. (2011) Hold the Croissant! The European Union Declares War on Obesity, *Journal of European Social Policy* 21, pp. 107–19.

Kurzer, P. and Cooper, A. (forthcoming) Issue Framing and Policy-Making in the EU: The Struggle to Enact the Consumer Information Regulation, *Journal of European Public Policy*.

Laffan, Brigid (2002) The European Commission: Promoting EU Governance, in J.R. Grote and B. Gbikpi (eds) *Participatory Governance: Political and Societal Implications*, Opladen, Germany: Leske + Budrich.

Lalis, G. (2007) Introductory Speech of Director Georgette Lalis on WHO IMPACT International Connference Developing Effective Legislation to Combat Counterfeit Medical Products, Lisbon.

Lambert, H. (2006) Accounting for EBM: Notions of Evidence in Medicine, *Social Science and Medicine* 62, pp. 2633–45.

Lamping, Wolfram (2005) European Integration and Health Policy: A Peculiar Relationship, in M. Steffen (ed.) *Health Governance in Europe: Issues, Challenges, and Theories*, London: Routledge, pp. 18–48.

Lamping, W. and Steffen, M. (2005) Conclusion: The New Politics of European Health Policy: Moving Beyond the Nation-State, in M. Steffen (ed.) *Health Governance in Europe: Issues, Challenges, and Theories*, London: Routledge, pp. 188–200.

Lamping, W. and Steffen, M. (2009) European Union and Health Policy: The Chaordic Dynamics of Integration, *Social Science Quarterly* 90(5), pp. 1361–79.

Lampland, M. and Star, S.L. (eds) (2009) *Standards and Their Stories: How Quantifying, Classifying, and Formalizing Practices Shape Everyday Life,* Ithaca, NY: Cornell University Press.

Landelius, A.-C. (2001) *Om soft law på det sociala skyddsområdet: en EG rättslig studie* [Soft law on the social policy area: a EC legal study], Stockholm: Norstedts juridik AB.

Lang, T. (2006) Food, the Law and Public Health: Three Models of the Relationship, *Public Health* 120, pp. 30–41.

Lang, T. and Rayner, G. (2005) Obesity: A Growing Issue for European policy? *Journal of European Social Policy*, 15, pp. 301–27.

Lang, A. and Mertes, A. (2011) E-Health Policy and Deployment Activities in Europe, *Telemedicine Journal and E-Health* 17(4): 262–8.

Latour, B. (1983) Give Me a Laboratory and I Will Raise the World, in K. Knorr-Cetina and M. Mulkay (eds) *Science Observed: Perspectives on the Social Study of Science*, London and Beverly Hills: Sage, pp. 141–70.

Laugesen, M.J. and Vargas-Bustamante, A. (2010) A Patient Mobility Framework That Travels: European and United States-Mexican Comparisons, *Health Policy* 96(2–3), pp. 225–31.

Lazarou, J., Pomeranz, B.H. and Corey, P.N. (1998) Incidence of Adverse Drug Reactions in Hospitalized Patients, *Journal of the American Medical Association* 279(15), pp. 1200–5.

Lear, Julia, Mossialos, Elias and Karl, Beatrix (2010) EU Competition Law and Health Policy, in E. Mossialos, G. Permanand, R. Baeten and T.K. Hervey (eds) *Health Systems Governance in Europe: The Role of European Union Law and Policy*, Cambridge: Cambridge University Press, pp. 337–78.

Leifman, H. (2002) Trends in Population Drinking, in T. Norström (ed.) *Alcohol in Postwar Europe: Consumption, Drinking Patterns, Consequences and Policy Responses in 15 European countries*, Stockholm: National Institute of Public Health, Almqvist & Wiksell International, pp. 49–81.

Lelieveldt, H. and Princen, S. (2011) *The Politics of the European Union*, New York: Cambridge University Press.

Lenglet, A. and Hernandez Pezzi, G. (2006) Comparison of the European Union Disease Surveillance Networks Websites, *Euro Surveillance: bulletin européen sur les maladies transmissibles* [European communicable disease bulletin] 11(5), pp. 119–22.

Lewin, A., Lindstrom, L. and Nestle, M. (2006) Food Industry Promises to Address Childhood Obesity: Preliminary Evaluation, *Journal of Public Health Policy* 27, pp. 327–48.

Lewit, E.D. and Coate, D. (1982) The Potential for Using Excise Taxes to Reduce Smoking, *Journal of Health Economics* 1, pp. 121–45.

Liebfried, Stephan (2005) Social Policy: Left to the Judges and the Markets? in H. Wallace, W. Wallace and M. Pollack (eds) *Policy-Making in the EU*, 5th ed., Oxford: Oxford University Press, pp. 245–78.

Leibfried, S. and Pierson, P. (2000) Social Policy: Left to Courts and Markets? in H. Wallace, W. Wallace and M. Pollack (eds) *Policy-Making in the EU*, 4th ed., Oxford: Oxford University Press, pp. 267–92.

Liefferink, D. and Skou Andersen, M. (2002) Strategies of the Green Member States in EU Environmental Policy-Making, in A. Jordan (ed.) *Environmental Policy in the European Union: Actors, Institutions and Processes*, London: Earthscan, pp. 63–80.

Light, D.W. and Warburton, R. (2011) Demythologizing the High Costs of Pharmaceutical Research, *BioSocieties* 6(1), pp. 34–50.

Lindberg, Leon (1963) *The Political Dynamics of European Integration*, Stanford, CA: Stanford University Press.

Lipand, A. (2007) for the World Health Organization Tobacco Free Initiative, *Successful Use of Smoke-Free Policies in Tobacco Control in Estonia*, Geneva: World Health Organization.

Liverani, M. and Coker, R. (2012) Protecting Europe from Diseases: From the International Sanitary Conferences to the ECDC *Journal of Health Politics, Policy and Law*, doi: 10.1215/03616878–1813772.

Lobstein, T., Baur, L. and Uauy, R. (2004) Obesity in Children and Young People: A Crisis in Public Health, *Obesity Reviews* 5 (Supplement), pp. 4–85.

Lohr, K. and Field, M. (eds) (1992) A Provisional Instrument for Assessing Clinical Practice Guidelines, in M.J. Field and K.N. Lohr (eds) *Guidelines for Clinical Practice: From Development to Use*, Washington, DC: National Academy Press.

Lopez, A.D., Collishaw, N.E. and Piha, T. (1994) A Descriptive Model of the Cigarette Epidemic in Developed Countries, *Tobacco Control* 3, pp. 242–7.

Lubkin, G.P. (1996) Is Europe's Glass Half-Full or Half-Empty? The Taxation of Alcohol and the Development of a European Identity, Working paper, NYU School of Law, Jean Monnet Centre, available at: http://www.jeanmonnetprogram.org/papers/96/9607ind. html (accessed December 13, 2011).

McAviney, S. (2009) Ever Broader Border Controls? *Journal of Intellectual Property Law & Practice* 4(7), pp. 455–56.

MacDermid, J.C., Brooks, D., Solway, S., Switzer-McIntyre, S., Brosseau, L. and Graham, I.D. (2005) Reliability and Validity of the AGREE Instrument Used by Physical Therapists in Assessment of Clinical Practice Guidelines, *BMC Health Services Research* 5, p. 18.

McHale, J. (2010) Fundamental Rights and Health Care, in E. Mossialos, G. Permanand, R. Baeten and T.K. Hervey (eds) *Health Systems Governance in Europe: The Role of European Union Law and Policy*, Cambridge: Cambridge University Press, pp. 282–314.

McKee, D. and Stuckler, D. (2011) There Is an Alternative: Public Health Professionals Must Not Remain Silent at a Time of Financial Crisis, *European Journal of Public Health* 22(1), pp. 2–3.

McKee, M., Hervey, T.K. and Gilmore, A. (2010) Public Health Policies, in E. Mossialos, G. Permanand, R. Baeten and T.K. Hervey (eds) *Health Systems Governance in Europe: The Role of European Union Law and Policy*, Cambridge: Cambridge University Press, pp. 231–81.

McKee, M., Rosenmoller, M., MacLehose, L. and Zajac, M. (2004) The Process of Enlargement, in M. McKee, L. MacLehose and E. Nolte (eds) *Health Policy and European Union Enlargement*, Maidenhead: Open University Press.

McKee, M. and Ryan, J. (2003) Monitoring Health in Europe: Opportunities, Challenges and Progress, *European Journal of Public Health* 13 (Supplement 3), pp. 1–4.

McLean (2007) Commoditization of the International Teleradiology Market, *Journal of Health Services Research and Policy* 12(2), pp. 120–2.

MacLehose, L., Brand, H., Camaroni, I., Fulop, N., Gill, O.N., Reintjes, R., Schaefer, O., McKee, M. and Weinberg (2001) Communicable Disease Outbreaks Involving More Than One Country: Systems Approach to Evaluating the Response, *British Medical Journal (Clinical research ed.)* 323, pp. 861–3.

Majone, G. (1997) From the Positive to the Regulatory State: Causes and Consequences of Changes in the Mode of Governance, *Journal of Public Policy* 17(2), pp. 139–67.

Majone, G. (1994) The Rise of the Regulatory State in Europe, *West European Politics* 17(3), pp. 77–102.

Mamudu, H. and Studlar, D.T. (2009) Multilevel Governance and Shared Sovereignty: The European Union, Member States, and the FCTC, *Governance* 22, pp. 73–97.

Manchikanti, L., Singh, V., Derby, R., Helm, S., Trescot, A.M., Staats, P.S., Prager, J.P. and Hirsch, J.A. (2008) Review of Occupational Medicine Practice Guidelines for Interventional Pain Management and Potential Implications, *Pain Physician* 11, pp. 271–89.

Marchal, B. and Kegels, G. (2003) Health Workforce Imbalances in Times of Globalization: Brain Drain or Professional Mobility? *International Journal of Health Planning and Management* 18, pp. 89–101.

Mariotti, F., Kalonji, E., Huneau, J-F. and Margaritis, I. (2010) Potential Pitfalls: Health Claims from a Public Health Nutrition Perspective, *Nutrition Reviews* 68, pp. 624–38.

Marks, Harry (1997) *The Progress of Experiment: Science and Therapeutic Reform in the United States, 1900–1990*, Cambridge: Cambridge University Press.

Marmot, M., Friel, S., Bell, R., Houweling, T.A.J. and Taylor, S. (2008) Closing the Gap in a Generation: Health Equity through Action on the Social Determinants of Health, *The Lancet* 372(9650), pp. 1661–9.

Marmor, T.R. and Lieberman, E.S. (2004) Tobacco Control in Comparative Perspective: Eight Nations in Search of an Explanation, in E.A. Feldman and R. Bayer (eds) *Unfiltered: Conflicts over Tobacco and Public Health*, Cambridge, MA: Harvard University Press.

Márquez, X. (2007) Technologies of State: The Technological Foundations of the Modern State. Unpublished manuscript.

Mars, M. and Scott, R.E. (2010) Global E-Health Policy: A Work in Progress, *Health Affairs* 29(2), pp. 237–43.

Marsden, T., Lee, R., Flynn, A. and Thankappan, S. (2010) *The New Regulation and Governance of Food: Beyond the Food Crisis?* New York: Routledge.

Martinsen, Dorte Sindbjerg (2005) Towards an Internal Health Market with the European Court, *West European Politics* 28(5), pp. 1035–56.

Martinsen, D.S. and Vrangbæk, K. (2008) The Europeanisation of Health Care Governance: Implementing the Market Imperatives of Europe, *Public Administration* 86(1), pp. 169–84.

Mastel, G. (1996) *American Trade Laws after the Uruguay Round*, Armonk, NY: M.E. Sharpe.

May, C. (2006) Mobilising Modern Facts: Health Technology Assessment and the Politics of Evidence, *Sociology of Health & Illness* 28, pp. 513–32.

Medicines Sans Frontières (2009) MSF Briefing Paper on the Quality of Medicines, Campaign for Access to Essential Medicines.

Médecins Sans Frontières (2010a) Anti-Counterfeiting Trade Agreement (ACTA) and Its Impact on Access to Medicines, MSF Campaign for Access to Essential Medicines, Geneva, October 2010.

Médecins Sans Frontières (2010b) Europe! Hands Off Our Medicine (Design by TaunusGrafik), available at: https://action.msf.org/en_CH (accessed October 2011).

Meins, Erika (2003) *Politics and Public Outrage: Explaining Transatlantic and Intra-European Diversity of Regulations on Food Irradiation and Genetically Modified Food*, London/Munich: Lit Verlag.

Mereckiene, J., Cotter, S., D'Ancona, F., Giambi, C., Nicoll, A., Levy-Bruhl, D., Lopalco *et al.* (2010) Differences in National Influenza Vaccination Policies Across the European Union, Norway and Iceland 2008–2009, *Eurosurveillance* 15(44).

Meunier, S. and Nicolaïdis, K. Who Speaks for Europe? The Delegation of Trade Authority in the EU, *Journal of Common Market Studies* 37(3), pp. 477–501.

Michalos, A.E. (2008) *Trade Barriers to the Public Good: Free Trade and Environmental Protection*, Montreal and Kingston: McGill-Queens University Press.

Mörth, U. (2003) Europeanization as Interpretation, Translation, and Editing of Public Policies, in K. Featherstone and C.M. Radaelli (eds) *The Politics of Europeanization*, Oxford: Oxford University Press, pp. 159–78.

Mörth, U. (ed.) (2004) *Soft Law in Governance and Regulation: An Interdisciplinary Analysis*, Cheltenham: Edward Elgar Publishing Limited.

Mossialos, E., Permanand, G., Baeten, R. and Hervey, T.K. (eds) (2010) *Health Systems Governance in Europe: The Role of EU Law and Policy*, Cambridge: Cambridge University Press.

Mounier-Jack, S. and Coker, R.J. (2006) How Prepared Is Europe for Pandemic Influenza? Analysis of National Plans, *The Lancet* 367(9520), pp. 1405–11.

Muraskin, W.A. (1998) *The Politics of International Health: The Children's Vaccine Initiative and the Struggle to Develop Vaccines for the Third World*, Albany, NY: State University of New York Press.

Mykhalovskiy, E. and Weir, L. (2004) The Problem of Evidence-Based Medicine: Directions for Social Science, *Social Science and Medicine* 59, pp. 1059–69.

Nestle, M. (2002) *Food Politics: How the Food Industry Influences Nutrition and Health*, Berkeley, CA: University of California Press.

Neuman, M., Bitton, A. and Glantz, S. (2002) Tobacco Industry Strategies for Influencing European Community Tobacco Advertising Legislation, *The Lancet* 359(9314), pp. 1323–30.

Nicolaïdis, K. and Schmidt, S.K. (2007) Mutual Recognition on Trial: The Long Road to Services Liberalization, *Journal of European Public Policy* 14(5), pp. 717–34.

Niemann, Arne (1998) The PHARE Programme and the Concept of Spillover: Neofunctionalism in the Making, *Journal of European Public Policy* 5(3), pp. 428–46.

Niemann, A. (2006) *Explaining Decisions in the European Union*, Cambridge: Cambridge University Press.

Nuckols, T.K., Lim, Y.W., Wynn, B.O., Mattke, S., Maclean, C.H., Harber, P., Brook *et al.* (2008) Rigorous Development Does Not Ensure That Guidelines Are Acceptable to a Panel of Knowledgeable Providers, *Journal of General Internal Medicine* 23, pp. 37–44.

Nunn, A., Fonseca, E. and Gruskin, S. (2009) Changing Global Essential Medicines Norms to Improve Access to AIDS Treatment: Lessons from Brazil, *Global Public Health* 4(2), pp. 1–17.

Obermaier, Andreas (2009) *The End of Territoriality? The Impact of ECJ Rulings on British, German and French Social Policy*, London: Ashgate.

O'Connell, J. (1993) Metrology: The Creation of Universality by the Circulation of Particulars, *Social Studies of Science* 23, pp. 129–73.

Ogien, A. (2010) La valeur sociale du chiffre: La quantification de l'action publique entre performance et démocratie, *Revue française de socio-économie* 5, pp. 19–40.

Oh, H., Rizo, C., Enkin, M. and Jadad, A. (2005) What Is eHealth? A Systematic Review of Published Definitions, *Journal of Medical Internet Research* 7, p. 1.

Ollenschläger, G., Marshall, C., Qureshi, S., Rosenbrand, K., Burgers, J., Makela, M. and Slutsky, J. (2004) Improving the Quality of Health Care: Using International Collaboration to Inform Guidelines Programmes by Founding the Guidelines International Network (G-I-N) *Quality & Safety in Health Care* 13(6): 455–60.

Oortwijn, W., Mathijssen, J., Stoiescu, D., ten Have, A., Banta, D. and Macleod, S. (2008) External Evaluation of the ECDC: Final Report, Rotterdam: ECORYS.

Organisation for Economic Co-operation and Development (OECD) (2004) *Towards High-Performing Health Systems*, Paris: OECD Publishing.

Organisation for Economic Co-operation and Development (OECD) (2010) *Health at a Glance: Europe 2010*, Paris: OECD Publishing.

Organisation for Economic Co-operation and Development (OECD) (2011) *Health at Glance 2011: OECD Indicators*, Paris: OECD Publishing.

Orren, K. and Skowronek, S. (2004) *The Search for American Political Development*, Cambridge: Cambridge University Press.

Orzack, L.H., Kaitin, K. and Lasagna, L. (1992) Pharmaceuticals in the European Community: Barriers to Single Market Integration, *Journal of Health Politics, Policy and Law* 17(4), pp. 847–68.

Österberg, E. and Karlsson, T. (eds) (2002) *Alcohol Policies in EU Member States and Norway: A Collection of Country Reports*, Helsinki: Stakes, available at: http://ec.europa.eu/health/ph_projects/1998/promotion/fp_promotion_1998_a01_27_en.pdf (accessed December 14, 2011).

Out of Step (2011) Shadow Report from EU Tobacco Control NGOs on the European Commissions Report Dancing the Tango, Brussels; Smokefree Partnership.

Oxfam (2009) Trading Away Access to Medicines: How the European Union's Trade Agenda Has Taken a Wrong Turn, available at: http://www.oxfam.org/en/policy/trading-away-access-medicines (accessed September 10, 2012).

Oxfam (2010) Anti-Counterfeiting Trade Agreement Could Endanger Lives of People Needing Affordable Medicines, Oxfam, 19 June.

Oxfam (2011a) Eye on the Ball: Medicine Regulation – Not IP Enforcement – Can Best Deliver Quality Medicines, 143 Oxfam Briefing Paper, Oxfam.

Oxfam (2011b) Oxfam Reaction to the May 2011 Proposal for a Regulation of the European Parliament and of the Council Concerning Customs Enforcement of Intellectual Property Rights (replacing Council Regulation 1383/2003), available at: http://www.oxfamsol.be/fr/IMG/pdf/Oxfam_Reaction_to_EC_proposal_for_new_regulation_on_customs_enforcement_of_IPR.pdf (accessed October 2011).

Page, E.C. (2001) The European Union and the Bureaucratic Mode of Production, in A. Menon (ed.) *From the Nation State to Europe: Essays in Honour of Jack Hayward*, Oxford: Oxford University Press, pp. 139–57.

Palm, Willy and Glinos, Irene A. (2010) Enabling Patient Mobility in the EU: Between Free Movement and Coordination, in E. Mossialos, G. Permanand, R. Baeten and T.K. Hervey (eds) *Health Systems Governance in Europe: The Role of European Union Law and Policy*, Cambridge: Cambridge University Press, pp. 509–60.

Palmer, M., Steffen, C., Iakovidis, I. and Giorgio, F. (2009) European Commission perspective: Telemedicine for the Benefit of Patients, Health Care Systems and Society, *Eurohealth* 15(1), pp. 13–15.

Parsons, C. (2003) *A Certain Idea of Europe*, Ithaca, NY: Cornell University Press.

Patashnik, E.M. (2008) *Reforms at Risk: What Happens* After *Major Policy Changes are Enacted*, Princeton, NJ: Princeton University Press.

Permanand, G. (2006) *EU Pharmaceutical Regulation: The Politics of Policy-Making*, Manchester: Manchester University Press.

Permanand, Govin and Mossialos, Elias (2005) Constitutional Asymmetry and Pharmaceutical Policy-Making in the European Union, *Journal of European Public Policy* 12(4), pp. 687–709.

Peters, B.G., Rhodes, R.A.W. and Wright, V. (2000) Staffing the Summit: The Administration of the Core Executive: Convergent Trends and National Specificities, in B.G. Peters, R.A.W. Rhodes and V. Wright (eds) *Administering the Summit: Administration of the Core Executive in Developed Countries*, Basingstoke: Macmillan, pp. 2–23.

Peto, R., Lopez, A.D., Boreham, J. and Thun, M. (2006) *Mortality from Smoking in Developed Countries 1950–2000*, 2nd revised ed., available at: http://www.ctsu.lox.ac.uk/tobacco/C4170.pdf (accessed September 11, 2012).

Pharmabiz (2010) WHO Executive Board Meet on Jan 18 to Focus on Funding Research for Neglected Disease, Pharmabiz, 18 January.

Pierson, P. (1994) *Dismantling the Welfare State? Reagan, Thatcher, and the Politics of Retrenchment*, Cambridge: Cambridge University Press.

Pirmohamed, M., James, S., Meakin, S., Green, C., Scott, A.K., Walley, T.J., Farrar, K., Park, B.K. and Breckenridge, A.M. (2004) Adverse Drug Reactions as Cause of Admission to Hospital: Prospective Analysis of 18,820 Patients, *British Medical Journal* 329(7456), pp. 15–19.

Pollack, M.A. (2003) *The Engines of European Integration: Delegation, Agency, and Agenda Setting in the EU*, Oxford: Oxford University Press.

Pollitt, C., Bathgate, K., Caulfield, J., Smullen, A. and Talbot, C. (2001) Agency Fever? Analysis of an International Policy Fashion, *Journal of Comparative Policy Analysis* 3, pp. 271–90.

Popkin, B.M., Adair, L.S. and Ng, S.W. (2012) Global Nutrition Transition and the Pandemic of Obesity in Developing Countries, *Nutrition Reviews* 70, pp. 3–21.

Porter, T.M. (1995) *Trust in Numbers: The Pursuit of Objectivity in Science and Public Life*, Princeton, NJ: Princeton University Press.

Press release (2004) Alcohol Taxation: Commission Launches Debate, IP/04/669, Brussels, 26 May.

Princen, S. (2007) Advocacy Coalitions and the Internationalization of Public Health Policies, *Journal of Public Policy* 27, pp. 13–33.

Princen, S. (2009) *Agenda-Setting in the European Union*, New York: Palgrave Macmillan.

Proctor, R. (1999) *The Nazi War on Cancer*, Princeton, NJ: Princeton University Press.

Rabinovich, L., Brutscher, P-B., de Vries, H., Tiessen, J., Clift, J. and Reding, A. (2009) The Affordability of Alcohol Beverages in the European Union, RAND Europe, Technical report.

Radaelli, C. (2003) The Europeanization of Public Policy, in K. Featherstone and C.M. Radaelli (eds) *The Politics of Europeanization*, Oxford: Oxford University Press, pp. 27–56.

Radaelli, Claudio (2008) Europeanization, Policy Learning, and New Modes of Governance, *Journal of Comparative Policy Analysis* 10, pp. 239–54.

Radaelli, C. and Pasquier, R. (2007) Conceptual Issues, in P. Graziano and M.P. Vink (eds) *Europeanization: New Research Agendas*, Basingstoke: Palgrave Macmillan, pp. 35–45.

Randall, Ed (2000) European Union Health Policy With and Without Design: Serendipity, Tragedy and the Future of EU Health Policy, *Policy Studies* 21(2), pp. 133–64.

Randall, E. (2001) *The European Union and Health Policy*, Basingstoke: Palgrave.

Rasmussen, M.K. (2011) Lobbying the European Parliament: A Necessary Evil, *CEPS Policy Brief* No. 242, May 2011.

Reintjes, R. (2012) Variation Matters: Epidemiological Surveillance in Europe, *Journal of Health Politics, Policy, and Law* 37(6), pp. 953–63.

Reintjes, R., Thelen, M., Reiche, R. and Csohan, A. (2007) Benchmarking National Surveillance Systems: A New Tool for the Comparison of Communicable Disease Surveillance and Control in Europe, *European Journal of Public Health* 17(4), pp. 375–80.

Reuters (2009) Brazil to Object to Dutch Seizure of Generic Drugs, Reuters, 23 January.

Rhodes, M. (1995) A Regulatory Conundrum: Industrial Relations and the Social Dimension, in S. Leibfried and P. Pierson (eds) *European Social Policy: Between Fragmentation and Integration*, Washington, DC: Brookings Institution, pp. 78–122.

Rigaud, A. and Craplet, M. (2004) The Loi Evin: A French Exception, *The Globe* no. 1–2, pp. 33–6, available at: http://www.ias.org.uk/resources/publications/theglobe/globe200401-02/gl200401-02_p33.html (accessed February 13, 2012).

Risse, T. (2000) Let's Argue! Communicative Action in World Politics, *International Organization* 54(1), pp. 1–39.

Rittberger, Berthold and Wonka, Arndt (2012) Introduction: Agency Governance in the European Union, *Journal of European Public Policy* 18, pp. 780–9.

Roemer, R. (1982) *Legislative Action to Combat the World Tobacco Epidemic*, Geneva: World Health Organization.

Room, R. (1999) The Idea of Alcohol Policy, *Nordic Studies on Alcohol and Drugs* 16 (English supplement), pp. 7–20.

Rothgang, H., Cacace, M., Frisina, L., Grimmeisen, S., Schmid, A. and Wendt, C. (eds) (2010) *The State and Healthcare: Comparing OECD Countries*, Basingstoke: Palgrave Macmillan.

Rumford, C. (2002) *The European Union: A Political Sociology*, Oxford: Blackwell Publishing, pp. 46–81.

Sabel, C.F. and Zeitlin, J. (2007) Learning from Difference: The New Architecture of Experimentalist Governance in the *European Union, European Law Journal* 14(3), pp. 271–327.

Sackett, D.L. and Rosenberg, W.M. (1995) The Need for Evidence-Based Medicine, *Journal of Research in Social Medicine* 88, pp. 620–4.

Sanchez-Salgado, R. (2007) *Comment l'Europe construit la société civile*, Paris: Dalloz.

Scharpf, F. (1997) *Games Real Actors Play: Actor-Centred Institutionalism in Policy Research*, Colorado/Oxford: Westview Press.

Scharpf, F.W. (2002) The European Social Model: Coping with the Challenges of Diversity, *Journal of Common Market Studies* 40(4), pp. 645–70.

Scharpf, Fritz W. (2008) Individualrechte gegen nationale Solidarität, in M. Höpner and A. Schäfer (eds) *Die Politische Ökonomie der europäischen Integration*, Frankfurt/New York: Campus, pp. 89–99.

Scheingold, S.A. (1971) *European Integration through Law*, New Haven, CT: Yale University Press.

Schmid, A. and Wendt, C. (2010) The Changing Role of the State in Healthcare Service Provision, in H. Rothgang, M. Cacace, L. Frisina, S. Grimmeisen, A. Schmid and C. Wendt (eds) *The State and Healthcare: Comparing OECD Countries*, Basingstoke: Palgrave Macmillan, pp. 53–71.

Scoggins, A., De Vries, H., Conklin, A. and Hatziandreu, E. (2009) *Analysis to Support the Impact Assessment of the Commissions Smoke-Free Initiatives,* Cambridge: RAND Europe.

Scott, J.C. (1998) *Seeing Like a State: How Certain Schemes to Improve the Human Condition Have Failed*, New Haven, CT: Yale University Press.

Scott, J. and Trubek, D.M. (2002) Mind the Gap: Law and New Approaches to Governance in the European Union, *European Law Journal* 8, pp. 1–18.

Sell, S. (2007) International Institutions, Intellectual Property an the HIV/AIDS Pandemic, in R. Ostergaard (ed.) *HIV/AIDS and the Threat to National and International Security*, Basingstoke: Palgrave Macmillan.

Sell, S. and Prakash, A. (2004) Using Ideas Strategically: The Contest between Business and NGO Networks in Intellectual Property Rights, *International Studies Quarterly* 48, pp. 143–75.

Seuba, X. (2009) Border Measures Concerning Goods Allegedly Infringing Intellectual Property Rights: The Seizures of Generic Medicines in Transit (Working paper) Geneva, International Centre for Trade and Sustainable Development: Programme on IPRs and Sustainable Development.

Shafey, O., Eriksen, M., Ross, H. and Mackay, J. (2009) *The Tobacco Atlas*, 3rd ed., Atlanta, GA: American Cancer Society, World Lung Foundation.

Shore, Cris (2000) *Building Europe: The Cultural Politics of European Integration*, New York: Routledge.

Sibille, B. (2010) Voir l'Europe pour la faire: Un système d'informations géographiques dans la gouvernance européenne, *Politique européenne* 31, pp. 147–72.

Silberschmidt, G. (2009) *The European Approach to Global Health: Identifying Common Ground for a US-EU Agenda*, Washington, DC: Center for Strategic and International Studies.

Simpura, J., Karlsson, T. and Leppänen, K. (2002) European Trends in Drinking Patterns and Their Socioeconomic Background, in T. Norström (ed.) *Alcohol in Postwar Europe*: *Consumption, Drinking Patterns, Consequences and Policy Responses in 15 European Countries*, Stockholm: National Institute of Public Health, Almqvist & Wiksell International, pp. 83–114

Sjöstedt, G. (1977) *The External Role of the European Community*, Farnborough: Saxon House, Swedish institute of international affairs.

Skogstad, G. (2006) Regulating Food Safety Risks in the Comparative Perspective, in C. Ansell and D. Vogel (eds) *What's the beef? The Contested Governance of European Food Safety*, Cambridge, MA: MIT Press, pp. 213–36.

Smith, A. (2004), *Le gouvernement de l'Union européenne: Une sociologie politique*, Paris: LGDJ.

Smith, Mitchell P. (2012) *Environmental and Health Regulation in the United States and the European Union: Protecting Public and Planet*, New York: Palgrave Macmillan.

Smith, R.D., Chanda, R. and Tangcharoensathien, V. (2009) Trade in Health-Related Services, *The Lancet* 373, pp. 593–601.

Smokefree Partnership (2009) Annual Report 2009, available at: http://www.smoke freepartnership.eu/IMG/pdf/Annual_Report_FINAL_DRAFT.pdf (accessed September 11, 2012).

Solomon, S.G., Murard, L. and Zylberman, P. (eds) (2008) *Shifting Boundaries of Public Health*, Rochester: University of Rochester University Press.

Sopal, J. (1995) The Medicalization and Demedicalization of Obesity, in D. Maurer and J. Sobal (eds) *Eating Agendas: Food and Nutrition as Social Problems*, New York: Aldine de Gruyter, pp. 67–90.

Sorenson, C., Naci, H., Cylus, J. and Mossialos, E. (2011) Evidence of Comparative Efficacy Should Have a Formal Role in European Drug Approvals, *British Medical Journal* 343(7822), pp. 514–17.

South Centre (2008) Ensuring Transparency and a Legitimate, Member-Driven Process in the SECURE Working Group, Submission by Brazil and Argentina to the World Customs Organisation (WCO) South Bulletin: Reflections and Foresights 25, 16 October, p. 14.

Spanish Presidency of the EU (2010) EU Comments and Proposals on the Revised Draft Global Code of Practice on the International Recruitment of Health Personnel, available at: http://www.who.int/healthsystems/workforce/European_Union.pdf (accessed January 10, 2012).

Ståhl, T., Wismar, M., Ollila, E., Lahtinen, E. and Leppo, K. (eds) (2006) *Health in All Policies: Prospects and Potentials*, Helsinki: Ministry of Social Affairs and Health.

Steffen, M. (2000) The Normalisation of AIDS Policies in Europe: Patterns, Path Dependency, and Innovation, in J.-P. Moatti, Y. Souteyrand, A. Prieur, T. Sandfort and P. Aggleton (eds) *AIDS in Europe: New challenges for the Social Sciences*, London: Routledge, pp. 207–22.

Steffen, Monika (ed.) (2005) *Health Governance in Europe: Issues, Challenges, and Theories*, New York: Routledge.

Steffen, M. (2012) The Europeanization of Public Health: How does it work? The Seminal Role of the AIDS Case, *Journal of Health Politics, Policy, and Law* 37(6), pp. 1056–87.

Stein, Hans (2003) The Open Method of Coordination in the Field of EU Health Care Policy, in Y. Jorens (ed.) *Open Method of Coordination: Objectives of European Health Care Policy*, Baden-Baden, Germany: Nomos, pp. 21–5.

Stone Sweet, A. (2004) *The Judicial Construction of Europe*, Oxford: Oxford University Press.

Strünck, C. (2005) Mix-Up: Models of Governance and Framing Opportunities in U.S. and EU Consumer Policy, *Journal of Consumer Policy* 28, pp. 203–30.

Stuckler, D., Basu, S., Suhrcke, M., Coutts, A. and McKee, M. (2009) The Public Health Effect of Economic Crises and Alternative Policy Responses in Europe: An Empirical Analysis, *The Lancet* 374, pp. 315–23.

Stuckler, D., Basu, S. and McKee, M. (2010a) Public Health in Europe: Power, Politics, and Where Next? *Public Health Reviews*, issue. 32, pp. 213–42.

Stuckler, D., Basu, S., McKee, M. and Suhrcke, M. (2010b) Responding to the Economic Crisis: A Primer for Public Health Professionals, *Journal of Public Health* 32(3), pp. 298–306.

Studlar, D.T. (2002) *Tobacco Control: Comparative Politics in the United States and Canada*, Peterborough, Canada: Broadview Press.

Studlar, D.T. (2004) Tobacco Control Policy Instruments in a Shrinking World: How Much Policy Learning? in D. Levi-Faur and E. Vigoda (eds) *Public Policy and Public Management in a Globalized World: Policy Learning and Policy Emulation Across Countries and Regions*, New York: Marcel Dekker.

Studlar, D.T. (2009) Tobacco Control Policy in Western Europe: A Case of Protracted Paradigm Change, in G. Capano and M. Howlett (eds) *European and North American Experiences of Policy Change: Policy Drivers and Policy Dynamics*, London: Routledge.

Studlar, D.T., Christensen, K. and Sitasari, A. (2011) Tobacco Control in the EU-15: The Role of Member States and the European Union, *Journal of European Public Policy* 18, pp. 727–44.

Sutton, C. and Nylander, J. (1999) Alcohol Policy Strategies and Public Health Policy at an EU-level: The Case of Alcopops, *Nordisk Alkohol and Narkotikatidskrift*, vol. 16, English supplement, pp. 74–91.

Sverdrup, U. (2006) Administering Information: Eurostat and Statistical Integration, in M. Egeberg (ed.), *Multilevel Union Administration: The Transformation of Executive Politics in Europe*, New York: Palgrave Macmillan, pp. 103–23.

Szilágyi, T. (2006) *Hungry for Hungary: Examples of Tobacco Companies Expansionism: Case Studies from Hungary*, Érd, Hungary: Health 21 Hungarian Foundation.

Talbot, C. (2004) The Agency Idea: Sometimes Old, Sometimes New, Sometimes Borrowed, Sometimes Untrue, in C. Pollitt and C. Talbot (eds) *Unbundled Government: A Critical Analysis of the Global Trend to Agencies, Quangos and Contractualisation*, London: Routledge, pp. 3–21.

Tallberg, J. (2003) The Agenda Shaping Powers of the Council Presidency, in O. Elgström (ed.) *European Union Council Presidencies: A Comparative Perspective*, London: Routledge, pp. 18–37.

Tellez, V. (2009) The Changing Global Governance of Intellectual Property Enforcement: A New Challenge for Developing Countries Attack Dutch Seizure of Generic Medicincs, in X. Li and C. Correa (eds) *Intellectual Property Enforcement: International Perspectives*, Cheltenham: Edward Elgar.

Thatcher, M. (2007) Internationalisation and Economic Institutions: Comparing European Experiences, Oxford: Oxford UnTiessen, J., Hunt, P., Celia, C., Faxekas, M., De Vries, H., Staetsky, L., Diepeveen, S. *et al.* (2010) *Assessing the Impacts of Revisiting the Tobacco Products Directive: Study to Support a DG SANCO Impact Assessment,* Cambridge: RAND Europe.

Tigerstedt, C., Karlsson, T., Mäkelä, P., Österberg, E. and Tuominen, I. (2006) Health in Alcohol Policies: The European Union and Its Nordic Member States, in T. Ståhl, M. Wismar, E. Ollila, E. Lahtinen and K. Leppo (eds.) *Health in All Policies: Prospects and Potentials*, Helsinki: Ministry of Social Affairs and Health, pp. 111–27.

Tigerstedt, C. and Törrönen, J. (2007) *Comparative Research Strategies and Changes in Drinking Cultures*, SoRAD Forskningsrapport no. 45.

Timmermans, S. and Berg, M. (1997) Standardization in Action: Achieving Local Universality through Medical Protocols, *Social Studies of Science* 27, pp. 273–305.

Timmermans, S. and Berg, M. (2003) *The Gold Standard: A Challenge of Evidence-Based Medicine and Standardization in Health Care*, Philadelphia, PA: Temple University Press.

Timmermans, S. and Epstein, S. (2010) A World of Standards but Not a Standard World: Toward a Sociology of Standards and Standardization, *Annual Review of Sociology* 36, pp. 69–89.

Timmermans, S. and Kolker, E.S. (2004) Evidence-Based Medicine and the Reconfiguration of Medical Knowledge, *Journal of Health and Social Behavior* 45 (Special Issue), 177–93.

Timmermans, S. and Mauck, A. (2005) The Promises and Pitfalls of Evidence-Based Medicine, *Health Affairs* 24, pp. 18–28.

Topping, A. (2011) Body Blow for Butter-Loving Danes as Fat Tax Kicks In, *Guardian*, 2 October, available at: http://www.guardian.co.uk/world/2011/oct/02/denmark-fat-tax-obesity (accessed July 13, 2011).

Trubek, L. (2007) Regulation through Information: The Fight Against Cancer in the EU and US, Paper presented at the annual meeting of The Law and Society Association, TBA, Berlin, Germany, July 25, 2007.

Trubek, L., Nance, M. and Hervey, T. (2008) The Construction of Healthier Europe: Lessons from the Fight Against Cancer, *Wisconsin International Law Journal*, 26(3), pp. 804–44.

Trubek, L.G., Rees, J.V., Hoflund, A.B., Farquhar, M. and Heimer, C.A. (2008) Health Care and New Governance: The Quest for Effective Regulation – Introduction, *Regulation & Governance* 2, pp. 1–8.

Ugland, T. (2003) A Case of Strange Bedfellows: An Institutional Perspective on French-Swedish Cooperation on Alcohol Control, *Scandinavian Political Studies* 26(3), pp. 269–86.

Ugland, T. (2011) Alcohol on the European Union's Political Agenda: Getting Off the Policy Roller-Coaster? Oslo: Norwegian Institute for Alcohol and Drug Research (SIRUS).

UNITAID (2009) UNITAID Statement on Dutch Confiscation of Medicines Shipment UNITAID online, 4 March.

United Nations (2011a) Non-Communicable Diseases Deemed Development Challenge of Epidemic Proportions in Political Declaration Adopted During Landmark General Assembly Summit, GA 111/38, New York, 19 September, available at: http://www.un.org/News/Press/docs/2011/ga11138.doc.htm (accessed January 10, 2012).

United Nations (2011b) Political Declaration of the High-level Meeting of the General Assembly on the Prevention and Control of Non-communicable Diseases, A/66/L.1, New York, 16 September.

Valor Economico (2009) Apreensão de genéricos na Holanda preocupa o Brasil Valor Economico, Sao Paulo, 23 January 23.

Van de Gronden, J. (2009) The Services Directive and Services of General (Economic) Interest, in M. Krajewski, U. Neergaard, and J. van de Gronden (eds) *The Changing Legal Framework for Services of General Interest in Europe: Between Competition and Solidarity*, The Hague, the Netherlands: T.M.C. Asser.

Van den Gronden, Johan Willem, Szyszczak, Erika, Neergaard, Ulla B. and Krajewski, Markus (eds) (2011) *Health Care and EU Law*, The Hague, the Netherlands: T.M.C. Asser Press.

Van der Wees, P.J., Hendriks, E.J., Custers, J.W., Burgers, J.S., Dekker, J. and de Bie, R.A. (2007) Comparison of International Guideline Programs to Evaluate and Update the

Dutch Program for Clinical Guideline Development in Physical Therapy, *BMC Health Services Research* 23, p. 191.

Van Schaik, L.G. (2009) The European Union: A Healthy Negotiator? A Study on Its Unity in External Representation and Its Performance in the World Health Organization, Research report, Laxenburg: International institute for advanced system analysis.

Van Schaik, L. (2011) The EU's Performance in the World Health Organization: Internal Cramps after the Lisbon Cure, *Journal of European Integration* 33(6), pp. 699–713.

Vauchez, A. (2012) Keeping the Dream Alive: The European Court of Justice and the Transnational Fabric of Integrationist Jurisprudence, *European Political Science Review* 4(1), pp. 51–71.

Verschuuren, M., Badeyan, G., Carnicero, J., Gissler, M., Asciak, R.P., Sakkeus, L., Stenbeck, M. and Devillé (2008) The European Data Protection Legislation and Its Consequences for Public Health Monitoring: A Plea for Action, *European Journal of Public Health* 18(6), pp. 550–1.

Virchow, R. (1848) Der Armenarzt, *Medicinske Reform* 18, pp. 125–7.

Vlayen, J., Aertgeerts, B., Hannes, K., Sermeus, W. and Ramaekers, D. (2005) A Systematic Review of Appraisal Tools for Clinical Practice Guidelines: Multiple Similarities and One Common Deficit, *Int J Qual Health Care* 17, pp. 235–42.

Wagner, Caroline, Dobrick, Katharina and Verheyen, Frank (2010) EU Cross-Border Health Care Survey 2010: Patient Satisfaction, Quality, Information and Potential, Scientific Institute for TK for Benefit and Efficiency in Health Care, WINEG Wissen 02, Hamburg.

Wall Street Journal (2009) India Prepares EU Trade Complaint, *Wall Street Journal*, 6 August.

Watine, J., Friedberg, B., Nagy, E., Onody, R., Oosterhuis, W., Bunting, P.S., Charet, J.C. and Horvath, A.R. (2006) Conflict between Guideline Methodologic Quality and Recommendation Validity: A Potential Problem for Practitioners, *Clinical Chemistry* 52, pp. 65–72.

Weiler, Joseph (1982) Community, Member-States and European Integration, *Journal of Common Market Studies* 21(1), pp. 39–56.

Weir, L. and Mykhalovskiy, E. (2009) *Global Public Health Vigilance: Creating a World on Alert*, London: Routledge.

Weissman, R. (1996) Long, Strange Trips: The Pharmaceutical Industry Drive to Harmonize Global Intellectual Property Rules and the Remaining WTO Legal Alternatives Available to Third World Countries, *Pennsylvania Journal of International Economic Law*, pp. 1069–125.

Weisz, G., Cambrosio, A., Keating, P., Knaapen, L., Schlich, T. and Tournay, V.J. (2007) The Emergence of Clinical Practice Guidelines, *Milbank Quarterly* 85, pp. 691–727.

Welshman, J. (1996) Images of Youth: The Issue of Juvenile Smoking, 1880–1914, *Addiction* 91, pp. 1379–86.

Wendt, A. (1999) *Social Theory of International Politics*, New York: Cambridge University Press.

White Paper (2007) *Together for Health: A Strategic Approach for the EU 2008–2012*, Commission for the European Community.

Wiechoczek, O. (2006) *The EU's Contribution to Global Governance: The Case of Global Infectious Diseases*, Thesis presented for the degree of Master of European Studies, College of Europe.

Wilensky, H.L. (2002) *Rich Democracies: Political Economy, Public Policy and Performance*, Berkeley, CA: University of California Press.

Wismar, M., Maier, C.B., Glinos, I.A., Dussault G. and Figueras, J. (eds) (2011a) *Health Professional Mobility and Health Systems: Evidence from 17 European Countries*, Observatory Studies Series 23, Brussels: European Observatory on Health Systems and Policies.

Wismar, M., Palm, W., Figueras, J., Ernst, K. and van Ginneken, E. (eds) (2011b) *Cross-Border Health Care in the European Union*, Observatory Studies Series 22, Brussels: European Observatory on Health Systems and Policies.

World Bank (2003) The Economics of Tobacco Use & Tobacco Control in the Developing World, Background Paper for the High level Round Table on Tobacco Control and Development Policy, Brussels, 3–4 February.

World Health Organization (n.d.) History of the Development of the ICD, available at: http://www.who.int/classifications/icd/en/HistoryOfICD.pdf (accessed February 17, 2012).

World Health Organization (1995) *Defining and Measuring the Social Accountability of Medical Schools*, Geneva: World Health Organization.

World Health Organization (2003) Tobacco & Health in the Developing World, Background Paper for the High level Round Table on Tobacco Control and Development Policy, Brussels, 3-4 February.

World Health Organization (2004) Equitable Access to Essential Medicines: A Framework for Collective Action, Geneva: WHO Policy Perspectives on Medicines.

World Health Organization (2006) The World Health Report 2006: Working Together for Health, Geneva: World Health Organization.

World Health Organization (2008) *WHO European Action Plan for Food and Nutrition Policy 2007–2012*, available at: http://www.euro.who.int /data/assets/ pdf_file/0017/ 74402/ E91153.pdf (accessed July 13, 2011).

World Health Organization (2010) International Recruitment of Health Personnel: Global Code of Practice, Resolution adopted by the 63rd World Health Assembly, A63/8, Geneva, 21 May.

World Health Organization (2011) Framework Convention on Tobacco Control: Status of Payments of Voluntary Assessed Contributions as of 15 July 2011, available at: http://www.who.int/fctc/cop/VAC_15_July_2011_rev.pdf (accessed January 10, 2012).

World Trade Organization (1994) *Uruguay Round Agreement: Decision on Professional Services*, available at: http://www.wto.org/english/docs_e/legal_e/51-dsprf_e (accessed September 11, 2012).

World Trade Organization (2001) Declaration on the TRIPS Agreement and Public Health, adopted on November 14, 2001, WT/MIN(01)/DEC/2, Doha, 20 November.

World Trade Organization (2010a) European Union and a Member State: Seizure of Generic Drugs in Transit, Dispute settlement: dispute DS408, available at: http://www.wto.org/english/tratop_e/dispu_e/cases_e/ds408_e.htm (accesssed October 2010).

World Trade Organization (2010b) European Union and a Member State: Seizure of Generic Drugs in Transit, Dispute settlement: dispute DS409, available at: http://www.wto.org/english/tratop_e/dispu_e/cases_e/ds409_e.htm (accesssed October 2010).

World Trade Organization (2010c) URUGUAY ROUND AGREEMENT: TRIPS. Part III: Enforcement of Intellectual Property Rights, available at: http://www.wto.org/english/docs_e/legal_e/27-trips_05_e.htm#Footnote14 (accessed January 24, 2010).

Wyszewianski (2009) Basic Concepts of Healthcare Quality, in E.R. Ransom (ed.) *The Healthcare Quality Book*, Chicago, IL: Health Administration Press, pp. 25–42.

Yataganas, X.A. (2001) Delegation of Regulatory Authority in the European Union: The Relevance of the American Model of Independent Agencies, 3/01 ed. NYU Jean Monnet Program working papers series, New York.

Zacher, W. and Keefe, T.J. (2008) *The Politics of Global Health Governance*, Basingstoke: Palgrave Macmillan.

Zacher, M.W. and Keefe, T.J. (2011) *The Politics of Global Health Governance: United by Contagion*, New York: Palgrave Macmillan.

Zanon, Elisabetta (2011) Health Care Across Borders: Implications of the EU Directive on Cross-border Health Care for the English NHS, *Eurohealth* 17(2–3), pp. 34–6.

Zatoński, W. (2003) *Democracy Is Healthier: A Nation's Recovery: Tobacco Control in Poland*, Warsaw: Health Promotion Foundation.

Zeitlin, Jonathan, Pochet, Philippe and Magnusson, Lars (eds) (2005) *The Open Method of Co-Ordination in Action: The European Employment and Social Inclusion Strategies*, Oxford: Peter Lang.

Zourek, H. (2007) Introductory Speech of Director General Heinz Zourek on the First Parliamentary Symposium Putting an End to Drug Counterfeiting, Brussels.

Zuiderent-Jerak, T. (2007) Preventing Implementation: Exploring Interventions with Standardization in Healthcare, *Science as Culture* 16, pp. 311–29.

Index

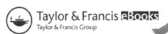